HISTAMINE
RECEPTORS

Monographs of the Physiological Society of Philadelphia

Volume 1
IMMUNOPHARMACOLOGY
Proceedings of the Conference on Immunopharmacology
Philadelphia, January 27-28, 1975
Marvin E. Rosenthale and Herbert C. Mansmann, Jr., Editors

Volume 2
NEW ANTIHYPERTENSIVE DRUGS
Proceedings of the A.N. Richards Symposium
King of Prussia, Pennsylvania, May 19-20, 1975
Alexander Scriabine and Charles S. Sweet, Editors

Volume 3
PROSTAGLANDINS IN HEMATOLOGY
Proceedings of the International Symposium on Prostaglandins in Hematology
Philadelphia, March 4-5, 1976
M.J. Silver, J.B. Smith and J.J. Kocsis, Editors

Volume 4
PATHOPHYSIOLOGY AND THERAPEUTICS OF MYOCARDIAL ISCHEMIA
Proceedings of the A.N. Richards Symposium
Philadelphia, May 6-7, 1976
Allan M. Lefer, Gerald J. Kelliher and Michael J. Rovetto, Editors

Volume 5
HISTAMINE RECEPTORS
Proceedings of the A.N. Richards Symposium
Philadelphia, March 21-22, 1977
Tobias O. Yellin, Editor

HISTAMINE RECEPTORS

Proceedings of the A.N. Richards Symposium
Philadelphia, March 21-22, 1977

Edited by
Tobias O. Yellin, Ph.D.
Head, Gastrointestinal Pharmacology
ICI Americas, Inc.
Wilmington, Delaware

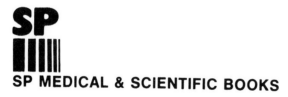

SP MEDICAL & SCIENTIFIC BOOKS

New York • London

SPECTRUM PUBLICATIONS, INC.
175-20 Wexford Terrace, Jamaica, New York 11432

Library of Congress Cataloging in Publication Data
Main entry under title:

Histamine receptors.

Includes index.
1. Histamine receptors. I. Yellin, Tobias O.
QP801.H5H57   612'.0157   78-13215
ISBN 0-89335-065-6

List of Contributors

GEOFFREY ALLAN, Ph. D.
Department of Pharmacology
Cornell University Medical College
New York, N. Y.

G. BARBIN, M. D.
Unité de Neurobiologie (U. 109)
Centre Paul Broca de l'I.N.S.E.R.M.
Paris, France

THOMAS BERGLINDH, Ph. D.
Department of Physiology and
  Medical Biophysics
Biomedicum
Uppsala
Sweden

JAMES W. BLACK, F.R.S.
Wellcome Research Laboratories
Beckenham, Kent
England

MICHAEL J. BRODY, Ph. D.
Department of Pharmacology
College of Medicine
The University of Iowa
Iowa City, Iowa

S. H. BUCK, M. S.
Department of Pharmacology
University of Arizona
College of Medicine
Tucson, Arizona

K. T. BUNCE, Ph. D.
The Research Institute
Smith Kline and French
  Laboratories Limited
Welwyn Garden City
Hertfordshire
England

SIDNEY COHEN, M. D.
Gastrointestinal Section
Hospital of the University of Pennsylvania
Philadelphia, Pennsylvania

CYRUS R. CREVELING, Ph. D.
National Institute of Arthritis, Metabolism,
  and Digestive Diseases
National Institute of Health
Bethesda, Maryland

JOHN W. DALY, Ph. D.
National Institute of Arthritis, Metabolism,
  and Digestive Diseases
National Institute of Health
Bethesda, Maryland

C. ROBIN GANELLIN, Ph. D.
The Research Institute
Smith Kline and French
  Laboratories Limited
Welwyn Garden City
Hertfordshire
England

LIST OF CONTRIBUTORS

M. GARBARG, Ph. D.
Unité de Neurobiologie (U. 109)
Centre Paul Broca de l'l.N.S.E.R.M.
Paris,
France

JACK PETER GREEN, M. D., Ph. D.
Department of Pharmacology
Mount Sinai School of Medicine
of the City University of New York
New York, New York

MARTIN D. GREEN, Ph. D.
Department of Pharmacology
School of Medicine and the
Brain Research Institute
University of California
Los Angeles, California

VERNON R. GRUND, Ph. D.
College of Pharmacology
University of Cincinnati
Cincinnati, Ohio

PAUL H. GUTH, M. D.
Medical and Research Services
VA Wadsworth Hospital Center
Los Angeles, California

H. L. HAAS, M. D.
Neurophysiologisches Laboratorium
Neurochirurgische Universitatsklinik
Zurich, Switzerland

M. J. HUGHES, Ph. D.
Texas Tech University
School of Medicine
Department of Physiology
Lubbock, Texas

DONALD B. HUNNINGHAKE, M. D.
Department of Pharmacology
School of Medicine
University of Minnesota
Minneapolis, Minnesota

CARL LYNN JOHNSON, Ph. D.
Department of Pharmacology
University of Cincinnati
College of Medicine
Cincinnati, Ohio

E. M. JOHNSON, Jr., Ph. D.
Department of Pharmacology
Washington University
Meddell School
St. Louis, Mo.

HEIKKI KARPPANEN, M. D.
Department of Pharmacology
University of Oulu
Oulu, Finland

MARK KNEUPFER, B. A.
Department of Pharmacology
College of Medicine
The University of Iowa
Iowa City, Iowa

JOHN J. KRANTZ, M. D.
Gastrointestinal Section
Hospital of the University of Pennsylvania
Philadelphia, Pennsylvania

CHI-HO LEE, M. D.
Department of Pharmacology
Cornell University Medical College
New York, New York

JOAN LEE, B. S.
Imperial Chemical Industries Ltd.
Pharmaceuticals Division
Department of Biochemistry
Alderley Park, Macclesfield
Cheshire, England

SARAH FRYER LEIBOWITZ, Ph. D.
The Rockefeller University
New York, New York

ROBERTO LEVI, Ph. D.
Department of Pharmacology
Cornell University Medical College
New York, N. Y.

**LAWRENCE M. LICHTENSTEIN,
M. D., Ph. D.**
Clinical Immunology Division
Department of Medicine
The Johns Hopkins University
School of Medicine at
The Good Samaritan Hospital
Baltimore, Maryland

PETER LOMAX, M. D., D. Sc.
Department of Pharmacology
School of Medicine and the
  Brain Research Institute
University of California
Los Angeles, California

RALPH LYDIC, M. S.
Texas Tech University
School of Medicine
Department of Psychology
Lubbock, Texas

ELIZABETH T. McNEAL, B. S.
National Institute of Arthritis, Metabolism,
  and Digestive Diseases
National Institute of Health
Bethesda, Maryland

JOHN H. McNEILL, Ph. D.
Division of Pharmacology and Toxicology
Faculty of Pharmaceutical Sciences
University of British Columbia
Vancouver, Canada

JOHN MAJOR, Ph. D.
Imperial Chemical Industries Limited
Pharmaceuticals Division
Department of Biochemistry
Alderley Park, Macclesfield
Cheshire, England

KARL JOHAN ÖBRINK, M.D.
Department of Physiology and
  Medical Biophysics
Biomedicum
Uppsala
Sweden

DR. ILARI PAAKKARI
Department of Pharmacology
University of Oulu
Oulu, Finland

DR. PIRKKO PAAKKARI
Department of Pharmacology
University of Oulu
Oulu, Finland

DR. J. M. PALACIOS
Unité de Neurobiologie (U. 109)
Centre Paul Broca de l'I.N.S.E.R.M.
Paris, France

M. E. PARSONS, Ph. D.
The Research Institute
Smith Kline and French
  Laboratories Limited
Welwyn Garden City
Hertfordshire
England

MARSHALL PLAUT, M. D.
Clinical Immunology Division
Department of Medicine
The Johns Hopkins University
  School of Medicine at
  The Good Samaritan Hospital
Baltimore, Maryland

TH. T. QUACH, Ph. D.
Unité de Neurobiologie (U. 109)
Centre Paul Broca de l'I.N.S.E.R.M.
Paris, France

G. VICTOR ROSSI, Ph. D.
Department of Biological Sciences
Philadelphia College of Pharmacy
  and Science
Philadelphia, Pennsylvania

WALDEMAR ROSZKOWSKI, M. D.
Clinical Immunology Division
Department of Medicine
The Johns Hopkins University
  School of Medicine at
  The Good Samaritan Hospital
Baltimore, Maryland

PETER SCHOLES, Ph. D.
Imperial Chemical Industries Limited
Pharmaceuticals Division
Department of Biochemistry
Alderley Park, Macclesfield
Cheshire, England

J. C. SCHWARTZ, Ph. D.
Unité de Neurobiologie (U. 109)
Centre Paul Broca de l'I.N.S.E.R.M.
Paris, France

RICHARD A. SHAFFER, MED. TECH.
Department of Pharmacology
College of Medicine
The University of Iowa
Iowa City, Iowa

LIST OF CONTRIBUTORS

ESTHER SMITH, M. S.
University of California at Los Angeles
School of Medicine
Los Angeles, California

WILLIAM J. SNAPE, JR., M.D.
Gastrointestinal Section
Hospital of the University of Pennsylvania
Philadelphia, Pennsylvania

M. R. STRAIT, Ph. D.
Department of Pharmacology
College of Medicine
The University of Iowa
Iowa City, Iowa

SUBHASH C. VERMA, Ph. D.
L. M. School of Pharmacy
Ahmebabed
India

MICHAEL WALTERS
Imperial Chemical Industries Limited
Pharmaceuticals Division
Department of Biochemistry
Alderley Park, Macclesfield
Cheshire, England

HAREL WEINSTEIN, D. Sc.
Department of Pharmacology
Mount Sinai School of Medicine
   of the City University of New York
New York, New York

P. WOLF, M. D.
Neurophysiologisches Laboratorium
Neurochiurgische Universitatsklinik
Zurich, Switzerland

T. O. YELLIN, Ph. D.
Biomedical Research Department
Pharmaceuticals R & D
ICI Americas Inc.
Wilmington, Delaware

JAMES H. ZAVECZ, Ph. D.
Biomedical Research Department
Pharmaceuticals R & D
ICI Americas Inc.
Wilmington, Delaware

A SHORT PHARMACOLOGIC HISTORY OF HISTAMINOLOGY

DISCOVERY OF HISTAMINE
HENRY HALLETT DALE   —1910

DISCOVERY OF ANTIHISTAMINES
DANIELE BOVET   —1937

DISCOVERY OF H_2—BLOCKERS
JAMES WHYTE BLACK   —1972

Preface

OPENING REMARKS, A. N. Richards Symposium on Histamine Receptors

Professor Black, distinguished speakers and guests, Ladies and Gentlemen,
    Before I make my opening remarks, I want to offer a number of personal acknowledgments. First of all, I would like to pay tribute to the speakers for the trouble they took to come here, for the honor they do us in being here, and for the enrichment they are about to give us. Second, I want to thank the drug industry, very much, for its essential support of this symposium. I particularly want to express my personal appreciation to SKF Laboratories for their extraordinary help through the courtesy of Dr. Lee Greene and Dr. Allen Misher here in the States and Dr. Bill Duncan in England. And likewise, my thanks to ICI in the persons of Dr. Henry Freedman and Dr. Ralph Giles in the U.S. and Dr. Brian Newbould in the U.K. Finally, but not least, I want to thank Victor Rossi of the Philadelphia College of Pharmacy and Science (which was co-sponsor of the symposium) and the officers of the Society, Connie Harakal, Ted Pruss, Allan Lefer, Grace Fisher, Warren Chernick, Alan Freeman, Gerald Kelliher and Jay Roberts for the latitude they accorded me in organizing this meeting.
    Now I would like to briefly introduce our subject. Histamine was fished out of a wonderful, old gemisch called ergot extract and studied pharmacologically by Dale and his coworkers, who held their interest in histamine for decades. At once, Dale recognized that the pharmacologic activity of histamine and more especially its effects in toxic doses resembled the symptoms of certain pathological conditions, notably anaphylactic shock. The work on the possible pathophysiologic role of histamine took impetus

and special interest as it spanned World War I with its terrible toll of traumatic shock victims.

During this period, the founder of our society, Alfred Newton Richards, made important contributions to histaminology in Dale's laboratory. In their classic paper of 1918, Dale and Richards traced the vasodilatory activity of histamine to the capaillaries and suggested "that the current conception of the peripheral resistance to blood flow, as determined almost exclusively by the tone of the arterioles, allows too little importance to capillary tone as a factor." Such basic pharmacology gave rise, eventually, to the physiologic theory that histamine is involved in control of the microcirculation. Similarly, Popielski's discovery, two years later, that histamine stimulates gastric secretion led eventually to the theory that endogenous histamine plays a role in the control of gastric function.

Returning to Dale's main thesis, by 1929, when there was no doubt remaining that histamine was a natural constituent of practically all living mammalian tissues, Dale's proposal that histamine played a role in the pathology resulting from traumatic injury and antigen-antibody reactions was the reigning dogma, but nonetheless only a theory. The theory could not be proved because the Law of Medicinal Biology remained unfulfilled. It is this law which puts the physiologist and physiological chemist in the debt of pharmacologists like Jim Black and medicinal chemists like Robin Ganellin and simply states: If you can't block it, you don't know it.

Thus, the most convincing evidence for Dale's theory came later, in 1937, with the advent of the antihistamines discovered by Bovet. But whereas antihistamines proved useful as tools for delineating the pathophysiologic role of histamine, they did nothing to promote other physiological theories of histamine, notably its possible role in gastric secretion. Consequently, histaminology has contributed relatively little to our understanding of biology in the years since antihistamines entered medicine, until recently.

There is a law in Camelot, that after the Winter comes the Spring. And in April of 1972, Black and his coworkers, in England, called an end to the Winter of histaminology by their invention of H_2-receptor blockers. I need not dwell on Black's work in as much as this entire symposium is a celebration of his fundamental contribution to histaminology. Suffice it to say that the field is in Spring again and that histamine is entering physiology. The most encouraging development in this regard is the linkage of H_2-receptors, in a variety of tissues, to a key enzymic reaction, namely, the formation of cyclic AMP. This thread binds together histaminologists of every discipline, in a sort of way that was not possible before Black's great taxonomic work.

The purpose of this symposium is to recapitualte and enlarge upon the tremendous progress of histaminology since the Spring of '72. But in conclusion, I think I must say something modest on behalf of all the speakers and it is this: We still know practically nothing about histamine receptors as such, and in this sense, the title of this symposium is only a prayer, to be answered, perhaps, by the present generation of histaminologists.

T. O. YELLIN

PHILADELPHIA, PENNSYLVANIA
21 MARCH 1977

Contents

PREFACE

1. Histamine—A Review of Physiology and
   Pharmacology   1
   G. V. Rossi

PART I — GASTROINTESTINAL HISTAMINE RECEPTORS

2. The Riddle of Gastric Histamine   23
   J. W. Black

3. Histamine As a Physiological Stimulant of
   Gastric Parietal Cells   35
   T. Berglindh and K. J. Öbrink

4. Studies on Metiamide and Acid
   Secretion in the Isolated Whole
   Rat Stomach   57
   M. E. Parsons and K. T. Bunce

5. Esophageal Histamine Receptors   69
   S. Cohen, J. J. Kravitz,
   and W. J. Snape, Jr.

CONTENTS

6. Imidazoline Stimulants of
Gastric Secretion   79
   T. O. Yellin, S. H. Buck, and
   E. M. Johnson, Jr.

PART II — CARDIOVASCULAR HISTAMINE RECEPTORS

7. Histamine—Drug-Disease Interactions
and Cardiac Function   99
   R. Levi, J. H. Zavecz,
   C. H. Lee, and G. Allan

8. Histamine Receptors in Vascular
Smooth Muscle: Mechanisms of
Vasodilatation   115
   M. J. Brody, M. Kneupfer,
   M. R. Strait, and R. A. Shaffer

9. H_1- and H_2- Histamine Receptors in the
Gastric Microcirculation   131
   P. H. Guth and E. Smith

10. Characteristics of H_1- and H_2-
Histamine Receptors Which Mediate
the Chronotropic Response of
Rabbit Atrial Muscle   143
   M. J. Hughes and R. Lydic

PART III — NEURAL HISTAMINE RECEPTORS

11. Histamine Receptors in Mammalian
Brain: Characteristics and Modifications
Studied Electrophysiologically and
Biochemically   161
   J. C. Schwartz, J. M. Palacios,
   G. Barbin, T. T. Quach, M. Garbarg,
   H. L. Haas, and P. Wolf

12. Histamine Activation of Adenylate
Cyclase in Brain: An H_2-Receptor and
Its Blockade by LSD   185
   J. P. Green, C. L. Johnson,
   and H. Weinstein

13. Histamine Receptors in the
Central Thermoregulatory Pathways   211
   P. Lomax and M. D. Green

14. Histamine: Modification of
Behavioral and Physiological Components
of Body Fluid Homeostasis   219
   S. F. Leibowitz

15. Studies on the Nature of Cerebral
Receptors Mediating the Hypotensive
Effect of Clonidine in Rats   255
   H. Karppanen, I. Paakkari,
   and P. Paakkari

PART IV — HISTAMINE RECEPTORS LINKED TO NEUCLEOTIDE CYCLASES

16. Cardiac Histamine Receptors and
Cyclic AMP: Differences between
Guinea Pig and Rabbit Heart   271
   J. H. McNeill and S. C. Verma

17. Prostaglandin and Histamine Effects
on Cyclic AMP Levels in Parietal Cells   285
   P. Scholes, J. Lee, J. Major,
   and M. Walters

18. Accumulation of Cyclic AMP in
Brain Tissue: Role of H_1- and H_2-
Histamine Receptors   299
   J. W. Daly, E. T. McNeal,
   and C. R. Creveling

19. Histamine Receptors and Cyclic
Nucleotides in Adipose Tissue   325
   V. R. Grund and D. B. Hunninghake

PART V — HISTAMINE RECEPTORS IN IMMUNE REACTIONS

20. Modulation of Inflammation by
Histamine Receptor-Bearing Cells   351
   M. Plaut and L. M. Lichtenstein

CONTENTS

21. Lymphocyte Subpopulations Bearing
Histamine Receptors   361
M. Plaut and W. Roszkowski

PART VI — MEDICINAL CHEMISTRY

22. Chemical Development and Properties
of Histamine H_2-Receptor Agonists
and Antagonists   377
C. R. Ganellin

Index   **415**

1

Histamine—A Review of Physiology and Pharmacology

G. Victor Rossi
Department of Biological Sciences
Philadelphia College of Pharmacy and Science
Philadelphia, Pennsylvania

HISTORICAL PERSPECTIVE

Histamine was synthesized 70 years ago as a venture in chemistry; exploration of its role in health and disease continues to provide scientific adventure. The relatively simple organic molecule, β-imidazolylethylamine, was prepared chemically by Windaus and Vogt (1907) before its discovery in nature. Three years later the biological activity of this amine began to unfold when it was identified by Barger and Dale (1910) as a uterine stimulant in extracts of ergot. Despite demonstrations of a fascinating range of pharmacologic effects, there was no evidence of physiologic significance during this early period inasmuch as the substance had not been isolated from animal tissue. Barger and Dale (1911) recovered from intestinal mucosa a base indistinguishable in its pharmacologic properties from synthetic β-imidazolylethylamine; however, the suspicion long persisted that the amine was not a product of living tissue but was formed by the action of bacterial enzymes on the amino acid histidine, as had been demonstrated by Ackermann (1910) and confirmed by Mellanby and Twort (1912). Prior to 1912 the compound under consideration was referred to in the literature by the chemical name, β-imidazolylethylamine, or by the empirical terms ergamine and histidine-base; the designation *histamine* first appeared in publications by Führner (1912) and Fröhlich and Pick (1912).

That histamine is present normally in many body tissues and is not exclusively a product of bacterial decarboxylation of histidine was reported by Abel and Kubota (1919), but it was not until 1927 that Best and Dale and their co-workers (1927) succeeded in isolating crystalline histamine picrate from ox lung, liver, and muscle by a procedure that precluded histamine formation by putrefactive processes.

In pioneering investigations published during the decade from 1910 to 1920, Dale in conjunction with Richards and Laidlaw (review by Dale, 1953) revealed the diverse effects of histamine on the smooth musculature in various species and speculated with remarkable prescience on the relationships of this ubiquitous amine to inflammatory and anaphylactic phenomena. Throughout this period there emerged conflicting humoral and cellular theories on the nature of *anaphylatoxin.* Lewis (1927) proposed that a histamine-like "H-substance" was liberated from cells upon injury or in response to the interaction of antigen and antibody. Forcible evidence that histamine was indeed the postulated "H-substance" was provided by Bartosch and his co-workers (1932) and by Dragstedt and Gebauer-Fuelnegg (1932) who identified quantitatively the presence of this amine in perfusates of sensitized tissues exposed to specific antigen.

Acknowledgement of histamine as a major if not the sole mediator of allergic and hypersensitivity phenomena provided strong impetus in the search for clinically useful inhibitors of histamine activity. The era of synthetic histamine antagonists was opened by Bovet and Staub (1937) by their demonstration of selective blockade of histamine toxicity in guinea pigs by a phenolic ether derivative (compound 929F) developed earlier by Fourneau (1933). During the post-World War II period the physician was provided with a multiplicity of antihistaminic agents. Clinical experimentation established their usefulness in the palliation of local and systemic allergic disorders, in the prophylaxis and relief of motion sickness and other vestibular disturbances, and as adjuncts in the treatment of parkinson's disease.

It soon became apparent that the mechanistic classification of "antihistamine" represented an oversimplication in that many drugs to which this term was applied possessed, in addition to histamine-blocking activity, a variety of pharmacologic properties including anticholinergic, adrenolytic, local anesthetic, cardiac depressant and central nervous sytem suppressant activity. And in several situations the clinical utility of these drugs was apparently related to properties other than histamine antagonism. Further, it was obvious early on that the therapeutic efficacy of antihistamines fell short of expectations based on a unipolar theory of the biochemical mediation of anaphylaxis. In the drama of allergy, histamine shares the stage with other players, some of which have dominant roles.

One aspect of histamine pharmacology that received little attention in the thorough investigations of Dale and his colleagues was the response of the gastric secretory apparatus to this amine. Popielski (1920) and Keeton and his co-workers (1920) discovered the powerful stimulant effect of histamine on gastric secretion in experimental animals, and a similar action in humans was demonstrated by Carnot and his associates (1922). The concept that histamine functions as a local agent in excitation of the acid-secreting cell, whatever the nature of the preceding stimulus, was first formulated by Babkin (1938). During the next several decades the concept gained general but by no means universal currency. Ivy and Bachrach (1966) reviewed the impressive evidence supporting the view that histamine is the final chemostimulant of the parietal cell. But failure of pharmacologic agents, including conventional antihistaminic drugs, to selectively block the parietal cell response to histamine denied, for many years, examination of critical agonist/antagonist relationships in the gastric secretory process.

Ash and Schild (1966) characterized the biological loci with which histamine interacts; they designated as H_1 receptors those reactive sites involved in responses to histamine that are blocked by mepyramine and related antihistaminic agents, and as nonH_1 receptors (later termed H_2 receptors) those which mediate responses to histamine that are refractory to mepyramine. Reevaluation of correlations among chemical structure and biological activity in a series of imidazole derivatives led, in 1972, to development of the first histamine H_2-receptor antagonist burimamide by Black and his co-workers (1972).

Pathology is perturbed physiology; a role in disease is a logical extrapolation of a presumed function in health. To discern the role in the natural economy played by an endogenous bioactive substance it is of critical importance to be able to effectively eliminate the reactant from the organism or to selectively deny access of the agonist to its target sites. The ubiquity of histamine precludes the endocrinologist's ablative approach. Potent histamine-releasing agents, such as compound 48/80, have provided valuable insights into the nature of cellular storage mechanisms and the role of this amine in inflammatory and immune processes. The early antihistaminic agents served to further characterize the nature of histamine-effector cell interactions and to define the relative importance of histamine among the biochemical mediators of allergic and anaphylactic states. But neither tool proved adequate to pharmacological dissection of the precise roles of this autocoid. Understanding of the significance of histamine in health and disease has advanced phenomenally since the introduction of histamine H_2-receptor antagonists. However, the number of questions continues to exceed the number of definitive answers.

BIOSYNTHESIS AND CATABOLISM

Almost all of the histamine found in animal tissues appears to be formed in the cells by decarboxylation of the amino acid L-histidine. Although the intracellular formation of histamine in intact man has not been established conclusively, *in vitro* conversion of *L*-histidine to the corresponding amine has been demonstrated in fetal and adult human tissues (Lindell and Westling, 1966). Mammalian tissues contain at least two enzymes capable of decarboxylating this amino acid. One is the diffusely distributed enzyme aromatic *L*-amino acid decarboxylase, which has a relatively low affinity for *L*-histidine, and the other is a selective histidine decarboxylase. It is this specific decarboxylase that is most abundant in histamine-rich mast cells and in certain rapidly growing tissues such as fetal rat liver. Both enzymes require pyridoxal-5-phosphate as cofactor and are inhibited by compounds such as semicarbazide that combine with this cofactor. There is no evidence that tissue histamine is derived from smaller molecules or that it is synthesized by nonenzymatic processes.

Although exogenous histamine can be taken up by a variety of different cell types, it is unlikely that dietary sources or histamine formed in the gut by bacterial decarboxylation of histidine contribute significantly to the endogenous histamine pool. Intralumenal histamine is largely inactivated *in situ* by conversion to N-acetylhistamine and any traces of the amine absorbed from the intestine confront efficient catabolic systems before reaching the systemic circulation.

Metabolic pathways for the biotransformation of histamine have been established in detail, largely by the comprehensive researches of Schayer and his associates (1956; Schayer, 1959). A major pathway of histamine metabolism in many species, including man, involves ring N-methylation to form 1-methyl-4-(β-aminoethyl) imidazole through transfer of a methyl group from S-adenosylmethionine in the presence of the enzyme imidazole-N-methyltransferase. Methylhistamine is, to a large extent, subsequently deaminated by monoamine oxidase to form 1-methylimidazole-4-acetic acid, the principal urinary metabolite of histamine in man. A secondary catabolic route involves oxidative deamination by diamine oxidase to form imidazole acetic acid, a large fraction of which is conjugated with ribose forming 1-ribosyl-imidazole-4-acetic acid. This reaction appears unique in that histamine is the only known endogenous compound to be metabolized by conjugation with ribose. The purpose of ribose conjugation is not clear inasmuch as imidazole acetic acid is excreted by the kidney as readily as the ribosyl derivative. Only a small percentage of parenterally administered ^{14}C-labeled histamine appears unchanged in the urine.

The body possesses an amazing capacity to inactivate histamine. Studies with labeled histamine have demonstrated that within minutes after intravenous administration histamine has largely disappeared from the plasma and appears in almost all tissues as metabolites. Blockade of one pathway with metabolic inhibitors shifts histamine catabolism to an alternate route. Beaven (1976), in his recent comprehensive review of histamine, remarked that a capacity for rapid degradation of histamine appears necessary because of the potentially lethal amounts of this amine stored in the tissues of most species and, further, that the existence of alternate metabolic pathways provides an adaptable system.

Schayer and Reilly (1973) found that burimamide but not metiamide markedly altered the distribution of injected ^{14}C-histamine in mice and rats; burimamide-treated animals evidenced increased isotopically labeled histamine in the blood and kidneys but a decrease in the heart. It is interesting to note that burimamide is a rather potent catecholamine-releasing agent whereas metiamide is only weakly active in this respect and that burimamide, but not metiamide, possesses considerable α-adrenoceptor blocking activity (Brimblecombe *et al.,* 1976).

DISTRIBUTION AND STORAGE

Feldberg (1956) stated that histamine has been found in all body tissues examined with the possible exception of cartilage and bone. He further noted that histamine occurs in many physiologic and pathologic fluids such as blood, plasma, gastric juice, bile, urine, sputum, blister fluid, and pus. An extensive survey of the histamine content of mammalian organs and body fluids, published 10 years later by Vugman and Rocha et Silva (1966), reinforced Feldberg's generalization that "histamine is very widely distributed in the body." There are, however, marked variations in the histamine concentration among different tissues within any one species, and enormous interspecies differences in the histamine content of any particular organ. For example, high concentrations of histamine are present in the liver of the rabbit, dog, and horse, as compared to the relatively small amounts found in the liver of the rat and guinea pig. In man, the concentration of this amine is particularly high in the skin, gastrointestinal mucosa, lungs, and bone marrow. Lesser, but significant amounts of histamine are also found in peripheral nerves, particularly adrenergic fibers, and in the central nervous system. In the brain, the pattern of distribution of histamine is similar to that of 5-hydroxytryptamine, namely a relatively high concentration in some regions of the brain stem such as the hypothalamus and thalamus, and low levels in the cerebellum and cerebral cortex (White, 1973).

The investigations of Schayer (1961) and Kahlson and Rosengren (1965) have suggested that steady-state levels do not reflect accurately the functional status of histamine in any particular tissue. Some tissues possess the capacity to synthesize and metabolize histamine at remarkably high rates. Induced or nascent histamine, formed locally in response to exogenous or endogenous stimuli that evoke histidine decarboxylase activity, is not stored in the cell but is available, presumably, for physiologic reaction and subsequent rapid inactivation and elimination. Thus, the histamine content of any tissue is not a reliable index of the rate of turnover of this amine and there is no consistent relationship between histamine content and histamine-forming capacity.

A major locus of stored histamine in mammalian tissue is the mast cell. These metachromatic cells, first described by Ehrlich (1877), are associated with connective tissue elements throughout the body. Mast cells are also a principal depot for heparin, a sulfated mucopolysaccharide that imparts to these cells the characteristic property of metachromasia. In man, almost all of the histamine in the blood is found in the basophilic leukocytes, the cytological counterpart of the mast cell in the tissues. In certain other species, the histamine repository function of the basophils is assumed by blood platelets and eosinophils.

A considerable fraction of the histamine contained in some areas of the body, notably the epidermis, the brain, and the stomach, is not associated with mast cells. In the gastrointestinal tract, histamine is present in at least three cell types—mast cells, cells of the amine precursor uptake and distribution (APUD) system, and a nonmast cell-nonAPUD system. Nonmast cell histamine has a more rapid turnover than that sequestered within the mast cell; this finding has led to the suggestion that the former may be of greater physiological significance. Further, histidine decarboxylase activity associated with nonmast cell systems is inducible, being subject to activation by such stimuli as gastrin, insulin, and 2-deoxyglucose.

Histamine in mast cells is highly concentrated in subcellular particles that have a greater density than mitochondria. These histamine-containing granules also contain large amounts of heparin and, in the mouse and rat, 5-hydroxytryptamine. The precise nature of histamine binding to subcellular fractions remains to be determined, but there is considerable evidence that the amine is held within the membrane-limited granule by electrostatic forces (Green, 1962; Green and Day, 1963). This may involve an ionic linkage between the primary amino group of the histamine side-chain and the sulfate or carboxyl moieties of heparin. Hydrogen bonding may reinforce the molecular association. Green (1967) has further suggested that protamine in the mast cell granule may complex with the electron-rich carbon of the imidazole ring.

HISTAMINE RELEASE

Since publication of the classical paper by MacIntosh and Paton (1949) on the liberation of endogenous histamine by certain organic bases, the nature and mechanism of physical and chemical agents that release stored histamine have been extensively explored. Histamine release has been the subject of innumerable experimental articles as well as several comprehensive surveys and symposia (Rocha e Silva, 1955; Paton, 1956; Uvnas, 1963; Rothschild,

1966; Goth, 1973; McIntire, 1973), and will be considered only briefly in this review. Goth (1973) has grouped the many diverse substances that can release histamine into three broad categories depending on their chemical nature and mode of action. These classes are: (1) *basic compounds,* e.g., compound 48/80, stilbamidine, *d*-tubocurarine, (2) *macromolecular compounds,* e.g., dextran, polyvinylpyrrolidone, ovomucoid, and (3) *enzymes and venoms,* e.g., phospholipase A, chymotrypsin, cobra venom.

It is well established that histamine release by basic compounds is not simply a displacement of the amine from its binding site. At least two different mechanisms have been identified and the process may vary not only with the particular compound but with the species involved. One process, typified by the action of low concentrations of compound 48/80 on rat mast cells, involves activation of an energy-requiring system that culminates in histamine release and degranulation without disruption of the cell membrane. Histamine release by compound 48/80 exhibits many of the characteristics of anaphylactic histamine release including temperature and pH optima, a requirement for calcium, and susceptibility to anoxia and metabolic inhibitors. In contrast, histamine release by aliphatic amines such as decylamine involves a nonspecific detergent-like action with morphological evidence of discontinuities in the plasma membrane. Despite intensive study the mechanism by which macromolecular compounds such as dextran evoke the release of histamine in certain species remains unclear; proposals relating to the intervention of specific antibodies, phosphatides or other cofactors are intriguing but not firmly supported (Goth, 1973).

PHARMACOLOGIC ACTIONS OF HISTAMINE

Pharmacologic actions of histamine are manifested principally on vascular smooth muscle, extravascular smooth muscle, and exocrine glands, notably the acid secreting cells of the gastric mucosa. In addition histamine exerts important effects on the myocardium, adrenal medulla, and certain neural processes.

Striking species differences exist in responsiveness to histamine; the mouse and rat are highly resistant to this amine, whereas the guinea pig and man are extraordinarily sensitive. Further, among various animal species there are notable qualitative differences in the response of certain effector organs. For example, the rat uterus *in vitro* and *in vivo* is relaxed by histamine in contrast to the myometrial contractile response observed in most other mammals. The overall vascular effects of histamine in most species, including man, lead to a fall in systemic blood pressure, whereas in the rabbit this amine generally evokes a vasopressor response.

Cardiovascular System

Following the observation by Schmidt-Mulheim (1880) that intravenous injection of Witte's peptone (a preparation obtained by peptic digestion of bovine blood fibrin) into an anesthetized dog evoked a dramatic reduction of arterial blood pressure, there appeared in the literature sporadic reports of "depressor substances" associated with extracts of a variety of mammalian tissues. Popielski (1920) proposed that a substance to which he applied the name "vasodilatin" was a common denominator in the blood pressure reducing action of tissue extracts. Subsequent separation of histamine from a host of animal tissues coupled with the finding that the purified compound essentially reproduced the vascular responses to various tissue extracts identified histamine as the hypothetical principle "vasodilatin."

The classic studies of Dale and Richards (1918) demonstrated that small doses of histamine in anesthetized cats and dogs cause constriction of certain arteries and veins but general dilation of small blood vessels and that these responses are independent of vascular innervation. Dilation of microcirculatory vessels and an increase in the permeability of the microvasculature are among the most characteristic effects of histamine observed in essentially all species, although less consistently in the rabbit (Rocha e Silva, 1966a). Distention of the capillaries and postcapillary venules, which are essentially devoid of contractile elements, is attributable both to the relaxant effect of histamine on terminal arterioles with consequent increased perfusion of the capillary bed and to outflow impedance as a result of histamine-induced constriction of the larger veins. It is probable that the transudation of plasma and plasma macromolecules in respone to exposure to histamine occurs largely at the level of the postcapillary venules, and that this phenomenon is due in part to increased hydrostatic pressure as a result of venoconstriction and also to a direct action of histamine to enlarge the endothelial intercellular spaces (Haddy, 1960).

Intradermal injection of histamine provides a dramatic illustration of the regional vascular effects of this potent vasoactive substance. Lewis (1927) described the characteristic sequence of local changes that follows introduction of small amounts of histamine into the skin; the "triple response" includes (1) an initial circumscribed area of erythema caused by dilation of microcirculatory vessels in direct contact with the injected amine solution; (2) an irregular red flare, surrounding the initial erythema, representing arteriolar dilation mediated by the mechanism of an axon reflex involving peripheral sensory nerves, and (3) a wheal or bleb of edema fluid that develops as a consequence of the increased permeability of small blood vessels exposed to histamine and which occupies and obscures the original red spot. This triad of reactions may also be induced by intradermal injection of specific antigen in sensitized individuals, by local application of heat or the introduction of chemicals that liberate endogenous histamine from the dermis.

Dale and Laidlaw (1910) and Dale and Richards (1918) demonstrated dose-dependent depressor responses to intravenous histamine in anesthetized dogs and cats. Large intravenous doses of histamine in these species produce a steep fall in systemic blood pressure, followed shortly by an intermediate and incomplete recovery of arterial pressure mediated largely by reflex sympathetic discharge and adrenomedullary catecholamine release, and succeeded by a third phase during which the blood pressure declines slowly and, in some cases, irreversibly. Despite contraction of large arteries and veins, notably the pulmonary artery in the cat and suprahepatic vein in the dog, vasodepression is the dominant response to large doses of histamine due to marked dilation of small blood vessels with pooling of blood in the microcirculatory bed, escape of plasma from the vascular system in areas of increased permeability and consequent reduction of effective circulatory fluid volume. Arteriolar dilation and systemic hypotension also represent the predominant vascular responses to intravenous injection of histamine in man. Activation of baroreceptor reflexes in response to the fall in arterial pressure, venoconstriction with increased venous return, and direct inotropic and chronotropic effects result initially in cardiac acceleration and increased cardiac output following intravascular histamine in the dog. Compensatory reflex mechanisms are sufficient to prevent hypotension in man when histamine is infused intravenously in low concentrations at slow rates (Wakim *et al.,* 1949).

Folkow and his co-workers (1948) observed that the systemic hypotensive response to small amounts of histamine could be reduced or abolished by mepyramine and pharmacologically related histamine antagonists but, in confirmation of an earlier report by Staub (1939), found that the depressor effect of large intravascular doses of histamine was refractory to conventional antihistamines. Based on these observations, Folkow and his associates suggested the existence of two types of histamine-sensitive reactive sites. The development of burimamide provided a selective pharmacologic tool for testing the dual histamine-receptor hypothesis advanced by Folkow and co-workers (1948) and subsequently by Ash and Schild (1966). Black and his colleagues (1972) demonstrated that depressor responses to large doses of histamine, which are refractory to mepyramine, are blocked completely by a combination of mepyramine and burimamide. Further studies by Parsons and Owen (1973) and Powell and Brody (1973, 1976) strongly support the presence of both H_1 and H_2 receptors in the vasculature of the cat and dog and indicate that both receptor types mediate a common response to histamine, i.e., arteriolar dilation and reduction in systemic arterial pressure. Chipman and Glover (1976) observed that the vasodilator response to intraarterial infusion of histamine in the human forearm is only partially attenuated by mepyramine but is abolished completely by mepyramine and metiamide administered in combination; these investigators concluded that the peripheral circulatory response to histamine in the human is mediated both by H_1 and H_2 receptors.

Although the responsiveness of the isolated mammalian heart to histamine differs considerably among the various species, in general, low concentrations of the amine increase the frequency and amplitude of the beat (Bartlet, 1963). Mepyramine and related antishistamines have been reported to antagonize, to varying degrees, the positive chronotropic and inotropic responses to histamine in isolated perfused mammalian hearts. But inhibition of these cardiac responses to histamine is achieved only with concentrations of conventional antihistamines that depress the rate and force of myocardial contraction (Levi and Kuye, 1974), and which effects have been termed nonspecific (Trendelenburg, 1960). Detailed studies by Levi and his co-investigators (1976; Levi and Capurro, 1973) have led to proposals that H_2 receptors mediate the positive chronotropic and ventricular inotropic effects of histamine and that the negative dromotropic (impaired atrioventricular conduction) and possibly the atrial inotropic responses to histamine are subserved by H_1 receptors in the isolated guinea pig heart. Coronary vascular responses to histamine in the guinea pig heart appear to involve both types of histamine receptors; an initial H_1 receptor-mediated vasodilatation that is blocked by mepyramine and a secondary prolonged increase in coronary flow that is suppressed by burimamide and is, therefore, linked to H_2 receptors (Broadley, 1975). Cardiac arrhythmias induced by exogenous histamine or which occur during immediate hypersensitivity reactions, either *in vitro* or *in vivo,* are effectively controlled only by a combination of both H_1- and H_2-receptor antagonists (Levi and Capurro, 1973; Levi *et al.,* 1976).

Smooth Muscle

Nonvascular smooth muscle tone is generally increased by histamine due largely to direct musculotropic action and in part to stimulation of intrinsic neural fibers (Parrot and Thouvenot, 1966). Bioassay systems for the quantitation of histamine activity have been based on the exquisite sensitivity of the guinea pig ileum and bronchial musculature to this amine. Considerable variation in the responsiveness of extravascular smooth muscle to histamine is found not only among different tissues and different species but exists also among normal and disease states. For example, doses of histamine that exert relatively little effect on smooth musculature of the respiratory tract in the normal human may evoke intense bronchoconstriction in the patient with bronchial asthma. In general, smooth muscle of the urinary bladder, gallbladder, and iris is contracted weakly and inconsistently by histamine. And in some structures, for example, the rat uterus, cat trachea, and sheep bronchus, histamine causes smooth muscle relaxation.

Histamine-induced increases in smooth muscle tone in the guinea pig ileum and bronchi are blocked effectively by relatively low concentrations of mepyramine and thus are considered to be mediated by H_1 receptors (Ash and Schild, 1966); inhibition by histamine of uterine contractions in certain species is mepyramine-insensitive but is antagonized by burimamide and is regarded, therefore, as an H_2 receptor-mediated response (Black et al., 1972).

In most vascular beds, H_1 and H_2 receptors appear to function synergistically in smooth muscle relaxation; however, Turker (1973) has presented evidence that H_1 and H_2 receptors are involved in opposing physiological effects in the guinea pig pulmonary vasculature. Powell and Brody (1976) concluded that histamine-induced venoconstriction in the dog is mediated only by H_1 receptors. Analysis of agonist–antagonist relationships suggest the presence in guinea pig intestine (Bareicha and Rocha e silva, 1976) and in rat uterus (Verma and McNeill, 1976) of H_2 receptors that subserve smooth muscle relaxation. Generalizations with regard to their role in either inhibitory or excitatory processes are thus no more appropriate for the recently differentiated histamine receptor subtypes than for the multiple cholinoceptive or adrenoceptive loci.

Exocrine and Endocrine Glands

Histamine is a remarkably active stimulant of gastric acid secretion; in man, doses less than those required to produce a sustained reduction of arterial blood pressure, evoke a copious outflow of gastric juice (Ivy and Bachrach, 1966). This secretory response appears to represent a direct action of histamine on parietal cells. That the parasympathetic nervous system plays a permissive role in this process is evidenced by a substantial but incomplete reduction in the maximal secretory response to histamine following vagotomy in man. Histamine H_1-receptor antagonists attenuate histamine-induced gastric secretion only in doses sufficiently large to exert an antimuscarinic (atropine-like) effect.

Code (1965) stated that "no other chemostimulator is interposed between histamine and the parietal cell." Evidence that burimamide and metiamide function as competitive antagonists of histamine at H_2 receptors in the gastric mucosa, and the ability of these compounds to effectively reduce acid secretion irrespective of the nature of the primary stimulus (Black et al., 1972; Parsons, 1973) strongly support the statement by Code that "histamine is the final common local chemostimulator of the parietal cells of the gastric mucosa." It is pertinent to note, however, that the compounds designated as histamine H_2-receptor antagonists do not violate the dictum that drugs possess more than a single pharmacological action. The extent, if any, to which catecholamine-releasing activity and effects on gastric mucosal blood flow may contribute to suppression of histamine-induced parietal cell secretion by H_2-receptor antagonists will be considered by others in this symposium.

Compared to its action on parietal cells, the secretory stimulant effect of histamine on other types of exocrine glands (salivary, lachrymal, respiratory mucosal, pancreatic, and intestinal) is neither prominent nor consistent. Evocation of salivary secretion by histamine appears to be mediated largely through autonomic fibers, although histamine retains some salivary secretory stimulant activity after chronic denervation (Emmelin, 1966).

Adrenal medullary chromaffin cells are stimulated by histamine directly, as well as indirectly via the splanchnic nerves, to secrete the catecholamines epinephrine and norepinephrine. In most individuals, sympathoadrenal discharge is insufficient to counter the depressor response to intravenous histamine; however, in patients with functional chromaffinomas, histamine generally evokes a secondary elevation of blood pressure as a consequence of excess catecholamines released from the tumor cells.

Mechanisms

Molecular mechanisms by which histamine induces target cell responses require further exploration. Douglas (1968, 1974) has suggested that excitatory responses to histamine, involving, for example, autonomic postganglionic fibers and chromaffin cells of the adrenal medulla, are attributable to altered ionic fluxes subsequent to an increase in cell membrane permeability. Similarly, facilitation of calcium entry and reversible release of calcium from intracellular binding sites have been proposed as ionic links in the process of histamine excitation of smooth muscle and cardiac muscle contraction (Somlyo and Somlyo, 1970; 1976). An apparent association of electrolyte and biochemical alterations with the mechanical response to histamine is suggested by studies that demonstrate augmentation of ^{45}Ca influx (DeMello, 1976) and elevation of intracellular levels of cAMP (Klein and Levey, 1971) by concentrations of histamine that elicit a positive inotropic effect in mammalian hearts. Inhibition by burimamide of the stimulatory effect on cardiac muscle and cyclic nucleotide levels (McNeill and Verma, 1974) as well as the acceleration of calcium influx (Ledda *et al.*, 1976) indicate that these myocardial actions of histamine are mediated by H_2 receptors. Verma and McNeill (1976) provided experimental evidence that activation of H_2 sites in the rat uterus evokes norepinephrine release and β-adrenergic receptor-mediated myometrial relaxation and elevation of uterine levels of cAMP. Further studies appear necessary to establish whether the temporal relationships among ionic fluxes, cyclic nucleotide levels and altered contractile states also represent cause-event relationships among the biochemical and mechanical responses of cardiac and smooth muscle cells.

PHYSIOLOGIC AND PATHOPHYSIOLOGIC ROLES OF HISTAMINE

Discovery of the natural occurrence of a biologically active molecule and the existence of selective biochemical mechanisms for its synthesis and disposition leads inevitably to pursuit of the *raison d'etre*. Despite many years of penetrating inquiry, the physiological significance of histamine remains largely an enigma.

Gastric Secretion

Of the several intriguing hypotheses relative to the role of histamine in the natural economy, its critical position in the neurohumoral sequence involved in the regulation of gastric secretion has been most firmly established. That histamine is a powerful stimulus to the acid-forming cell of the gastric mucosa has been demonstrated in essentially all species examined, including man. Several investigators, including Code (1965), Ivy and Bachrach (1966), and Kahlson and Rosengren (1968) have marshalled the multidimensional evidence supporting the proposal that gastric secretion is a physiological function of histamine. A major weakness in this postulate has been the inability of conventional antihistaminic agents to block the parietal cell response to histamine, gastrin and other secretagogues.

The keystone of the histamine "final common pathway" hypothesis seemed to have been mortared in place by the demonstration that burimamide, a selective H_2-receptor antagonist, inhibited gastric secretion stimulated by histamine as well as by pentagastrin in the rat, cat, and dog (Black *et al.*, 1972), and in man (Wyllie *et al.*, 1972). Subsequent studies that buttress the concept that burimamide and metiamide inhibit histamine-stimulated acid secretion by competitive antagonism at H_2-receptor sites in the gastric mucosa have been summarized by Parsons (1973) and Brimblecome and associates (1976). Dousa and Code (1973) and other investigators have described activation of a histamine H_2-receptor-mediated adenylate cyclase system as a further step in the metabolic sequence culminating in the secretory activity of oxyntic cells. But there are few absolutes in biology and the complexity of physiological mechanisms continues to frustrate attempts to delineate specific and exclusive roles for biogenic amines. The finality with which the role of histamine in gastric secretion was espoused more than 20 years ago has been tempered by advances both in knowledge and humility.

Local Vasodilator Mechanisms

It is not surprising that the cellular localization of histamine in proximity to small blood vessels and the potent relaxant effect of this endogenous amine on the microcirculation have fostered speculation on the possible involvement of histamine in physiological vasodilator mechanisms. On the basis of considerable data, Whelan (1956) concluded that the release of stored histamine does not play a part in vasodilator phenomena in man. Subsequent studies by Schayer (1963, 1965) demonstrated that a variety of nonspecific stressors induce histidine decarboxylase activity, resulting in local adaptive increases in histamine synthesis. It has been suggested that this newly formed or *induced histamine* is not stored but is immediately available to promote local dilation of small blood vessels. Thus, histamine is viewed as an integral component of the mechanism through which the microcirculation functions autonomously. However, Zweifach (1973) has pointed out discrepancies between microcirculatory reactivity and histamine-forming capacity. While not precluding a role for histamine in circulatory homeostasis, in recent years attention in this sphere has shifted to other vasoactive autocoids, notably the kinins and prostaglandins.

Tissue Growth and Repair

An extraordinarily high histamine-forming capacity is characteristic of many tissues undergoing rapid growth (e.g., embryonic and malignant cells) or repair (e.g., wound and granulation tissue). Kahlson and Rosengren (1965, 1968) reported that inhibition of histidine decarboxylase activity retarded wound healing and arrested fetal development and, conversely, that facilitation of the rate of histamine formation accelerated reparative growth in skin wounds in rats. These findings have been interpreted as being indicative of a metabolic role for *nascent histamine* in tissue growth and repair beyond that explainable on the basis of assuring an adequate blood supply to rapidly growing or regenerating tissue. However, the precise contribution of induced or nascent histamine to cellular anabolism remains obscure.

Peripheral Nervous System

The flare component of the triple response to intracutaneous histamine has classically been attributed to activation of a local axon reflex. Lewis (1927) postulated that a histamine-like substance serves as an integral link in the mechanism of antidromic vasodilatation. Failure of antihistamines (H_1-receptors antagonists) to attenuate antidromic vasodilatation casts serious doubt on the critical involvement of histamine at the neuroeffector site

(Parrott, 1954), but does not preclude a role for this autocoid as an excitant in the neurovascular phenomenon.

Introduction of histamine into the superficial layers of the skin induces pruritus, and pain is elicited if the amine is injected more deeply (Keele and Armstrong, 1964). Chapman and co-workers (1961) demonstrated that cell injury and intracutaneous histamine promote the release of bradykinin or bradykinin-like polypeptides that possess extraordinary potency as vasodilators and as excitants of nociceptive afferents. Whether histamine can function directly as a pruritogenic agent or only indirectly via the intervention of polypeptides of the bradykinin type remains uncertain (Mountcastle, 1974).

Experimental evidence for the existence of histaminergic fibers in pathways that elicit active reflex vasodilatation in the skin and other organs has been documented by Beck (1965) and Tuttle (1967). Studies by Powell and Brody (1976), utilizing mepyramine and metiamide, provide further evidence that histamine mediates the active component of reflex vasodilatation and indicate that this mediation involves both H_1 and H_2 receptors.

Central Nervous System

More than 15 years ago, Erspamer (1961) remarked "Histamine in the CNS has been ignored for a long time by several investigators as a second-class amine. But this amine, however annoying the fact may be, has the same citizenship rights in the CNS as the catecholamines and 5-HT, whose function in the CNS is approximately as obscure as that of histamine." Recent observations relating to the selective distribution of histamine in the brain, the identification in brain tissue of specific enzymatic systems for histamine synthesis and catabolism, and the ability of histamine introduced intraventricularly or applied iontophoretically to profoundly alter central neuronal activity have been offered as evidence that histamine may have a function in the central nervous system, possibly as a neurotransmitter (Snyder and Taylor, 1972).

Rogers and co-workers (1975) found that histamine-induced stimulation of cAMP formation in guinea pig brain slices was inhibited in the presence of either H_1- or H_2-receptor antagonists. However, Phillis and associates (1975) reported that while metiamide selectively blocked the depressant effect of iontophoretically applied histamine on cerebral cortical neurons in the rat, comparable inhibition was achieved with conventional antihistaminic drugs only at dose levels that nonselectively blocked the action of norepinephrine, 5-hydroxytryptamine, and acetylcholine, as well as histamine. Regional differences in H_1- and H_2-receptor populations in peripheral systems are now well established; it is not surprising that a similar situation may apply to the highly specialized subunits of the central nervous system.

In many aspects, knowledge concerning histamine in the brain has advanced considerably since Erspamer (1961) chided aminologists on their relative neglect of this versatile amine; however, as several authors (Green, 1970; White, 1973; Beaven, 1976) have recently concluded, the data available to date are not sufficient to ascribe to histamine a definitive role in brain function.

Allergy and Anaphylaxis

Dale (1913) demonstrated the exquisite sensitivity to antigen of uterine smooth muscle isolated from sensitized guinea pigs, in agreement with the earlier findings of Schultz (1910) on guinea pig ileum. Progression of the anaphylactic sequence in intact sensitized guinea pigs injected with minute doses of specific antigen was described in detail by Weil (1912, 1914). And the striking resemblance of *in vitro* and *in vivo* models of anaphylaxis to the pharmacologic actions of an amine isolated from samples of ergot (Barger and Dale, 1910) did not escape the attention of these pioneer investigators. That histamine might be involved prominently in the mediation of allergic and anaphylactic phenomena (Dale and Kellaway, 1922) remained an intriguing supposition until Best and his associates (1927) established that this amine was in fact a component of healthy animal tissue and, most crucially, that is appeared in significant quantities in the effluate of sensitized tissues perfused with solutions of specific antigen (Bartosch *et al.*, 1932; Dragstedt and Gebauer-Fuelnegg, 1932).

During the next several decades, extensive studies on the cellular localization of histamine (Riley and West, 1952), mechanisms of its release by chemicals and antigen–antibody interaction (Paton, 1956), and modification by synthetic antihistamines of effector organ responses to this amine refined the histamine theory of anaphylaxis and defined its major limitations (Rocha e Silva, 1966b). Appearance on the scene of serotonin, bradykinin, kalidin, the prostaglandins, slow-reacting substance (SRS-A), eosinophil chemotactic factor (ECF-A), and platelet-activating factor (PAF) has clouded though not obscured the role of histamine in inflammatory and immune processes.

Acting on receptors of the H_1 type, histamine apparently functions as a major mediator of the dilatation and increase in permeability of the microvasculature characteristic of the inflammatory response. Acting on receptors of the H_2 type, histamine may also exert a modulating influence on inflammatory and immune reactions as suggested by observations that this amine is a potent inhibitor of antigen-induced IgE mediated release of histamine from basophilic leukocytes isolated from sensitized patients (Lichtenstein and Gillespie, 1973, 1975). Immunologic release of histamine and other chemical mediators from tissue mast cells and blood basophils is modulated through alterations in intracellular levels of cyclic nucleotides

(Ishizaka *et al.*, 1972; Bourne *et al.*, 1974; Plaut *et al.*, 1975; Kaliner and Austen, 1975). Busse and Sosman (1976) further demonstrated that histamine, acting via a metiamide-sensitive system, suppresses the release of a lysosomal enzyme, β-glucuronidase, from human polymorphonuclear leukocytes. These investigators propose that, depending upon the stage of inflammation, the cell type involved and whether H_1 or H_2 receptors are activated, histamine may exert either an amplifying or an inhibiting effect on the inflammatory response.

EPILOGUE

That the mammalian organism possesses specialized mechanisms for the synthesis, storage, release, and inactivation of the biologically active β-imidazolylethylamine is established unequivocally. New tools and methodologies have enabled characterization of different populations of histaminoceptive sites that subserve effector cell responses to this biogenic amine. And new insights into biochemical mechanisms by which histamine modulates its own functional availability have brought into sharper focus its critical involvement in physiologic and pathophysiologic processes. With apologies to Rudyard Kipling, the "who and what and when and how and where" of histamine are now reasonably well defined; it is the elusive "why?" that we continue to pursue relentlessly.

ACKNOWLEDGMENTS

The author gratefully acknowledges the capable assistance of David Morse, Reference Librarian at the Philadelphia College of Pharmacy and Science.

REFERENCES

Abel, J.J., and Kubota, S. (1919). On the presence of histamine (β-iminazolylethylamine) in the hypophysis cerebri and other tissues of the body and its occurrence among the hydrolytic decomposition products of proteins. *J. Pharmacol. Exper. Therap* **13**, 243–300.

Ackermann, D. (1910). Uber den bacteriellen Abbau des Histidins. *Ztschr. f. physiol. chem.* **65**, 504–510.

Ash, A.S.F., and Schild, H.O. (1966). Receptors mediating some actions of histamine. *Brit. J. Pharmacol. Chemotherap.* **27**, 427–439.

Babkin, B.P. (1938). The triple mechanism of the chemical phase of gastric secretion. *Am. J. Digest. Dis.* **5**, 467–472.

Bareicha, I., and Rocha e Silva, M. (1976). H_1- and H_2-receptors for histamine in the ileum of the guinea pig. *Gen. Pharmac.* **7**, 103–106.

Barger, G., and Dale, H.H. (1910). The presence in ergot and physiological activity of β-imidazolylethylamine. *J. Physiol. (Lond.)* **40**, 38–40.

Barger, G., and Dale, H.H. (1911). β-iminazolylethylamine, a depressor constituent of the intestinal mucosa. *J. Physiol. (London)* **41**, 499–503.

Bartlet, A.L. (1963). The action of histamine on the isolated heart. *Brit. J. Pharmacol. Chemotherap.* **21**, 450–461.

Bartosch, R., Feldberg, W., and Nagel, E. (1932). Das Freiwerden eines histaminähnlichen Stoffes bei der Anaphylaxie des Meerschweinchens. *Pflugers Arch. ges. Physiol.* **230**, 120–153.

Beaven, M.A. (1976) Histamine. *New Engl. J. Med.* **294**, 30–36, 320–325.

Beck, L. (1965). Histamine as the potential mediator of active reflex dilation. *Fed. Proc. 24*, 1298–1310.

Best, C.H., Dale, H.H., Dudley, H.W., and Thorpe, W.V. (1927). The nature of the vaso-dilator constituents of certain tissue extracts. *J. Physiol. (London)* **62**, 397–417.

Black, J.W., Duncan, W.A.M., Durant, G.J., Ganellin, C.R., and Parsons, M.E. (1972). Definition and antagonism of histamine H_2-receptors. *Nature (London)* **236**, 385–390.

Bourne, H.R., Lichtenstein, L.M., Henney, C.S., Melmon, K.L., Weinstein, Y., and Shearer, G.M. (1974). Modulation of inflammation and immunity by cyclic AMP. *Science* **184**, 19–28.

Bovet, D., and Staub, A.M. (1937). Action protectrice des éthers phénoliques au cours de l'intoxication histaminique. *C. R. Soc. Biol. (Paris)* **124**, 547–549.

Brimblecombe, R.W., Duncan, W.A.M., Owen, D.A.A., and Parsons, M.E. (1976). The pharmacology of burimamide and metiamide, two histamine H_2-receptor antagonists. *Fed. Proc.* **35**, 1931–1941.

Broadley, K.J. (1975). The role of H_1 and H_2 receptors in the coronary vascular response to histamine of isolated perfused hearts of guinea pigs and rabbits. *Brit. J. Pharmacol.* **54**, 511–521.

Busse, W.W., and Sosman, J. (1976) Histamine inhibition of neutrophil lysosomal enzyme release: an H_2 histamine receptor response. *Science* **194**, 737–738.

Carnot, P., Koskowski, W., and Libert, E. (1922). Action de l'histamine sur les sucs digestifs chez l'homme. *C. R. Soc. Biol. (Paris)* **86**, 670–673.

Chapman, L.F., Ramos, A.O., Goodell, H., and Wolff, H.G. (1961). Neurohumoral features of afferent fibers in man. Their role in vasodilation, inflammation and pain. *Arch. Neurol.* **4**, 617–650.

Chipman, P., and Glover, W.E. (1976). Histamine H_2-receptors in the human peripheral circulation. *Brit., J. Pharmacol.* **56**, 494–496.

Code, C.F. (1965) Histamine and gastric secretion: a later look 1955–1965. *Fed. Proc.* **24**, 1311–1321.

Dale, H.H. (1913). The effect of varying tonicity on the anaphylactic and other reactions of plain muscle. *J. Pharmacol. Exper. Ther.* **4**, 517–537.

Dale, H.H. (1953). "Adventures in Physiology." Pergamon Press, London.

Dale, H.H., and Kellaway, C.H. (1922). Anaphylaxis and anaphylatoxins. *Phil. Tr. Royal Soc. London B.* **211**, 273–315.

Dale, H.H., and Laidlaw, P.P. (1910). The physiological action of β-iminazolylethylamine. *J. Physiol. (London)* **41**, 318–344.

Dale, H.H., and Richards, A.N. (1918). The vasodilator action of histamine and some other substances. *J. Physiol. (London)* **52**, 110–166.

DeMello, W.C. (1976). On the mechanism of histamine action in cardiac muscle. *Eur. J. Pharmac.* **35**, 315–324.

Douglas, W.W. (1968). Stimulus-secretion coupling: the concept and clues from chromaffin and other cells. The First Gaddum Memorial Lecture. *Brit. J. Pharmacol.* **34**, 451–474.

Douglas, W.W. (1974). Involvement of calcium in exocytosis and the exocytosis-vesiculation sequence. *Biochem. Soc. symp.* **39**, 1–28.

Dousa, T.P., and Code, C.R. (1973). Stimulation of cyclic AMP formation in guinea pig gastric mucosa by histamine and N$\propto$-methylhistamine and their blockade by metiamide, in "International Symposium on Histamine H$_2$-Receptor Antagonists" (C.J. Wood, and M.A. Simkins, eds.), pp. 319–330. Smith Kline and French Laboratories, London.

Dragstedt, C.A., and Gebauer-Fuelnegg, E. (1932). Studies in anaphylaxis. I. The appearance of a physiologically active substance during anaphylactic shock. *Am. J. Physiol.* **102**, 512–521.

Ehrlich, P. (1877). Beiträge zur Kenntnis der Anilinfärbungen und iher Verwendung in der mikroskopischen Technik. *Arch. mikr. Anat.* **13**, 263–277.

Emmelin, N. (1966). Action of histamine upon salivary glands, in "Handbook of Experimental Pharmacology, Histamine and Antihistamines. Part 1. Histamine. Its Chemistry, Metabolism and Physiological and Pharmacological Actions" (O. Eichler and A. Farah, eds.), pp. 294–301. Springer-Verlag, New York.

Erspamer, V. (1961). Pharmacologically active substances of mammalian origin. *Ann. Rev. Pharmacol.* **1**, 175–218.

Feldberg, W. (1956). Distribution of histamine in the body, in "Ciba Foundation Symposium on Histamine" (G.E.W. Wolstenholme and C.M. O'Connor, eds.), pp. 4–13. Little, Brown and Co., Boston.

Folkow, B., Haeger, K., and Kahlson, G. (1948). Observations on reactive hyperemia as related to histamine, on drugs antagonizing vasodilation induced by histamine and on vasodilator properties of adenosine triphosphate. *Acta Physiol. Scan.* **15**, 264–278.

Fourneau, E., and Bovet, D. (1933). The "sympathicolytic" action of a new derivative of dioxane. *Arch. int. pharmacodyn.* **46**, 178–191.

Fröhlich, A., and Pick, E.P. (1912). Die Folgen der Vergiftung durch Adrenalin, Histamine, Pituitrin, Pepton, sowie der anaphylaktischen Vergiftung in Bezug auf das vegetative Nervensystem. *Arch. Exp. Path. Pharm.* **71**, 23–61.

Fühner, H. (1912). Das Pituitrin und seine wirksamen Bestandteile. *Münch. med. wochenschrift* **59**, 852–853.

Goth, A. (1973). Histamine release by drugs and chemicals. "International Encyclopedia of Pharmacology and Therapeutics. Histamine and Antihistamines." Section 74, Vol. 1, pp. 25–43.

Green, J.P. (1962). Binding of some biogenic amines in tissues. *Adv. Pharmacol.* **1**, 349–422.

Green, J.P. (1967). Uptake and binding of histamine. *Fed. Proc.* **26**, 211–218.

Green, J.P. (1970). Histamine, in "Handbook of Neurochemistry, Control Mechanisms in the Nervous System" (A. Lajtha, ed.), pp. 221–250. Plenum Press, New York.

Green, J.P., and Day, M. (1963). Biosynthetic pathways in mastocytoma cells in culture and *in vivo. Ann. N.Y. Acad. Sci.* **103**, 334–351.

Haddy, F.J. (1960). Effect of histamine on small and large vessel pressures in the dog foreleg. *Amer. J. Physiol.* **198**, 161–168.

Ishizaka, T., DeBernardo, R., Tomioka, H., Lichtenstein, L.M., and Ishizaka, K. (1972). Identification of basophil granulocytes as a site of allergic histamine release. *J. Immunol.* **108**, 1000–1008.

Ivy, A.C., and Bachrach, W.H. (1966). Physiological significance of the effect of histamine on gastric secretion, in "Handbook of Experimental Pharmacology. Histamine and Antihistaminics. Part 1. Histamine. Its Chemistry, Metabolism and Physiological and Pharmacological Actions" (O. Eichler and A. Farah, Eds.), pp. 810–891. Springer-Verlag, New York.

Kahlson, G., and Rosengren, E. (1965). Histamine. *Ann. Rev. Pharmacol.* **5**, 305–320.

Kahlson, G., and Rosengren, E. (1968). New approaches to the physiology of histamine. *Physiol. Rev.* **48**, 155–196.

Kaliner, M., and Austen, K.F. (1975). Immunologic release of chemical mediators from human tissues. *Ann. Rev. Pharmacol.* **15**, 177–189.

Keele, C.A., and Armstrong, D. (1964). "Substances Producing Pain and Itch" Williams & Wilkins Co., Baltimore.

Keeton, R.W., Luckhardt, A.B., and Koch, F.C. (1920). Gastrin studies: IV. The response of the stomach mucosa to food and gastrinbodies as influenced by atropine. *Am. J. Physiol.* **51**, 469–483.

Klein, I., and Levey, G.S. (1971). Activation of myocardial adenyl cyclase by histamine in guinea pig, cat and human heart. *J. Clin, Invest.* **50**, 1012–1015.

Ledda, F., Mantelli, L., and Mugelli, A. (1976). Blockade by burimamide of the restorative effect of histamine in tetrodotoxin-treated heart preparations. *Br. J. Pharmacol.* **57**, 247–249.

Levi, R., and Capurro, N. (1973). Histamine H_2-receptor antagonism and cardiac anaphylaxis, in "International Encyclopedia of Pharmacology and Therapeutics. Histamine and Antihistamines." Section 74, Vol. 1, pp. 175–183.

Levi, R., and Kuye, J.O. (1974). Pharmacological characterization of cardiac histamine receptors: sensitivity to H_1-receptor antagonists. *Eur. J. Pharmac.* **27**, 330–338.

Levi, R., Allan, G., and Zavecz, J.H. (1976). Cardiac histamine receptors. *Fed. Proc.* **35**, 1942–1947.

Lewis, T. (1927). "The Blood Vessels of the Human Skin and Their Responses," Shaw and Sons, Ltd., London.

Lichtenstein, L.M., and Gillespie, E. (1973). Inihibition of histamine release by histamine controlled by H_2 receptor. *Nature (London)* **244**, 287–288.

Lichtenstein, L.M., and Gillespie, E. (1975). The effects of the H_1 and H_2 antihistamines on "allergic" histamine release and its inhibition by histamine. *J. Pharmacol. Exper. Ther.* **192**, 441–450.

Lindell, S.E., and Westling, H. (1966). Histamine metabolism in man, in "Handbook of Experimental Pharmacology. Histamine and Antihistaminics. Part 1. Histamine. Its Chemistry, Metabolism and Physiological and Pharmacological Actions" (O. Eichler and A. Farah, eds.), pp. 734–788. Springer–Verlag, New York.

MacIntosh, F.C., and Paton, W.D.M. (1949). The liberation of histamine by certain organic bases. *J. Physiol. (London)* **109**, 190–219.

McIntire, F.C. (1973). Histamine release by antigen-antibody reactions, in "International Encyclopedia of Pharmacology and Therapeutics. Histamine and antihistamines." Section 74, Vol. 1, pp. 45–99.

McNeill, J.H., and Verma, S.C. (1974). Blockade by burimamide of the effects of histamine and histamine analogs on cardiac contractility, phosphorylase activation and cyclic adenosine monophosphate. *J. Pharmacol. Exper. Ther.* **188**, 180–188.

Mellanby, E., and Twort, F.W. (1912). On the presence of β-imidazolylethylamine in the intestinal wall; with a method of isolating a bacillus from the alimentary canal which converts histidine into this substance. *J. Physiol. (London)* **45**, 53–60.

Mountcastle, V.B. (1974). Pain and temperature sensibilities, in *Medical Physiology,* vol. 1. 13 ed., pp. 348–381. C.V. Mosby Company, St. Louis.

Parrot, J.L. (1954). The place of histamine in neurohumoral transmission. *Pharmacol. Rev.* **6**, 119–122.

Parrot, J.L., and Thouvenot, J. (1966). Action de l'histamine sur les muscles lisses, in "Handbook of Experimental Pharmacology. Histamine and Antihistaminics. Part 1. Histamine. It Chemistry, Metabolism and Physiological and Pharmacological Actions" (O. Eichler and A. Farah, eds.), pp. 202–224. Springer-Verlag, New York.

Parsons, M.E. (1973). The evidence that inhibition of histamine-stimulated gastric secretion is a result of blockade of histamine H_2-receptors, in "International Symposium on Histamine H_2-Receptor Antagonists" (C.J. Wood and M.A. Simkins, eds.), pp. 207–215. Smith Kline & French Laboratories, London.

Parsons, M.E., and Owen, D.A.A. (1973). Receptors involved in the cardiovascular responses to histamine, in "International Symposium on Histamine H_2-Receptor Antagonists" (C.J. Wood and M.A. Simkins, eds.), pp. 127–135. Smith Kline & French Laboratories, London.

Paton, W.D.M. (1956). The mechanism of histamine release, in "Ciba Foundation Symposium on Histamine" (G.E.W. Wolstenholme and C.M. O'Connor, eds.), pp. 59–73. Little, Brown and Co., Boston.

Phillis, J.W., Kostopoulos, G.K., and Odutola, A. (1975). On the specificity of histamine H_2-receptor antagonists in the rat cerebral cortex. *Can. J. Physiol. Pharmacol.* **53**, 1205–1209.

Plaut, M., Lichtenstein, L.M., and Henney, C.S. (1975). Modulation of immediate hypersensitivity and cell-mediated immunity: the role of histamine, in "Immunopharmacology" (M.E. Rosenthale and H.C. Mansmann, Jr., eds.), pp. 57–72. Spectrum Publications, New York.

Popielski, L. (1920). β-imidäzolylathylamin und die Organextratke. Erster Teil. β-imidazolyläthylamin als mächtiger Erreger der Magendrüsen. *Pfluger's Arch. ges. Physiol.* **178**, 214–236.

Powell, J.R., and Brody, M.J. (1973). Identification of two vascular histamine receptors in the dog, in "International Symposium on Histamine H_2-Receptor Antagonists" (C.J. Wood and M.A. Simkins, eds.), pp. 137–146. Smith Kline & French Laboratories, London.

Powell, J.R., and Brody, M.J. (1976). Identification and specific blockade of two receptors for histamine in the cardiovascular system. *J. Pharmacol. Exper. Ther.* **196**, 1–14.

Riley, J.F., and West, G.B. (1952). Histamine in tissue mast cells. *J. Physiol. (London)* **117**, 72P–73P.

Rocha e Silva, M. (1955). "Histamine, Its Role in Anaphylaxis and Allergy," pp. 37–105. Charles C. Thomas, Springfield.

Rocha e Silva, M. (1966a). Action of histamine upon the circulatory apparatus, in "Handbook of Experimental Pharmacology. Histamine and Antihistaminics. Part 1. Histamine. Its Chemistry, Metabolism and Physiological and Pharmacological Actions" (O. Eichler and A. Farah, eds.), pp. 238–294. Springer-Verlag, New York.

Rocha e Silva, M. (1966b). Release of histamine in anaphylaxis, in "Handbook of Experimental Pharmacology. Histamine and Antihistaminics. Part I. Histamine. Its Chemistry, Metabolism and Physiological and Pharmacological Actions" (O. Eichler and A. Farah, Eds.), pp. 431–480. Springer-Verlag, New York.

Rogers, M., Dismukes, K., and Daly, J.W. (1975). Histamine-elicited accumulations of cyclic adenosine 3', 5'-monophosphate in guinea-pig brain slices: effect of H_1- and H_2-antagonists. *J. Neurochem.* **25**, 531–534.

Rothschild, A.M. (1966). Histamine release by basic compounds, in "Handbook of Experimental Pharmacology. Histamine and Antihistaminics. Part I. Histamine. Its Chemistry, Metabolism and Physiological and Pharmacological Actions" (O. Eichler and A. Farah, eds.), pp. 386–430. Springer-Verlag, New York.

Schayer, R.W. (1959). Catabolism of physiological quantities of histamine in vivo. *Physiol. Rev.* **39**, 116–126.

Schayer, R.W. (1961). Significance of induced synthesis of histamine in physiology and pharmacology. *Chemotherapia* **3**, 128–136.

Schayer, R.W. (1963). Induced synthesis of histamine, microcirculatory regulation and the mechanism of action of the glucocorticoid hormones. *Prog. Allergy* **7**, 187–212.

Schayer, R.W. (1965). Histamine and circulatory homeostasis. *Fed. Proc.* **24**, 1295–1297.

Schayer, R.W., and Reilly, M.A. (1973). Effect of H_2-receptor antagonists on histamine metabolism, in "International Symposium on Histamine H_2-Receptor Antagonists" (C.J. Wood and M.A. Simkins, eds.), pp. 87–95. Smith Kline & French Laboratories, London.

Schayer, R.W., Cooper, J.A.D., Smiley, R.L., and Davis, K.J. (1956). Metabolism of C^{14}-histamine in man. *J. Appl. Physiol.* **9**, 481–483.

Schmidt-Mülheim, A. (1880). Beiträge zur Kenntnis des Peptons und seiner physiologischen Bedeutung. *Arch. Physiol.* 33–56.

Schultz, W.H. (1910). Physiological studies in anaphylaxis I. The reactions of smooth muscle of the guinea pig sensitized with horse serum. *J. Pharmacol. Exper. Ther.* **1**, 549–567.

Snyder, S.H., and Taylor, K.M. (1972). Histamine in the brain: a neurotransmitter? in "Perspectives in Neuropharmacology: A Tribute to Julius Axelrod" (Snyder, S.H., ed.), pp. 43–73. Oxford University Press, New York.

Somlyo, A.P., and Somlyo, A.V. (1970). Vascular smooth muscle. II. Pharmacology of normal and hypertensive vessels. *Pharmacol. Rev.* **22**, 249–353.

Somlyo, A.P., and Somlyo, A.V. (1976). Ultrastructural aspects of activation and contraction of vascular smooth muscle. *Fed. Proc.* **35**, 1288–1293.

Staub, A.M. (1939). Recherches sur quelque bases synthetiques antagonistes de l'histamine. *Ann. Inst. Pasteur.* **63**, 400–436.

Trendelenburg, U. (1960). The action of histamine and 5-hydroxytryptamine on isolated mammalian atria. *J. Pharmacol. Exper. Ther.* **130**, 450–460.

Türker, R.K. (1973). Presence of histamine H_2-receptors in the guinea-pig pulmonary vascular bed. *Pharmacology* **9**, 306–311.

Tuttle, R.S. (1967). Physiological release of histamine-^{14}C in the pyramidal cat. *Am. J. Physiol.* **213**, 620–624.

Uvnas, B. (1963). Mechanism of histamine release in mast cells. *Ann. N.Y. Acad. Sci.* **103**, 278–283.

Verma, S.C., and McNeill, J.H. (1976). The effect of histamine, isoproterenol and tyramine on rat uterine cyclic AMP. *Res. Comm. Chem. Path. Pharm.* **13**, 55–64.

Vugman, I., and Rocha e Silva, M. (1966). Biological determination of histamine in living tissues and body fluids, in "Handbook of Experimental Pharmacology. Histamine and Antihistaminics. Part 1. Histamine. Its Chemistry, Metabolism and Physiological and Pharmacological Actions" (O. Eichler and A. Farah, eds.), pp. 81–115. Springer-Verlag, New York.

Wakim, K.G., Peters, G.A., Terrier, J.C., and Horton, B.T. (1949). The effects of intravenously administered histamine on the peripheral circulation in man. *J. Lab. Clin. Med.* **34**, 380–386.

Weil, R. (1912). The nature of anaphylaxis and the relations between anaphylaxis and immunity. *J. Med. Res.* **27**, 497–527.

Weil, R. (1914). Studies in anaphylaxis. *J. Med. Res.* **30**(2), 87–111.

Whelan, R.F. (1956). Histamine and vasodilatation, in "Ciba Foundation Symposium on Histamine" (Wolstenholme, G.E.W. and O'Connor, C.M., eds.), pp. 220–234. Little, Brown and Co., Boston.

White, T. (1973). Effect of drugs on brain histamine, in "International Encyclopedia of Pharmacology and Therapeutics. Histamine and Antihistamines" Section 74, Vol. 1, pp. 101–107. Pergamon Press Ltd., Oxford.

Windaus, A., and Vogt, W. 91907). Synthese des Imidazolyläthylamins. *Berichte deutsch. chem. Gesellschaft* **40**, 3691–3695.

Wyllie, J.H., Hesselbo, T., and Black, J.W. (1972). Effects in man of histamine H_2receptor blockade by burimamide. *Lancet* **2**, 1117–1120.

Zweifach, B.W. (1973). Microcirculation. *Ann. Rev. Physiol.* **35**, 117–150.

PART I
GASTROINTESTINAL HISTAMINE RECEPTORS

2

The Riddle of Gastric Histamine*

James W. Black
Department of Pharmacology
University College London
London, England

The general biology of histamine has always been mysterious. The particular relation of histamine to the stomach has been especially teasing and enigmatic.

Babkin (1950) has pointed to the irony that the discovery in 1920 that histamine was a powerful stimulant of gastric acid secretion was made by Popielski, "...a man who spent practically his entire scientific career in contesting the theory that the digestive glands (particularly the pancreatic gland) may be regulated by hormonal...influences...." Vasodilatin, not histamine, was Popielski's main pursuit. He stoutly maintained that the secretory effect of a hydrochloric acid extract of the duodenal mucosa does not depend on its containing a specific hormone, secretin, but is due to the presence of a substance of unknown nature which he called vasodilatin. The secretagogue effect of vasodilatin on the pancreas he attributed to its power of lowering the blood pressure by vasodilation and of diminishing the coagulability of the blood, and he employed the same argument to explain the secretagogue effect of gastrin. Dale and Laidlaw (1910) thought that vasodilatin was identical to histamine and that the presence of histamine in tissues was the result of bacterial contamination. Even though he had got it right, Edkins' (1905) gastrin theory succumbed first to vasodilatin and then to histamine. As R. A. Gregory (1974) put it, "Edkins might be said to have had the unhappy distinction of being the first known victim of that ubiquitous enigma, histamine, years before its existence in the body and its powerful effect on gastric acid secretion was recognized."

Since those early days, histamine and gastrin have weaved in and out of scientific thought. Histamine as a pharmacological fact in the 1920's gave

---

*The 1977 A. N. Richards Memorial Lecture.

way, in the 1930's, to histamine the physiological entity, the gastric hormone. However, when Komarov (1938) discovered an antral extract, free of histamine but potent in stimulating acid secretion, the counter-attack began. The failure of the first antihistamines to inhibit histamine-stimulated secretion seriously undermined its position and the isolation and subsequent synthesis of gastrin by Gregory and his team (Gregory *et al.*, 1966) finally removed histamine's credentials.

Given then that the true gastric hormone has been identified, what, if any, physiological role is left for histamine in the stomach? Is it some kind of local hormone? The powerful pharmacological effects of histamine on the stomach are hard to ignore and Kahlson and his colleagues (Kahlson and Rosengren, 1972) have steadily worked up the hypothesis that histamine alone acts on the oxyntic cells and that gastrin acts indirectly by releasing histamine. Thirty years earlier, MacIntosh (1938) claimed a similar mechanism for the action of the vagus on oxyntic cell secretion.

I have tried to draw up a checklist of questions about formation, storage, release, and inactivation—questions which might determine the viability of the claim that histamine is a local hormone. However, the available information seems to me too uncertain to be the basis of any wide generalization. Disagreement about methods crops up again and again and I do not have the biochemical experience needed to guide me. Therefore, I want to examine now whether the more oblique methods of pharmacological analysis can side-step the contemporary difficulties in biochemical analysis. Can the newer histamine antagonists, such as metiamide, throw some light on the relations between histamine and the physiological control of gastric function?

Metiamide has been classified (by measuring its dissociation constant) as a simple, competitive, antagonist of histamine at H_2-receptors (Black *et al.*, 1973). The archetypes of H_2-receptor mediated systems are guinea pig atrial muscle and rat uterine horns. Both of these tissues are convenient for measuring apparent dissociation constants because, used as isolated tissues, they are robust, fast-responding, and reproducible. Metiamide also inhibits histamine-stimulated gastric acid secretion. This is a general phenomenon and has been shown in man, monkey, dog, cat, guinea pig, rat, mouse, frog, and chicken. Histamine-stimulated acid secretion cannot be inhibited by mepyramine, an H_1-receptor antagonist, so, presumably, H_2-receptors are involved in this process as well. However, clinching this classification by pharmacological measurement has not been straightforward, because no simple and reliable *in vitro* measuring system has been available for studying acid secretion. This is no academic point because metiamide also interacts with pentagastrin.

In every species tested, pentagastrin-stimulated acid secretion is as sensitive to inhibition by metiamide as is histamine. This would be the prediction of the

Kahlson hypothesis; pentagastrin releases histamine and the subsequent action of histamine at H_2 receptors is blocked by metiamide. Before accepting this, however, we must know that metiamide not only blocks H_2 receptors on oxyntic cells but that it has no other relevant actions. The most obvious of these other actions would be that metiamide interferes with the secretory process itself, perhaps at a subcellular level. At the very least there seems to be clear evidence against this possibility in some systems. Isolated stomach preparations of cat (Tepperman *et al.*, 1975) rat, or mouse readily secrete acid in response to histamine, pentagastrin, or acetylcholine; metiamide can annul the responses to histamine and pentagastrin without inhibiting the response to acetylcholine. Therefore, the anti-secretory action of metiamide may be selective but there is no reason to presuppose that this is due to a specific action at H_2 receptors. Although evidence that metiamide is a competitive antagonist of histamine at H_2-receptors in the gastric mucosa would not prove that this was the mechanism involved in the antagonism to pentagastrin, nevertheless, if evidence against this mode of action were to be found, this would imply that metiamide had other anti-secretory properties. Given, then, that it is important to find out the nature of the metiamide-histamine interaction, what is needed to see if there is simple competition at H_2 receptors?

An *in vitro* preparation, where acid secretion is measured directly and both agonists and antagonists can be allowed to come into concentration equilibrium, is essential. We can then conclude that metiamide behaves like a simple, competitive, antagonist of histamine at H_2-receptors if the following relations are found (all are necessary, and no one alone is sufficient): if metiamide shifts histamine dose-response curves, dextrad, in parallel without reduction of maximum responses; if the extent of the displacement of these curves, or dose-ratios, is a simple linear function of metiamide concentration as defined by the Schild equation; if the dissociation constant (or pA_2, its negative logarithm) for the metiamide-receptor interaction calculated from this equation is similar to that already found using atrial and uterine tissues; and, finally, if the estimated pA_2 is found to be independent of the relative activity of the agonist used to measure it.

Bunce and Parsons (1976) were the first to tackle the problem. They developed an isolated, lumen-perfused, rat stomach preparation which responded well to histamine stimulation. They found that metiamide at concentrations between $3 \times 10^{-6} M$ and $3 \times 10^{-5} M$ produced parallel displacement of histamine log dose-response curves. However, although the Schild plot was linear over this narrow range of metiamide concentration, its slope of 0.73 (with 95% confidence limits 0.58–0.88) was significantly different from unity. This then is not a satisfactory representation of the Schild equation for conditions of simple, competitive, antagonism. Therefore, if metiamide **is** a simple, competitive antagonist at H_2-receptors in the gastric mucosa, some other process must also be operating to distort the Schild relationship. If metiamide **is not** a competitive antagonist then it will be of little use for analyzing the gastrin/histamine relationship.

To try to resolve the question, the effects of metiamide have been tested in isolated mouse stomachs using a 1000 fold range of antagonist concentration (Angus *et al.*, 1978). Metiamide produced a parallel shift of histamine log dose-response curves and the Schild plot was linear with a slope not different from unity. The calculated pA_2 was 5.08 ($\pm$0.32) and this was not significantly different from the pA_2 (5.14 $\pm$0.31) found using dimaprit as agonist. Therefore metiamide meets the criteria for a simple competitive antagonist on that tissue. However these pA_2 values are nearly 1 log unit lower than those measured using atria and uterus. Moreover, the pA_2's for burimamide and cimetidine were equally low compared to these other tissues. Are the histamine receptors in the stomach different from those in atria and uterus? The results with atropine provide a clue. The pA_2 for the atropine/bethanechol interaction measured using acid secretion in the isolated mouse stomach was found to be 7.5; the pA_2 for the same interaction measured using muscle contraction in the same preparation gave a pA_2 of 8.4. Apparently the acid-secreting mouse stomach preparation tends to give low pA_2 values in general. The reasonable though provisional conclusion is that the histamine receptors in the stomach can be classified as H_2 receptors. The corollary, derived from risky circular reasoning, is that the effects of metiamide on the gastric mucosa may be interpreted as due to histamine H_2-receptor blockade.

Returning to the metiamide-pentagastrin interaction, the simplest hypothesis using this assumption is that the activity of pentagastrin somehow involves histamine receptors. There are three elementary ways in which the action of pentagastrin could depend on the activation of histamine receptors. The first is that pentagastrin activates histamine receptors directly. In this case, metiamide would act like a simple competitive antagonist of pentagastrin. There is now evidence in man (Thjodleifsson Wormsley, 1974), in rats (Lundell, 1975), and dogs (Fig.1; Black, 1973) with Heidenhain pouches, and in isolated mouse stomachs that although the pentagastrin log dose-response curves are displaced to the right by metiamide, the maximum responses are progressively reduced as the concentrations of antagonist are increased. Therefore the hypothesis that metiamide and pentagastrin act in simple competition can probably be rejected.

The second possibility is that there is an obligatory connection, in parallel, between gastrin and histamine receptors. In this model, histamine would play a necessary, permissive role in the action of the gastric hormone (including pentagastrin) and blockade of histamine receptors would therefore produce noncompetitive antagonism to pentagastrin. This I take to be the essence of the model proposed by Grossman and Konturek (1974). When there is no longer a receptor reserve, this hypothesis predicts that the pentagastrin log

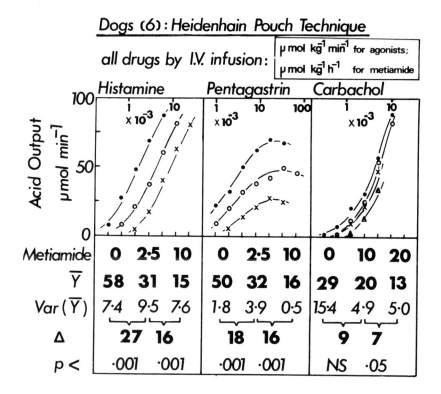

FIG. 1.   Noncompetitive antagonism of pentagastrin by metiamide (Black, 1973).

dose-response curves will be reduced in simple proportion without dextrad displacement. So far, all the reported pentagastrin log dose-response curves have been displaced to the right and proportionately reduced at the same time. The hypothesis cannot be rejected on this evidence, of course, but it is weakened at the first test.

In the third model, gastrin and histamine receptors are necessarily "connected" in series. This is the essence of the Kahlson–Rosengren–Svensson hypothesis (Kahlson *et al.*, 1973). An essential condition for the Grossman and Konturek hypothesis is that both receptors should be located on the same cell. The Kahlson hypothesis, however, explicitly locates the gastrin and histamine receptors on different cells. In this two-cell hypothesis, what would happen to pentagastrin dose-response curves during indirect antagonism— that is, when metiamide competitively antagonizes the histamine released from an adjacent cell by pentagastrin? If, in addition to the usual simplifying assumptions involved in applying the Law of Mass Action to drug-receptor interaction, we assume; (a) that the output of histamine secretion initiated by gastrin receptor occupancy follows the usual simple hyperbolic relationship/ and (b) that the amount of histamine secreted is in excess of the available histamine receptors then, in the presence of antagonist, the output maximum for histamine, determined by the gastrin interaction with its receptors, effectively prevents enough histamine arriving to overcome the blockade— consequently the maximum response is reduced. However, at low levels of receptor occupancy, the first stage can make enough histamine available for this second stage, and so the curve is displaced to the same extent that the histamine dose-response curve would have been shifted. This combination of progressive dextrad displacement plus reduction of the maximum is characteristic of this model of indirect antagonism.

Therefore, the simplest possible model of indirect antagonism in a sequential system behaves like the general case of the pentagastrin–metiamide interaction. This coincidence does not make it true but the verisimilitude reinforces the hypothesis and, as it were, keeps it alive.

The conclusion, at this stage then, is that no decisive answer can be obtained from examination of the effect of metiamide and, presumably, H_2-receptor blockade on agonist dose-response curves. The model system involving a *series* connection, via different cells, between gastrin and histamine is perhaps marginally more attractive as fewer simplifying assumptions have to be made. Is there, then, some other way of trying to distinguish the one and two-cell hypothesis?

The two cell hypothesis is quite explicit on one point: the relatively slow rate of histamine synthesis demands that preformed histamine be stored, bound in granules, and in special histamine cells, while H^+ ions are secreted instantly by the parietal cells. There is evidence from other secretory processes, salivation, for example (Martinez and Petersen, 1972), that not all secretory processes are equally dependent on the short-term supply of calcium ions. Therefore, as far as acid secretion is concerned, the two-cell hypothesis predicts that pentagastrin might be more sensitive to calcium than histamine.

Using isolated mouse stomachs, Welch and I (Black and Welch, 1977) have found that calcium-free solutions have a differential effect; pentagastrin responses are significantly reduced after 60 minutes in Ca^{2+}-free solution while histamine responses are still relatively well maintained. If calcium deprivation is the essential feature in this experiment, the same effect should be produced by calcium-ion antagonism. Manganese ions antagonize the effects of calcium on histamine-release from rat peritoneal mast cells and we found that adding 1 mM $MnCl_2$ led to a reduction in the size of the pentagastrin responses without significant reduction in the histamine responses. However, incubation with higher concentrations of $MnCl_2$ (5 mM) also reduced the histamine responses. The addition of 5 mM Mg^{2+} was found to have the same effect. However, 20 mM Mg^{2+} ions not only produced a significant inhibition of pentagastrin responses, there was now also a very significant potentiation of histamine responses and incubation with 10 mM Mg^{2+} gave intermediate responses. The control experiments, replacing Na^{2+} ions with glucose, had no effect on the responses to either stimulant. Although we have no explanation for this potentiating action of Mg^{2+}, the clear distinction between the two agonists suggests that different processes are involved in each.

This difference, however, is not completely incompatible with a one-cell hypothesis. For example, pentagastrin might act at receptors on the cell membrane to open Ca^{2+} channels while histamine could act at some Ca^{2+}-rich subcellular site, mitochondria for example, to release intracellular Ca^{2+}. However, it would be a strain on the imagination to see how gastrin and histamine receptors linked in parallel could behave in this way.

Another conclusion can perhaps be drawn from these simple experiments. The calcium dependence of the agonists implies that raising the intracellular Ca^{2+} concentration is needed for stimulus-secretion coupling. Therefore, raising the intracellular Ca^{2+} ion concentration by, for example, exposure to the calcium inophore A23187 should not only stimulate acid secretion but should do so beyond both histamine and gastrin receptors (and therefore be refractory to blockade by metiamide) if the action is in parietal cells. However, if the coupling is mainly to the secretion of histamine from cells anterior to parietal cells, then this response should be blockable by metiamide. We have found that isolated mouse stomachs secrete acid in response to equilibration with A23187 with a much slower time course than the response to histamine or pengastrin. Subsequent addition of metiamide during the plateau of secretion produced prompt inhibition. The log dose-response curves to A23187 which have been incubated either alone or with different concentrations of metiamide were displaced to the right with a reduction of the maximum response reminiscent of the effect of metiamide on pentagastrin log dose-response curves. There is no immediately obvious way of reconciling these observations with a one-cell hypothesis, but the accommodation is easy with the alternative hypothesis.

In summary, the pharmacological properties of metiamide point to it being a competitive antagonist of histamine at H_2-receptors in the gastric mucosa. The pattern of displacement of pentagastrin dose-response curves by metiamide are like those due to indirect competitive antagonism. The selective calcium dependence of pentagastrin tentatively points to the involvement of a different type of secretory process from that with histamine. All of the above plus the susceptibility to blockade by metiamide of secretion induced by a calcium ionophore point to the conclusion that histamine and H_2-receptor activation are somehow involved in the pharmacological mode of action of gastrin and therefore, presumably, involved in the physiologcial control of gastric acid secretion.

What are the implications of this thesis that histamine is necessarily involved in the regulation of gastric function? I would like to consider for a few moments what I imagine to be the real riddle of gastric histamine: If histamine is involved in the physiology of gastric acid secretion, if gastrin acts indirectly, where, if any, is the biological advantage over a direct action by the gastric hormone?

Gastrin is a true hormone with highly selective actions. Pharmacological studies have shown that rates of administration of gastrin which stimulate acid and pepsin secretion have hardly any other actions than on the upper gastrointestinal tract so that it can circulate in the blood with safety; that is not so with histamine. Vasodilatation and altered vascular permeability, hallmarks of the acute inflammatory reaction, which, for example, can regulate the flow of macromolecules into tissue spaces, are well-known actions that can be produced by histamine. Although these vascular actions of histamine can be blocked by a combination of H_1-receptor and H_2-receptor antagonists, the functional relationship of histamine to inflammation is still a controversial subject. If histamine is involved in inflammation, the modern consensus is that its action is early, brief, and probably irrelevant. Histamine is now massively outgunned in interest by prostaglandins, kinins, slow-reacting substances, lysosomal enzymes, lymphokines, and many other immunological factors.

However, the interaction of H_2-receptor antagonists alone with non-invasive inflammatory reactions perhaps points to a different story. In the first paper on burimamide (Black et al., 1972), there was a throwaway line near the end, namely, that "other experimental inflammatory reactions...can be inhibited by burimamide...." Behind that statement there were some experiments by Parsons where ultraviolet radiation was focussed, for 30 seconds, on to the shaved backs of guinea pigs. The areas were examined 2 and 5 hours later and an inflammatory reaction was recorded, using bias-free procedures, on a nominal scale. Treatment beforehand with mepyramine produced the well-known effect, i.e., the inflammation was suppressed at 2 hours but not at 5 hours. This is the kind of result that has contributed to the present view of the relative unimportance of histamine in inflammation. However, highly significant suppression of the inflammatory reaction was found with burimamide at *both* 2 and 5 hours and the combination with mepyramine was no better than burimamide alone.

More recently Brimblecombe and his colleagues (Brimblecombe et al., 1976) have shown an interaction between cimetidine and heat-induced inflammation in the hind paw of rats—a scalding reaction in which the paw volume was measured over a period of 4 hours. Treatment with cimetidine alone at either 50 or 250 mg/kg produced a very significant suppression of these changes.

Two points should be noted about these experiments: burimamide and cimetidine do *not* have general anti-inflammatory actions; for example, they do not suppress the inflammatory reaction to the injection of carageenin or turpentine in the rat paw; and, second, although there are no a priori grounds for assuming that this effect of these drugs is necessarily a consequence of their H_2-receptor antagonist properties (indeed, I suspect we will find it very difficult to either prove or disprove that this *is* the way they are acting) nevertheless these are unusual actions of drugs which are otherwise fairly selective antagonists of histamine-specific sites. Therefore, I am tempted to conclude that in the acute inflammatory reaction, as in the gastric secretory process, the role of histamine may need to be reassessed yet again.

If I concede this point to myself, I can see no reason why I should not also concede that those more-chronic processes which Schayer (1961) and Kahlson have shown to be associated with a high level of induced histidine decarboxylase activity may, indeed, be dependent on the continuous production and release of histamine. I am thinking here about cell growth and tissue repair.

Here then is some light-hearted speculation: animals may be discriminating about the quantity of food they eat but they show less judgment about its quality. The stomach acting as hopper and mill needs defense mechanisms against mechanical damage and bacterial invasion. The release of histamine in the submucosa, synchronized by gastrin to the ingestion of food, protects the stomach wall by inducing a complex pattern of vascular, humoral, and cellular events and, linked to these, the secretion of hydrochloric acid protects both stomach and host by sterilizing the gastric contents.

A few years ago Lewis Thomas (1971) gave a characteristically brilliant lecture on the "adaptive aspects of inflammation." He wrote, "Perhaps the inflammatory reaction should be regarded as a defense of an individual against all the rest of nature, symbolizing his individuality and announcing his existence as an entity.... There are as many such reactions of defense, as many pronouncements of entity, of individual integrity, as there are organisms in nature. They represent, obviously, a great natural force for the preservation of species, for protection against all kinds of foreignness." In short, Thomas looked at inflammation as the opposite of symbiosis.

At this we cannot fail to be struck by the relation of the stomach to individual identity and aggression. Wolf and Wolff's (1943) study of the gastric function of Tom, who suffered from a chronic gastric fistula, showed that acid secretion and mucosal reddening were often linked to emotional situations producing reddening of the face. For example, on one occasion Tom had been doing some piecework house cleaning after hours. The doctor who had hired him came to pay him off and insinuated that Tom's charges were excessive and that he worked slowly. Tom became angry and hostile and, "his face was red and his collar seemed too tight. The gastric mucosa became hyperaemic and engorged and acid production more than doubled. Vigorous contractions started and his stomach presented an appearance of overactivity similar to but less marked than that encountered in experimentally induced gastritis." On another occasion a similar "stomach-and-face" reaction was produced after a fruitless fight with a secretary in the clinic whom he particularly disliked.... "I wish I could get my hands on her neck" he said! Histamine may thus be involved not only in local defense reactions but also in the complex behavior patterns establishing one's individuality, as in Thomas' conception.

I think it is appropriate to end this A. N. Richards Lecture as I began, with the significance of histamine-induced vasodilatation, because it was the problems of the vascular actions of histamine and the nature of wound shock that first took Newton Richards to London (Bronk, 1976). He had already been Professor of Pharmacology here at the University of Pennsylvania for some years when the war time—that is the first world war—British Medical Research Committee cabled him for help to work with Henry Dale at the National Institute of Medical Research. The collaboration with Dale on histamine was brief but fruitful before the United States entered the war and Richards was called to join the armed forces. However, Richards' outstanding ability made enduring contributions to the subject of this present Symposium.

REFERENCES

Angus, J.A., Black, J.W., and Stone, M. (1978). Comparative assay of histamine H_2-receptor antagonists using the isolated mouse stomach. *Brit. J. Pharmacol.* **62**, 445–446 P.

Babkin, B.P. (1950). Histamine as a stimulant of gastric secretion, in "Secretary Mechanism of the Digestive Glands." Harper, New York.

Black, J.W. (1973). Speculation about the nature of the antagonism between metiamide and pentagastrin, in "International Symposium on Histamine H_2-Receptor Antagonists." (C.J. Wood and M.A. Simkins, eds.),pp. 219–221. SK&F Labs, Welwyn Garden City, U.K.

Black, J.W., Duncan, W.A.M., Durant, L.J., Ganellin, C.R., and Parsons, M.E. (1972). Definition and antagonism of histamine H_2-receptors. *Nature (London)* **236**, 385–390.

Black, J.W., Duncan, W.A.M., Emmett, J.C., Ganellin, C.R., Heselbo, T., Parsons, M.E., and Wyllie, J.A. (1973). Metiamide—an orally active histamine H_2-receptor antagonist. *Agents and Actions* **3**, 133–137.

Black, J.W., and Welch, L.A. (1977). Are gastrin receptors located on parietal cells? *Brit. J. Pharmacol.* **59**, 476P.

Brimblecombe, R.W., Farrington, H.E., Lavender, M.K., and Owen, D.A.A. (1976). Histamine H_2-receptor antagonists and thermal injury in rats. *Burns* **3**, 8–13.

Bronk, D.W. (1976). Alfred Newton Richards (1876–1966). *Persp. Biol. med.* **19**, 413–422.

Bunce, K.T., and Parsons, M.E. (1976). A quantitative study of metiamide, a histamine H_2-antagonist, on the isolated whole rat stomach. *J. Physiol. (London)* **258**, 453–465.

Dale, H.H., and Laidlaw, P.P. (1910). The physiological action of β-imidazolylethylamine. *J. Physiol. (London)* **41**, 318–344.

Edkins, J.S. (1905). On the chemical mechanism of gastric secretion. *Proc. Royal Soc.* **B76**, 376.

Gregory, R.A. (1974). The Bayliss-Starling Lecture 1973. The gastrointestinal hormones: a review of recent advances. *J. Physiol. (London)* **241**, 1–32.

Gregory, R.A., Tracy, H.J., and Grossman, M.I. (1966). Human gastrin: Isolation, structure, and synthesis. *Nature (London)* **209**, 583.

Grossman, M.I., and Konturek, S.J. (1974). Inhibition of acid secretion in dog by metiamide, a histamine antagonist acting on H_2-receptors. *Gastroenterology* **66**, 517–521.

Kahlson, G., and Rosengren, E. (1972). Histamine: entering physiology. *Experientia* **28**, 993–1002.

Kahlson, G., Rosengren, E., and Svensson, S.E. (1973). Histamine and gastric secretion with special reference to the rat, in "International Encyclopedia of Pharmacology and Therapeutics," Vol 1, Section 39A, *Pharmacology of Gastrointestinal Motility and Secretion* (G. Peters, ed.), pp. 41–102. Pergamon Press, New York.

Komarov, S.A. (1938). Gastrin. *Proc. Soc. Exp. Biol.* **38**, 514–516.

Lundell, L. (1975). Displacement by metiamide of the dose-response curves to pentagastrin and methacholine in the conscious rat. *Brit. J. Pharmacol.* **54**, 507–509.

MacIntosh, F.C. (1938). Histamine as a normal stimulant of gastric secretion. *Quart. J. Exp. Physiol.* **28**, 87–98.

Martinez, J.R., and Petersen, O.H. (1972). The importance of extracellular calcium for acetylcholine-evoked salivary secretion. *Experientia* **28**, 167–168.

Schayer, R.W. (1961). Significance of induced synthesis of histamine in physiology and pathology. *Chemotherapia* **3**, 128–136.

Tepperman, B.L., Schofield, B., and Tepperman, F.S. (1975). Effect of metiamide on acid secretion from isolated kitten fundic mucosa. *Can. J. Physiol. Pharmacol.* **53**, 1141–1146.

Thjodleifsson, B., and Wormsley, K.G. (1974). Aspects of the effect of metiamide on pentagastrin-stimulated and basal gastric secretion of acid and pepsin in man. *Gut* **16**, 501–508.

Thomas, L. (1971). Adaptive aspects of inflammation, in "International Congress Series," Vol. 229, *Immunopathology of Inflammation.* (B.K. Forscher and J.C. Houck, eds.), pp. 1–10. Excerpta Medica, Amsterdam.

Wolf, S., and Wolff, H.G. (1943). "Human Gastric Function: an Experimental Study of a Man and His Stomach." Oxford University Press, Oxford, England.

3

Histamine As a Physiological Stimulant of Gastric Parietal Cells

Thomas Berglindh and Karl Johan Öbrink
Department of Physiology and Medical Biophysics
Biomedicum, Uppsala, Sweden

INTRODUCTION

Ever since the days of Pavlov, the physiological stimulation of gastric secretion has been divided into three different phases, the cephalic, the gastric, and the intestinal phase. Pavlov showed that the vagus nerve was involved in the cephalic phase, whereas the gastric phase was thought to result from absorbed food stuffs. A major step in the development of gastric physiology was taken in 1905 when Edkins proposed that food liberated a humoral substance from the pyloric part of the stomach, which he called gastrin. It was soon shown that the extracts he made contained histamine, and when Popielski, in 1920, showed the very strong potency of histamine as a stimulant of gastric secretion, gastrin, and histamine were believed to be identical. In 1938, however, it was clearly demonstrated by Komarov that gastrin was not histamine. Komarov succeeded in making an extract from the antrum which did not contain histamine but was still a potent secretagogue for acid secretion. Another important step occurred when Uvnas (1942) found that the cephalic phase in effect was not very different from the gastric one, because stimulation of the vagus resulted in liberation of gastrin from the antrum. By this time it was also shown that the liberation of gastrin during the gastric phase could be due to local reflexes, e.g., due to distention.

Thus, the situation was that two potent humoral stimulants were implicated in gastric acid secretion, gastrin, and histamine. The question arose—and is still not answered— do they both or does only one of them act as a normal physiological stimulant for acid gastric secretion?

EVIDENCE FOR AND AGAINST HISTAMINE
AS A NORMAL STIMULATOR OF GASTRIC
SECRETION

There is a vast literature on this topic. There are many works for and equally as many against the hypothesis. The reader is referred to reviews by Code (1965), Waton (1971), Kahlson *et al.* (1973), and Lin (1974).

Some important milestones in the dispute will be mentioned. The development of the "classical" antihistamines was expected to prove whether or not histamine was a physiological and final mediator. We know that they failed to inhibit gastric secretion, and histamine seemed to drop out of the picture. We ought, however, to mention that Linde (1950) succeeded in getting an inhibition by antihistamine when animals were pretreated with a detergent. Another piece of evidence against histamine as the universal mediator for gastric secretion is the fact that some species respond very poorly to histamine, e.g., rats. On the other hand, the discovery of histidine decarboxylase in the gastric mucosa of the rat and the finding that gastrin activates this enzyme to form histamine seemed to favor the hypothesis. The work of Kahlson and co-workers (1973) should be consulted. However, with secretin it was possible to inhibit the gastrin-induced acid secretion in the rat but not histidine decarboxylase activity and histamine release (Johnson, 1971). Again, this was a piece of evidence against the hypothesis.

In recent years, there have been experiments that strongly favor the idea that histamine is a normal physiological stimulator. We should mention the work of Kasbekar, Ridley, and Forte (1969), where they exhausted an isolated gastric preparation, which then could be stimulated by no secretagogue other than histamine. However, the most important tool in this research has probably been the H_2 blockers, which are discussed in the following section.

CHANGES OF HISTAMINE SENSITIVITY
DURING GROWTH

As mentioned above, some species do respond more weakly to histamine than others. This also holds for the isolated stomach of rats which seem to be totally refractive to histamine. It was therefore sensational when Parsons (1975) (see also Bunce and Parsons, 1976) reported a successful method for stimulating the isolated rat stomach with histamine using immature rats weighing between 38–42 grams, which normally corresponds to an average age of about 3 weeks. This stimulated the experiments of Ekelund and Obrink (1976) who used rats of different ages and body weights. They found a potent stimulating effect of histamine when using small rats weighing approximately

20–40 grams, but the sensitivity decreased in larger animals and for rats weighing 150–200 grams the response was down to almost nil. These experiments are in some respects similar to the findings by Forte *et al.* (1975) on piglets. The reason why the sensitivity changes with age is unknown.

THE PARIETAL CELL RECEPTORS

As already mentioned, a new tool in the exploration of the histamine problem was provided when the H_2-receptor antagonists were discovered. Up until now, three different H_2 antagonists have been studied, burimamide, metiamide, and cimetidine (Black *et al.*, 1972, 1973; Brimblecombe *et al.*, 1975). Metimide has been shown to inhibit acid secretion stimulated by all the common secretagogues, as well as by a meal (Grossman and Konturek, 1974). This speaks in favor of histamine being the final mediator and supports the idea that the secretagogues work in a sequential fashion, at least in part. However, in spite of new tools, we are still facing a very complex stimulatory pattern. In animal experiments a cephalic stimulation can be blocked by vagus denervation; atropine will counteract the effects of a cholinergic drug but also, to some degree, inhibit histamine and gastrin stimulation (Hirschowitz and Sachs, 1969); gastrin but not histamine stimulation is inhibited by secretin (Johnson, 1971); and now H_2-receptor blockers inhibit not only histamine stimulation but also that induced by gastrin. Since it has been suggested that histamine acts as an activator of adenyl cyclase and that H_2-receptor antagonists competitively inhibit the histamine effect on this receptor (cf. Sung *et al.*, 1973), stimulants of acid secretion that act beyond this point should still be active. Cyclic AMP and the phosphodiesterase inhibitors belong to this group of stimulants (Shoemaker *et al.*, 1974).

Thus, what we still have to show is the target for each secretagogue and how, together they form the final response which we see in the intact animal. Accordingly, it seemed necessary to reduce the complexity of the gastric mucosa, and for that and other reasons a preparation of isolated gastric glands was developed (Berglindh and Obrink, 1976).

ISOLATED GASTRIC GLANDS

In a well-functioning isolated cell system a more direct study of possible sequential stimulation can be performed. If a gastric secretagogue stimulated acid secretion via release of a second substance in the vicinity of the parietal cell, and the latter activated the receptors on the parietal cell, this should not be seen as a response in an isolated cell system. The theory behind such an approach would be the following: normally, the mediator would be

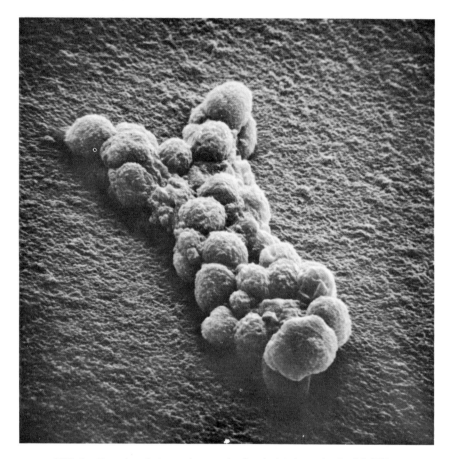

FIG. 1.   Scanning electron micrograph of an isolated gastric gland (x960).

transported in the narrow extracellular space in a concentration high enough to stimulate the receptors on the parietal cells, whereas in the case of an isolated cell system, which is suspended in a large volume of extracellular fluid, the released mediator would be infinitely diluted. Thus, in an isolated cell system only the direct, unmediated effect of added secretagogues would be recorded.

For many years, attempts have been made to separate cells from the mammalian gastric mucosa in a viable and functional state. Only recently, however, have some successful reports on stimulation of isolated parietal cells appeared (Michelangeli, 1974; Soll, 1977).

A quite different approach has been attempted in our laboratory, i.e., the disintegration of the mammalian gastric mucosa into functional units. Such functional units are the glands, containing acid-secreting parietal cells, and pepsin-secreting chief cells. As compared with totally isolated parietal

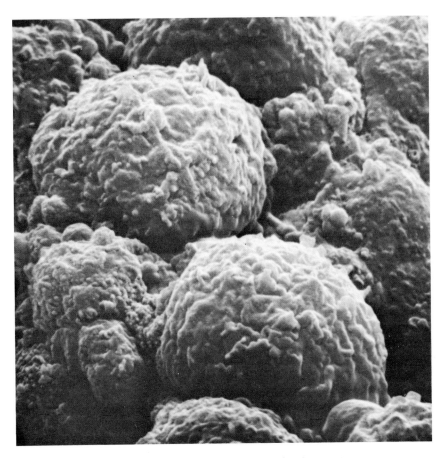

FIG. 2.   A close-up of the same gland as in Fig. 1 (x4800).

cells, several advantages of an isolated gland system could be recognized. Thus, the parietal cells keep their normal pronounced polarity with a basal and apical surface, and the cell contacts are not broken, which means that there can exist a cell coupling.

The method used to prepare isolated glands from the rabbit gastric mucosa has been described thoroughly elsewhere (Berglindh and Obrink, 1976). The technique involves a collagenase enzyme treatment of minced pieces of gastric mucosa for approximately 90 minutes at 37°C. To obtain glands, however, one very important prerequisite must be fulfilled; the stomach must be made edematous *in situ* by high pressure perfusion of saline through gastric arterial vessels. This step induces a mechanical separation of the glands which greatly facilitates the collagenase treatment. After separation, the glands appear highly viable as detected by the dye-exclusion technique and electrolyte-content measurements. Also, the intracellular morphology is not significantly different from that seen in the intact gastric mucosa (Berglindh and Obrink, 1976).

In the scanning electron microscope the appearance of an isolated gastric gland in low magnification is shown in Fig. 1. A higher magnification is shown in Fig. 2. The size of a gland is approximately 0.6 × 0.05 mm. It is obvious that the basal membrane structure reveals a rather rough texture.

FUNCTIONAL STUDIES OF ISOLATED GLANDS

Cell activity (mostly parietal) was determined by oxygen consumption using a Warburg technique, and acid secretion was indirectly determined by the use of the weak base aminopyrine (AP), which was ^{14}C labeled. The methods were described by Berglindh et al. (1976) and Berglindh (1977a). AP will accumulate in acid compartments according to the well known pH-partition hypothesis. Fig. 3 schematically shows the theoretical accumulation sites for AP. AP will mainly enter through the large basal surface of the parietal cells. Even in resting glands there is an AP accumulation (Berglindh et al., 1976), most of which might accumulate in the tubulo-vesicles of the resting parietal cell as indicated on the right hand side of the picture. In a

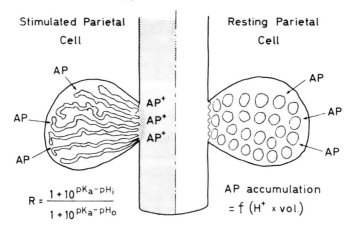

$$R = \frac{1 + 10^{pKa - pH_i}}{1 + 10^{pKa - pH_o}}$$

AP accumulation
= f (H⁺ × vol.)

FIG. 3.   Schematical illustration for the use of aminopyrine (AP) as an indirect tool to measure acid in isolated gastric glands. AP is a weak base ($pK_a = 5$), which is unionized and lipid soluble at neutral pH, and will therefore rapidly penetrate biological membranes. If AP enters an acid compartment it will be ionized and trapped, and thus an accumulation of the substance can be detected. As seen from the formula at the left hand side, the accumulation ratio R depends on the pK_a of AP as well as the pH inside (pH_i) and outside (pH_o) the accumulation compartment. However, an increased accumulation ratio does not necessarily mean that the acidity has increased, but could be due to an increased accumulation space, as indicated in the figure.

stimulated state the vesicles fuse and form the intracellular canaliculi. These have contact with the glandular lumen, which accordingly forms an additional site for accumulation. Even if the accumulation ratio for the weak base is dependent only on the internal pH, the amount of AP accumulated in the glands will depend also on the volume of the acid loci.

RESPONSES TO HISTAMINE

Through a number of investigations, the effects of histamine on the glandular parietal cell activity have been studied (Berglindh and Obrink, 1976); Berglindh et al., 1976; Berglindh 1977a; Berglindh 1977b). The addition of histamine will progressively increase both oxygen consumption and AP accumulation up to new steady-state levels within approximately 30 minutes, a time-response relationship of the same type as that seen in vivo. When using steady-state respiratory values obtained at different histamine concentrations, a dose-response curve of the normal sigmoid type is obtained, with an ED_{50} of approximately $3 \times 10^{-6} M$. The presence of an H_2-receptor antagonist such as burimamide or cimetidine causes a parallel shift of the response curve to the right, showing competitive antagonism. The histamine-stimulated AP accumulation is likewise antagonized. Finally, histamine changes the intracellular morphology of the parietal cells from a resting state to a secretory one. The histamine response is not inhibited by atropine except at very high concentrations, an effect which is probably nonspecific. Thus, the direct effect of histamine on the parietal cells of the isolated gastric glands, being exactly similar to that obtained in vivo, seems to prove the existence of histamine receptors on the parietal cells directly linked to acid secretion.

Having functional and easily accessible histamine receptors, and particularly since a number of investigations can be performed on the same gland population permitting direct comparison, it was of interest to further explore some of the characteristics. Thus, we have investigated the affinity constant for cimetidine, an H_2-receptor antagonist of the third generation (Brimblecombe et al., 1975). Cimetidine was a generous gift from Dr. Parsons (Smith Kline & French, Ltd. England). One way to perform such an analysis is by making a Schild plot (Arunlakshana and Schild, 1959), where the dose of the agonist alone and that which will produce the same response in the presence of an antagonist is determined. The following relation appears (see Sjostrand et al., 1977):

$$DR = \frac{[A]_B}{[A]_O} = 1 + \frac{[B]}{K_B} \text{ which will give the linear relationship}$$

$$\log(DR-1) = \log\left(\frac{[A]_B}{[A]_O} - 1\right) = \log[B] - \log K_B$$

where DR is the dose-ratio of $[A]_O$, the agonist concentration without antagonist and $[A]_B$, the concentration needed in the presence of antagonist B to give the same response. K_B is the reciprocal of the affinity constant for the antagonist used. All determinations were performed with oxygen consumption studies. Using two-point dose-response curves, where the agonist concentrations were chosen to give responses which would fall on the linear slope of the dose-response curve, it was possible to investigate K_B for cimetidine in the same gland population. A Schild plot of this kind is shown in Fig. 4, where log K_B was determined to be -6.22, corresponding to a K_B of 6.03 $\times 10^{-7} M$. This value is in the same range as reported earlier for the heart, uterus, and stomach using metiamide (Parsons, 1973; Bunce and Parsons, 1976). The affinity found here for cimetidine is in fact higher than the affinity for histamine itself since histamine in the gland preparation has a constant of about $3 \times 10^{-6} M$.

In the above determination of the affinity constant it was necessary not only to alter the concentration of the antagonist but also to increase the dose of the agonist simultaneously. However, there is a simpler way to determine the K_B, where the agonist concentration can be held constant and the decrease in response upon addition of increasing concentrations of the antagonist is

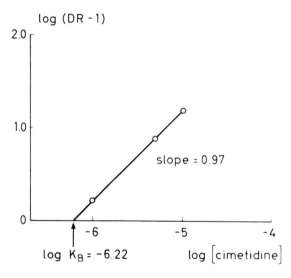

FIG. 4. Analysis of competitive antagonism of cimetidine on histamine-induced oxygen consumption. The plotted values are calculated as described in the text and they show a linear correlation, when plotted according to the Eq. $\log ([A]_B/[A]_O - 1) = \log [B] - \log K_B$. $[A]_B/[A]_O =$ DR (dose ratio). Log $K_B = -6.22$ corresponding to $K_B = 6.03 \times 10^{-7} M$. The slope was close to 1, indicating a one-to-one competition at the receptor site. All data were obtained from the same gland population.

recorded. As will be shown in Appendix 1, the following relation could be arrived at:

$$\frac{E_{AB}}{E_A} = \frac{1}{1 + \dfrac{[B]}{K_B/(1 - E_A)}}$$
(Appendix 1; eq. 7)

where E_A is the response to a chosen concentration of agonist A and E_{AB} is the response to the same concentration of the agonist in the presence of an antagonist in a concentration of $[B]$. Both E_A and E_{AB} are expressed as fractions of the maximal response. Thus, to determine the affinity constant for the antagonist, all we have to know is the maximal response to the agonist and then pick any agonist concentration for the experiment (preferably around ED_{50}). If from Appendix 1, eq. 7, E_{AB}/E_A is plotted as a function of log $[B]$ we will obtain the typical S-shaped curve as seen in Fig. 5, where the point of inflection will correspond to a dose value equal to $K_B/(1-E_A)$. From the Appendix 1, eq. 9, we get:

$$\log \left(\frac{E_A}{E_{AB}} - 1 \right) = \log B - \log K_B/(1 - E_A)$$

(Appendix 1; eq. 9)

This leads to the Schild-type plot in the lower part of fig. 5. In this particular experiment the histamine concentration used corresponded to 65% of the maximal response ($E_A = 0.65$). Since log $K_B/1-E_A$, in this case, was -5.22, log K_B will be -5.68 and $K_B = 2.09 \ 10^{-6}M$. Thus, this particular gland population had a lower affinity constant for cimetidine than the former. Preliminary results indicate, however, that there is no general discrepancy in the results between the two methods used here to determine K_B.

GASTRIN

When trying to study the effects of gastrin, the physiological relevance of the isolated gastric glands was for the first time challenged. With pentagastrin no responses were ever recorded in terms of change in oxygen consumption or AP-accumulation, regardless of concentration (Berglindh et al., 1976). These negative results are in sharp contrast to the results obtained in vivo where both gastrin and pentagastrin have a potent and well-documented effect on acid secretion. Two obvious explanations could immediately be offered; either the gastrin receptors on the parietal cells had been destroyed during the separation procedure, or gastrin receptors are not normally present on the parietal cells. This was discussed at some length by Berglindh et al. (1976). To

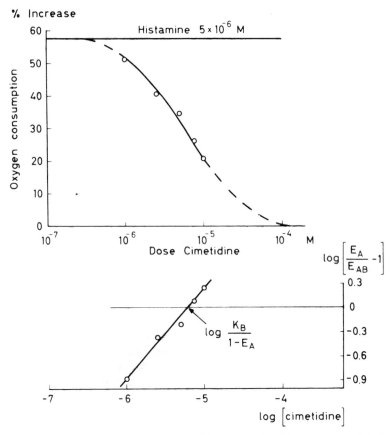

FIG. 5. A different approach to study competitive antagonism. The upper part of the figure shows the increase in oxygen consumption above basal, induced by histamine $5 \times 10^{-6} M$, and the decrease in that response following addition of increasing concentrations of cimetidine. The lower part shows the linear correlation obtained following analysis of the above data according to Appendix 1. K_B is calculated from the value E_A, which in this particular gland population was 0.65. This will make log $K_B = -5.68$, corresponding to $K_B = 2.09 \times 10^{-6} M$.

somewhat test the possibility that the receptors were destroyed, the following approach was applied. Normally, minced pieces of rabbit gastric mucosa will respond poorly to addition of secretagogues, but pieces of a mucosa, which previously were made edematous by a high pressure perfusion, will respond. This discrepancy indicates that the perfused mucosa is more permeable and that a mechanical separation of the glands has started. As shown in Fig. 6, such a preparation responded to secretagogues like histamine, carbachol, and db-cAMP, whereas no responses were obtained to pentagastrin in concentrations of $10^{-8} M$ or $10^{-6} M$. Likewise, pentagastrin $5 \times 10^{-5} M$ was without effect (Berglindh, unpublished results). In this case the negative response to pentagastrin cannot be explained by destruction due to collagenase digestion of gastrin receptors. Preliminary results show that this nonresponsiveness also holds for porcine gastrin I (kindly supplied by Dr. Grossman, CURE, VAC, Los Angeles), which did not stimulate the glandular parietal cells within a concentration span of 10^{-12}–$10^{-6}M$. Accordingly, if there exist gastrin receptors on the parietal cell, they cannot per se induce a secretory response in the glands. Whether they perhaps could be involved in some type of interaction with other secretagogues remains to be elucidated.

CHOLINERGIC STIMULATION

Cholinergic receptors on the glandular parietal cells can be activated by addition of acetylcholine or carbachol (Berglindh *et al.,* 1976; Berglindh, 1977b). The stimulation is, however, of a transient type. There is a rapid rise in both oxygen consumption and AP accumulation with a peak value after approximately 15 minutes, followed by a rapid and pronounced decline. Such a rapid transient response to cholinergic stimulation has not been reported from *in vivo* studies, but could be detected in the experiment with the minced pieces of gastric mucosa (Fig. 6). Atropine was a potent inhibitor of the

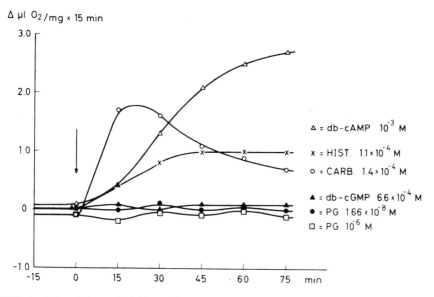

Δ μl O_2/mg × 15 min

Legend:
Δ = db-cAMP 10^{-3} M
x = HIST. 1.1×10^{-4} M
o = CARB. 1.4×10^{-4} M
▲ = db-cGMP 6.6×10^{-4} M
• = PG 1.66×10^{-8} M
□ = PG 10^{-6} M

FIG. 6.   Minced pieces of rabbit gastric mucosa, obtained after high pressure perfusion, were divided into seven Warburg flasks and the basal oxygen consumption was studied for 15 minute. At the arrow the substances listed were added, and the respiratory response in each preparation was correlated to a control flask with untreated mucosal pieces. PG, pentagastrin; CARB, carbachol. Note the nonresponsiveness also to db-cGMP.

cholinergic responses, indicating a true receptor mediated stimulation, whereas burimamide was without any effect (Berglindh, 1977a).

In vivo, gastric secretion is always supported by a cholinergic background from the vagus nerve. In fact, vagotomy of the stomach will act as a competitive inhibitor of histamine-stimulated secretion (Andersson and Grossman, 1965; Hirschowitz and Hutchison, 1975). Thus, to mimic *in vivo* conditions, the glandular response to histamine was investigated in the presence of carbachol. Fig. 7 presents the dose-response curves for histamine and histamine + carbachol, which clearly show that the response to histamine is potentiated in the presence of a cholinergic drug, as could be expected from the *in vivo* findings. In the dog, atropine will to some degree inhibit histamine stimulation (Hirschowitz *et al.,* 1972). As stated before, histamine stimulation of the glands was very insensitive to atropine. However, studying the effect of atropine on glands stimulated with a combination of histamine and

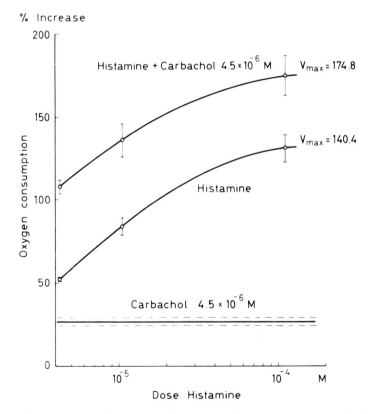

FIG. 7.   Dose-response respiratory curves for histamine alone and in the presence of carbachol. The response to carbachol alone is also presented (mean ±S.E., n = 4). The calculated maximal response (V_{max}) to histamine + carbachol was significantly higher than the corresponding additive effect of histamine and carbachol. The vertical bars indicate mean ±S.E., n = 4.

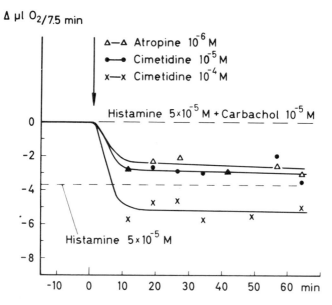

FIG. 8.   The respiratory response induced by a combination of histamine and carbachol and its time-dependent inhibition by atropine and cimetidine, which were added at the arrow. The hatched line indicates the response induced by histamine alone.

cholinergic stimuli, similar to the *in vivo* situation, explains how the histamine effect could appear to be sensitive to atropine. An experiment of this kind is shown in Fig. 8, where addition of atropine $10^{-6} M$ rapidly decreased the respiration down to a new steady state. In fact, atropine and cimetidine ($10^{-5} M$) appear to affect the response in a very similar manner, and neither of them down to the level of the pure histamine effect.

It is noteworthy that no transient response of carbachol was seen in the presence of histamine. The rapid phase of the carbachol response could, however, be seen when carbachol was added to glands pre-stimulated with histamine (Berglindh, 1977b). From these results it appears that a/ histamine stimulation is potentiated by a cholinergic background, b/ the cholinergic responses of the transient type are "normalized" in the presence of histamine, and accordingly c/ the reason that no "clean" cholinergic response ever is seen *in vivo* might be due to presence of histamine at the parietal cell level.

RELATIONSHIP BETWEEN HISTAMINE AND cAMP

Histamine has been shown to activate adenyl cyclase from the rabbit gastric mucosa, an effect which was inhibited by H_2-receptor blockers (Sung *et al.,* 1973), and also to dose-dependently increase the cAMP-content of gastric mucosa (Karppanen and Westermann, 1973). Exogenous cAMP or the more lipid soluble derivative, dibutyryl-cAMP (db-cAMP), has been shown to induce acid secretion (Harris and Alonso, 1965; Fromm *et al.*, 1975). In the isolated gland preparation, db-cAMP was the most potent of all secretagogues investigated, and the responses were in all respects qualitatively indistinguishable from those of histamine (Berglindh *et al.*, 1976; Berglindh, 1977a; Berglindh, 1977b). Of special interest is that the db-cAMP-induced response could be potentiated by carbachol in the same way as the histamine response (Berglindh, 1977b), indicating that the interaction between histaminic and cholinergic stimulation lies beyond the receptor level.

A more direct coupling between histamine and cAMP can be studied using phosphodiesterase inhibitors. An analysis of the kinetics of cAMP formation, accumulation, and breakdown will show (Appendix 2) that simultaneous stimulation of adenyl cyclase and inhibition of phosphodiesterase activity by nature will give a higher response than the sum of the two treatments given separately. If such a potentiation is not achieved, nothing can be said about involvement of cAMP in that particular process. In the gland preparation, the presence of a phosphodiesterase inhibitor such as aminophylline definitely potentiated the histamine-induced parietal cell respiration and AP accumulation (Berglindh, 1977b).

In conclusion, considering a possible sequential stimulation of acid secretion by secretagogues, in light of the concept: "Isolated glands will only respond to the direct effect of secretagogues," showed that histamine was the only *complete* secretagogue for the glandular parietal cells, whereas cholinergic drugs, although they induce a transient response, seem to serve as modulators for the histamine response. Gastrin itself was without any effect on the parietal cells as judged by the methods used to study the isolated glands. If gastrin receptors are present on the parietal cell, they most likely do not take part in any activation of the H^+ pump. Thus, the lack of response to gastrin found in the glands and the inhibition of gastrin-induced acid secretion *in vivo* by H_2-receptor antagonists (cf. Black *et al.*, 1972, 1973) are both consistent with the concept that the gastrin stimulating pathway goes via release of histamine (cf. Kahlson *et al.*, 1973).

HISTAMINE UPTAKE

Finally, we present some recent observations which could cast new light on the histamine story. Uptake of histamine has been noted in the stomach (Navert *et al.*, 1969), as well as in the heart (Moroni *et al.*, 1977). In both cases metabolism of the added ^{14}C labeled histamine was detected, indicating that the uptake mechanism might be a way of histamine destruction. The

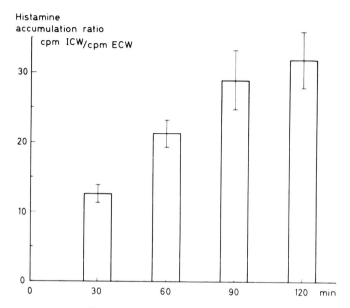

FIG. 9. Accumulation of ^{14}C histamine in isolated gastric glands. Before determination of radioactivity, the glands were washed three times in histamine-free medium. The accumulation is expressed as cpm in intracellular water/cpm in extracellular water. The vertical lines indicate mean ±S.E., n = 4.

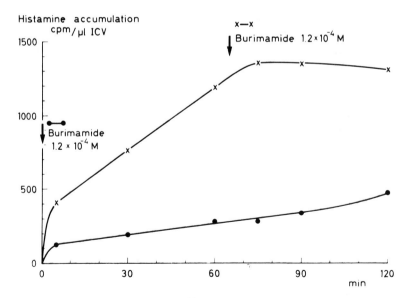

FIG. 10. The effect of burimamide on the ^{14}C histamine uptake in isolated gastric glands. To one fraction of the gland population (•–•), burimamide 1.2×10^{-4} M was added simultaneously with histamine. To the other, burimamide was added at 65 minute. The accumulation is expressed as cpm/μl intracellular water.

49

uptake might, however, also lead to a storage of histamine, which in turn could be released upon activation of the storage sites. As for the localization of uptake sites, Weinshelbaum and Ferguson (1971) showed that ^{3}H labeled histamine could be found in endocrine-like cells in the dog and mouse stomach.

Naturally, it was of interest to study whether a histamine uptake mechanism was present also in the isolated glands. Thus, together with Dr. L. Lundell (Dept. of Physiol., Lund) we have studied the distribution of ^{14}C histamine (spec. act. 18 mCi/mmol, Radiochemical Center, Amersham). Addition of ^{14}C histamine at a concentration of 10^{-6} M revealed a potent time-dependent accumulation (Fig. 9). The accumulation was expressed as the ratio: histamine per μl intracellular water/histamine per μl extracellular water. Thus, the ratio of 31.9 obtained after 2 hours incubation must be regarded as very high considering the fact that histamine most likely is concentrated only in a small fraction of the intracellular water. The accumulation showed some type of saturation with time. Whether this is a physiological phenomena or an unspecific effect is uncertain at present stage. The accumulated histamine was very firmly bound and could not be washed off (all samples were washed three times in histamine-free solutions before counting bound histamine). Whether the histamine, in spite of this, could be receptor associated was investigated by addition of the H_2-receptor antagonist burimamide.

Addition of a high dose of the H_2-blocker did not lower the glandular histamine content, but inhibited further uptake, as evident from Fig. 10. If burimamide was present from the start, the uptake was throughout much less than normal. The effect of burimamide could either be a simple competition of uptake sites (comparable with addition of cold histamine), or could be an effect on an H_2-receptor regulating the uptake.

For histamine to be the final mediator of acid secretion in all species, an uptake mechanism would be utterly important since only in the rat, mouse, and hamster has a high enough intramucosal histamine forming capacity (histidine decarboxylase) been found (Aures et al., 1969). The possible importance of the highly potent histamine uptake process found in the isolated gastric glands must await further exploration, but it might add an additional dimension, and probably confusion, to the "everlasting" problem of gastric histamine.

APPENDIX 1

There are several ways in which competitive and noncompetitive inhibition can be graphically presented. See the short review by Öbrink (1976). Below will follow a modification of evaluating the competitive antagonism according to Arunlakshana and Schild (1959). The assumptions and the mathematical background (see Sjöstand *et al.*, 1977) is the following: If a receptor R reacts with an agonist A, the complex RA is formed which causes an effect E_A. E_A is directly proportional to the ratio RA/R_t, where R_t is the total concentration of the receptor. E_A is consequently expressed as a fraction of the maximal response. When an antagonist B reacts competitively, RB is formed causing in itself no reaction.

According to the law of mass action

$$K_A [RA] = [A] [R] = [A] (R_t — [RA] — [RB])$$ (1)
$$K_B [RB] = [B] [R] = [B] (R_t — [RA] — [RB])$$ (2)

where K_A and K_B are, respectively, the reciprocals of the affinity constants of A and B for the receptor. In the absence of B ($RB = 0$), eq. 1 gives

$$\frac{[RA]}{R_t} = \frac{1}{1 + \dfrac{K_A}{[A]}} = E_A$$ (3)

The dose of A which results in $E = 0.5$ equals, according to eq. 3, $[A] = K_A$. If B is given along with A, eq. 1 and 2 combine (after division of eq. 1 with eq. 2, solving RB and substituting it into eq. 1 to:

$$K_A [RA] = [A] (R_t - [RA] - [RA] \frac{K_A [B]}{K_B [A]})$$ (4)

In order to evaluate the potency of the antagonist, K_B should be determined. The greater the potency, the smaller is K_B. Normally such determinations are made so that for each concentration of B, the dose of A $[A]$ is increased to $[A]_B$ so as to give the same response as it did without any B added (see Sjöstrand *et al.*, 1977). This procedure necessitates at least two determinations for each dose of B with two different doses $[A]_B$ so that an interpolation makes it possible to estimate which $[A_B]$ corresponds to the preset E_A. In the procedure to be described, it is possible, however, to make only one determination of each dose of B, and still analyze the value of K_B.

Suppose that E_A is determined for a certain dose $[A]$ with no B present. Now by keeping the dose $[A]$ unchanged and adding B we obtain an effect E_{AB}, which is a fraction of E_A.

By rearranging eq. 4 we get

$$E_{AB} = \frac{[RA]_{AB}}{R_t} = \frac{1}{1 + \dfrac{K_A}{[A]} (1 + \dfrac{[B]}{K_B})}$$ (5)

From eq. 3 we get that

$$\frac{K_A}{[A]} = \frac{1}{E_A} - 1 \qquad (6)$$

By inserting eq. 6 into eq. 5 we arrive at

$$\frac{E_{AB}}{E_A} = \frac{1}{\left(1 + \dfrac{(1 - E_A)\,[B]}{K_B}\right)} \qquad (7)$$

or

$$\frac{E_A}{E_{AB}} = 1 + \frac{[B]\,(1 - E_A)}{K_B} \qquad (8)$$

By plotting E_{AB}/E_A against log $[B]$ from eq. 7 we will arrive at the typical S-shaped curve in the upper part of Fig. 5, where the blocker cimetidine is given in increasing doses but the agonist, histamine, is given at a constant dose. The point of inflection corresponds to a value on the abscissa equal to log $[K_B/(1-E_A)]$. A more potent antagonist would shift the curve to the left and a less potent one to the right.

A Schild-type plot of the eq. 8 gives

$$\log \left(\frac{E_A}{E_{AB}} - 1\right) = \log [B] - \log \left(K_B/(1 - E_A)\right) \qquad (9)$$

which is represented in the lower part of Fig. 5, where the two variables are

log $[B]$ and log $\left(\dfrac{E_A}{E_{AB}} - 1\right)$. The intercept on the abscissa for

$$\log \left(\frac{E_A}{E_{AB}} - 1\right) = 0 \text{ equals log } \frac{K_B}{1 - E_A}$$

In the special case where the dose of A is chosen so that it corresponds to ED_{50}, then $E_A = 0.5$ and $K_B/(1-E_A) = 2K_B$. The method should be reliable provided the response is directly proportional to RA/R_t. If not, some care has to be taken. Probably, good advice is to keep E_A as close as possible to 0.5.

APPENDIX 2

cAMP is formed from ATP:

$$ATP \rightarrow cAMP \rightarrow 5'\text{-AMP}$$

or schematically

$$A \xrightarrow{k_1} B \xrightarrow{k_2} C$$

with the rate constants k_1 (adenyl cyclase) and k_2 (phosphodiesterase).

If we assume the concentration of ATP to be large in comparison to cAMP and that the reactions are of the first order, then

$$\frac{d[B]}{dt} = k_1[A] = \text{constant } (p) \tag{1}$$

$$-\frac{d[B]}{dt} = k_2[B] \tag{2}$$

This gives

$$-\frac{d[B]}{dt} = k_2[B] - k_1[A] = k_2[B] - p \tag{3}$$

Solving $[B] = f(t)$ for $[B] = 0$ when $t = 0$ gives

$$[B] = \frac{k_1}{k_2}[A] \, (1 - e^{-k_2 t}) \tag{4}$$

For a fixed time (t = constant) and for a constant k_2, $[B]$ = constant × k_1. The relation $[B] = f(k_2)$ when k_1 is constant is not meaningfully solved in an explicit form. In this context we therefore will demonstrate the effect on $[B]$ by changes of k_1 and k_2 simply by inserting some arbitrary figures in eq. 4.

If $A = 1$, $t = 1$, and if k_1 changes from 1 to 10 and k_2 from 10 to 1 then B changes in the following way:

	$k_1 = 1$	$k_1 = 10$
$k_2 = 10$	0.10	1.00
$k_2 = 1$	0.63	6.32

From this it is possible to calculate the effect of the changes in k. For instance, a stimulation of k_1 from 1 to 10 for a constant k_2 of 10, results in an increase of B from 0.10 to 1.00 Thus, a change in only k_1 (1 → 10) when $k_2 = 10$ results in an increase in B that is = 0.90. A change in only k_2 when $k_1 = 1$ results in an increase in $B = 0.53$. Together that gives 0.90 + 0.53 = 1.43. If, however, we stimulate the adenyl cyclase (increase in k_1) and inhibit the phosphodiesterase (decrease in k_2) simultaneously to the same extent as in the given example the increase in B will not be 1.43 but 6.32 – 0.10 = 6.22. By choosing other figures for k_1 and k_2 the discrepancy between the additive and the combined effect will differ.

Thus, a simultaneous treatment by an adenyl cyclase stimulator and a phosphodisterase inhibitor should by nature give a higher effect than the sum of the two treatments given separately. Whether this should be called synergism, potentiation or the like could be discussed. At any rate, there is nothing mysterious behind such a result. On the contrary if the combined action of two drugs only results in an additive effect it is not likely that these drugs are working on a sequential reaction as the one treated in this appendix.

ACKNOWLEDGMENTS

This study was supported by the Swedish Medical Research Council (Proj. No 151). We are indebted to Dr. H. F. Helander for preparing the scanning electron micrographs and to Miss Elisabet Bergqvist for skillful technical assistance.

REFERENCES

Andersson, S., and Grossman, M.I. (1965). Effect of vagal denervation of pouches on gastric secretion in dogs with intact or resected antrums. *Gastroenterology* **48**, 449–462.

Arunlakshana, O., and Schild, H.O. (1959). Some quantitative uses of drug antagonists. *Brit. J. Pharmacol.* **14**, 48–58.

Aures, D., Davidson, W.D., and Hakanson, R. (1969). Histidine decarboxylase in gastric mucosa of various mammals. *Eur. J. Pharmacol.* **8**, 100–107.

Berglindh, T., and Öbrink, K.J. (1976). A method for preparing isolated glands from the rabbit gastric mucosa. *Acta Physiol. Scand.* **96**, 150–159.

Berglindh, T., Helander, H.F., and Öbrink, K.J. (1976). Effects of secretagogues on oxygen consumption, aminopyrine accumulation and morphology in isolated gastric glands. *Acta Physiol. Scand.* **97**, 401–414.

Berglindh, T. (1977a). Effects of common inhibitors of gastric acid secretion on secretagogue-induced respiration and aminopyrine accumulation in isolated gastric glands. *Biochim. Biophys. Acta* **464**, 217–233.

Berglindh, T. (1977b). Potentiation by carbachol and aminophylline of histamine- and db-cAMP-induced parietal cell activity in isolated gastric glands. *Acta Physiol. Scand.* **99**, 75–84.

Black, J.W., Duncan, W.A.M., Durant, C.J., Ganellin, C.R., and Parsons, E.M. (1972). Definition and antagonism of histamine H_2-receptors. *Nature (London)* **236**, 385–390.

Black, J.W., Duncan, W.A.M., Emmet, J.C., Ganellin, C.R., Hesselbo, T., Parsons, M.E., and Wyllie, J.H. (1973). Metiamide—an orally active histamine H_2-receptor antagonist. *Agents and Actions* **3/3**, 133–137.

Brimblecombe, R.W., Duncan, W.A.M., Durant, C.J., Emmet, J.C., Ganellin, C.R., and Parsons, M.E. (1975). Cimetidine-a non-thiourea H_2-receptor antagonist. *J. Int. Med. Res.* **3**, 86–92.

Bunce, K.T., and Parsons, M.E. (1976). A quantitative study of metiamide, a histamine H_2-antagonist, on the isolated whole rat stomach. *J. Physiol.* **258**, 453–465.

Code, C.F. (1965). Histamine and gastric secretion: a later look, 1955–1965. *Fed. Proc.* **24**, 1311–1333.

Edkins, J.S. (1905). On the chemical mechanism of gastric secretion. *Proc. Roy. Soc., Ser. B* **76**, 376.

Ekelund, M., and Öbrink, K.J. (1976). Histamine sensitivity of isolated gastric mucosae from growing rats. *Acta Physiol. Scand.* **96**, 3A.

Forte, J.G., Forte, T.M., and Machen, T.E. (1975). Histamine-stimulated hydrogen ion secretion by in vitro piglet gastric mucosa. *J. Physiol.* **244**, 15–31.

Fromm, D., Schwartz, J.H., and Quijano, R. (1975). Effects of cyclic adenosine 3':5'-monophosphate and related agents on acid secretion by isolated rabbit gastric mucosa. *Gastroenterology* **69**, 453–462.

Grossman, M.I., and Konturek, S.J. (1974). Inhibition of acid secretion in dog by metiamide, a histamine antagonist acting on H_2 receptors. *Gastroenterology* **66**, 517–521.

Harris, J.B., and Alonso, D. (1965). Stimulation of the gastric mucosa by adenosine-3',5'-monophosphate. *Fed. Proc.* **24**, 1368–1376.

Hirschowitz, B.I., and Sachs, G. (1969). Atropine inhibition of insulin-, histamine-, and pentagastrin-stimulated gastric electrolyte and pepsin secretion in the dog. *Gastroenterology* **56**, 693–702.

Hirschowitz, B.I., Hutchison, G., and Sachs, G. (1972). Kinetics of atropine inhibition of histamine-stimulated gastric secretion in the dog. *Am. J. Physiol.* **222**, 1316–1321.

Hirschowitz, B.I., and Hutchison, G.A. (1975). Effects of vagotomy on urecholine-modified histamine dose responses in dogs. *Am. J. Physiol.* **228**, 1313–1318.

Johnson, L.R. (1971). Control of gastric secretion: no room for histamine? *Gastroenterology* **61**, 106–118.

Kahlson, G., Rosengren, E., and Svensson, S.E. (1973). Histamine and gastric secretion with special reference to the rat, in "Int. Encycl. Pharmacol. Ther." P. Holton, ed. Section 39(a). Vol. 1. Pharmacology of gastrointestinal motility and secretion, pp. 41–102. Pergamon Press, Oxford.

Karppanen, H.O., and Westermann, E. (1973). Increased production of cyclic AMP in gastric tissue by stimulation of histamine$_2$ (H_2)-receptors. *Naunyn-Schmiedeberg's Arch. Pharmacol.* **279**, 83–87.

Kasbekar, D.K., Ridley, H.A., and Forte, J.G. (1969). Pentagastrin and acetylcholine relation to histamine in H^+ secretion by gastric mucosa. *Am. J. Physiol.* **216**, 961–967.

Komarov, S.A. (1938). Gastrin. *Proc. Soc. Exptl. Biol. Med.* **38**, 514–516.

Lin, T.M. (1974). Possible relation of gastrin and histamine receptors in gastric hydrochloric acid secretion. *Med. Clin. N. Am.* **58**, 1247–1275.

Linde, S. (1950). Studies on the stimulation mechanism of gastric secretion. *Acta Physiol. Scand.* **21** suppl. 74.

Michelangeli, F. (1974). Secretory properties of isolated oxyntic cells from gastric mucosa. *Proc. Int. Union. Physiol. Sci.* Vol. XI.XXVI. Int. Congress, New Delhi **397**, 133.

Moroni, F., Fantozzi, R., Masini, E., and Mannaioni, P.F. (1977). The influence of catecholamines and serotonin on histamine uptake and metabolism by guinea pig atrium. *European J. Pharmacol.* **41**, 59–63.

Navert, H., Flock, E.V., Tyce, G.M., and Code, C.F. (1969). Metabolism of exogenous histamine-^{14}C during gastric secretion in dogs. *Am. J. Physiol.* **217**, 1823–1829.

Öbrink, K.J. (1976). Theoretical considerations concerning gastric inhibition. *Scand. J. Gastroenterol.* **11**, 7–13.

Parsons, M.E. (1973). The evidence that inhibition of histamine-stimulated gastric secretion is a result of the blockade of histamine H_2-receptors, in "International Symposium on Histamine H_2-Receptor Antagonists." (C.J. Wood, and M.A. Simkins, eds.), pp. 207–217. Welwyn Garden City: Research and Development Division, Smith Kline and French Laboratories.

Parsons, M.E. (1975). Studies on gastric acid secretion using an isolated whole mammalian stomach *in vitro*. *J. Physiol.* **247**, 35P–36P.

Popielski, L. (1920). β-imidazolyläthylamin und die organextrakte; I. β-imidazolyläthylamin als mächtigen Erreger der Magendrüsen. Pflügers *Arch. Ges. Physiol.* **178**, 214–236.

Shoemaker, R.L., Buckner, E., Spenney, J.G., and Sachs, G. (1974). Action of burimamide, a histamine antagonist, on acid secretion *in vitro*. *Am. J. Physiol.* **226**, 898–902.

Sjöstrand, S.E., Ryberg, B., and Olbe, L. (1977). Analysis of the actions of cimetidine and metiamide on gastric acid secretion in the isolated guinea pig gastric mucosa. *Naunyn-Schmiedeberg's Arch. Pharmacol.* **296**, 139–142.

Soll, A.H. (1977). The physiology of the isolated mammalian parietal cell: actions and interactions of secretagogues, in "Hormonal Receptors in Digestive Tract Physiology," INSERM Symposium No. 3. (S. Bonfils, P. Fromageot, and G. Rosselin, eds.) pp. 406–407. Elsevier/North-Holland Biomedical Press, Amsterdam.

Sung, C.P., Jenkins, B.C., Burns, L.R., Hackney, V., Spenney, J.G., Sachs, G., and Wiebelhaus, V.D. (1973). Adenyl and guanyl cyclase in rabbit gastric mucosa. *Am. J. Physiol.* **225**, 1359–1363.

Uvnäs, B. (1942). The part played by the pyloric region in the cephalic phase of gastric secretion. *Acta Physiol. Scand.* **4** suppl., 13.

Waton, N.G. (1971). Histamine and the parietal cell. *Dig. Dis.* **16**, 921–938.

Weinshelbaum, E.I., and Ferguson, D.J. (1971). Localization of tritium from histamine in gastric mucosa *in vivo*. *Histochemie* **26**, 9–18.

4

Studies on Metiamide and Acid Secretion in the Isolated Whole Rat Stomach

M. E. Parsons and K. T. Bunce
The Research Institute
Smith Kline and French Laboratories Limited
Welwyn Garden City
Hertfordshire

INTRODUCTION

In vivo, histamine H_2-receptor antagonists have been shown to inhibit gastric acid secretion stimulated by a wide variety of gastric secretagogues. These results could be interpreted as indicating that the antagonists are nonspecific antisecretory agents, although evidence from studies on nongastric tissues such as the heart and uterus establish that they are specific competitive histamine H_2-receptor antagonists. Alternatively, the secretory studies could provide important evidence to support the hypothesis that histamine is the final common mediator for all secretory stimulants. *In vivo* studies on the control of gastric acid secretion are complicated by modulating influences such as vagal and local cholinergic tone and endogenous gastrin release. A clearer view of the receptors involved (although not necessarily of the normal physiological control of secretion) could be obtained from *in vitro* studies. Until recently, entirely satisfactory mammalian gastric mucosal preparations have not been available.

The present paper describes studies carried out using an isolated lumen-perfused whole stomach from an immature rat which responds in a dose-related manner to a variety of gastric secretagogues. Clearly, vascular and vagal nerve elements have been removed in this preparation although local nerve pathways will still be intact. The antrum is present in the preparation but in the absence of a blood supply any gastrin release is unlikely to play a significant contributory factor in secretagogue action.

METHODS

The method has been described in detail elsewhere (Bunce and Parsons, 1976). Essentially the stomach of an immature rat is removed and placed in an organ bath containing Krebs-Henseleit ringer solution at 37° C. The lumen of the stomach is continuously perfused at a rate of 1 ml per minute with unbuffered Krebs–Henseleit solution via cannulae placed in the pylorus and nonsecretory rumen. The effluent perfusate is passed over a microflow electrode system and the H^+ activity of the perfusate is continuously monitored. Drugs are added to the serosal solution and the response parameter measured is the amount of H^+ secreted at the peak minus the basal secretion. In the majority of the studies the agonist was washed out of the bath after the peak effect had been achieved. Antagonists were allowed to equilibrate for approximately one hour before their effects on the response to the agonist were studied. The agonist drugs used were histamine, pentagastrin, gastrin (synthetic human gastrin I), acetylcholine, dibutyryl cyclic adenosine 3′, 5′-monophosphate (db cAMP), and a phosphodiesterase inhibitor (I.C.I. 63,197.)

RESULTS

Basal Secretion

The mean spontaneous (basal) H^+ secretory rate from 36 experiments was 4.19 ± 0.31 (S.E. of mean) $\times 10^{-8}$ mol minute^{-1}. It has been shown previously that concentrations of metiamide up to 3×10^{-5} M do not inhibit this basal secretion (Bunce and Parsons, 1976). Further increase of the metiamide concentration to 10^{-4} M and 10^{-3} M still did not exert a significant inhibitory effect (Table I). The anticholinergic compound atropine at concentrations up to 10^{-5} M also did not exert a statistically significant inhibitory effect. However at both $10^{-4} M$ and $10^{-3} M$ a significant inhibition was obtained (Table I).

Characteristics of the Agonist Responses

Repeated Single Doses

One advantage of continuously recording the H^+ activity secreted by the stomach is that the agonist can be washed out of the bath when the peak response has been achieved and hence repeated doses of an agonist can be administered. Using histamine and dbcAMP as the secretory stimulants, responses remained stable over a 5-hour period, whereas the responses to

Table I
**A Comparison of Basal H^+ Secretion under Control Conditions and in the
Presence of Metiamide or Atropine[a]**

Control	Metiamide $10^{-4}M$		
4.08 ± 0.94	3.07 ± 0.71	$t = 0.86$	$p > 0.05$
$(n = 18)$	$(n = 18)$		
	$10^{-3}M$		
3.92 ± 0.37	3.02 ± 0.31	$t = 1.87$	$p > 0.05$
$(n = 14)$	$(n = 14)$		
	Atropine $10^{-5}M$		
4.28 ± 0.72	2.95 ± 0.35	$t = 1.66$	$p > 0.05$
$(n = 10)$	$(n = 10)$		
	$10^{-4}M$		
3.22 ± 0.17	2.29 ± 0.23	$t = 3.23$	$p < 0.01$
$(n = 12)$	$(n = 12)$		
	$10^{-3}M$		
3.19 ± 0.35	2.18 ± 0.22	$t = 2.43$	$p < 0.05$
$(n = 20)$	$(n = 20)$		

[a]Rate of acid secretion (mol $\times$ 10^{-8} /minute) Mean and S.E. of mean.

acetylcholine showed a slight tendency to increase over the same period. In
contrast, the response to pentagastrin showed a marked tachyphylaxis such
that over a 5-hour period during which five doses of pentagastrin were
administered the acid secretory response diminished by approximately 70%
(Bunce *et al.* 1976). The tachyphylaxis to gastrin was less marked than to
pentagastrin and the responses for four doses were sufficiently reproducible
for the construction of two 2-point dose-response curves. Like pentagastrin,
the response to the phosphodiesterase inhibitor, I.C.I. 63,197, exhibited
marked tachyphylaxis and it was impossible to give repeated administrations
of the compound, so that a single dose was used in each preparation for the
antagonist studies.

Continuous Stimulation by Infusion

Although the peak response to repeated administration of histamine and
dbcAMP did not show tachyphylaxis, the response to a single administration
was not sustained when the agonist was allowed to remain in contact with the
tissue. This "fade" occurred with all the agonists used. One possible
explanation for this was that the agonists were being in some way inactivated,
and therefore the effect of a constant infusion of the agonist into the serosal
bathing fluid was studied. Histamine was infused at a rate which maintained a
constant concentration of approximately 10^{-4} M in the bath and the secretory
response is shown in Fig. 1. Despite the continued application of the agonist,

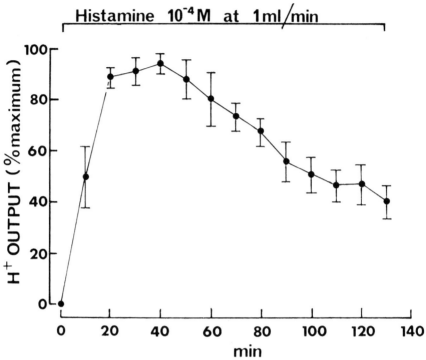

FIG. 1.   The acid response to an infusion of histamine. A solution of histamine at 10^{-4} M was infused into the organ bath at a rate of 1 ml/minute. The maximum output in each stomach was recorded as 100% and acid output was measured every 10 minutes and expressed as percentage of the maximum. Each point in the mean of five observations. Vertical bars shown the S.E. of the mean.

after the peak response had been obtained at 40 minutes, the response faded back to near basal levels after 130 minutes. Using dbcAMP by infusion, a different pattern was obtained (Fig. 2). A peak response was not achieved until 100 minutes after starting the infusion but only a slight fade occurred over the next 90 minutes.

Antagonist Studies with Metiamide

Histamine

The dose-response curve to histamine was linear over the dose range 10^{-5}–10^{-4} M. Metiamide produced a dose related parallel displacement of the histamine dose-response curve in the dose range 3×10^{-6}–3×10^{-5} M. The control curve and that obtained in the presence of $3 \times 10^{-5} M$ metiamide is shown in Fig. 3. From the measured dose ratios a linear regression of log (DR-1) on log [B] was obtained, where [B] is the concentration of the antagonist, and an empirical pA_2 value of 5.91 was calculated.

Gastrin

Secretory responses to gastrin were linear over the dose range 3×10^{-8}–3×10^{-7} M. Higher doses of gastrin gave submaximal responses. Metiamide at 10^{-5} and 3×10^{-5} M (Fig. 4) was an effective inhibitor of gastrin stimulated secretion although the pattern of the inhibition differed from that obtained when histamine was used as the agonist. Whereas metiamide produced a parallel displacement of the histamine dose-response curve, with gastrin a depressed maximum response was found in the presence of metiamide (Bunce *et al.* 1976) suggesting a noncompetitive type of antagonism and making the calculation of dose ratios for comparison with histamine impossible.

THE ACID RESPONSE TO AN INFUSION OF dbcAMP

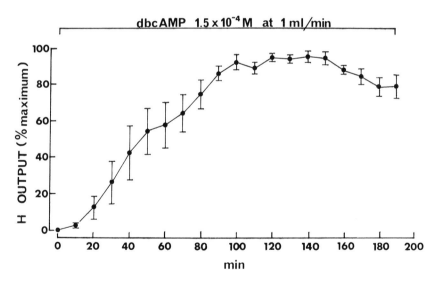

FIG. 2.   The acid response to an infusion of dbcAMP. A solution of dbcAMP at 1.5×10^{-4} M was infused into the organ bath at a rate of 1ml/minute. The maximum output in each stomach was recoreded as 100% and acid output was measured every 10 minutes and expressed as a percentage of the maximum. Each point is the mean of 5 observations. Vertical bars show the S.E. of the mean.

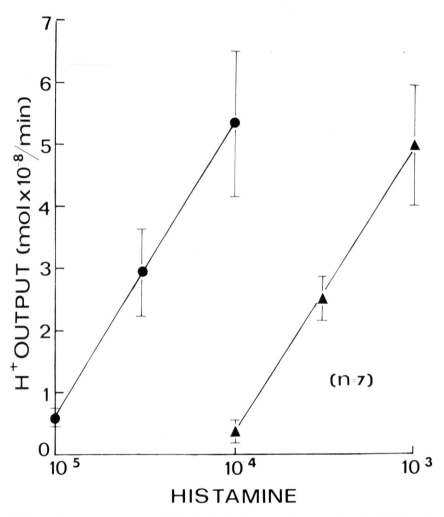

METIAMIDE $3\times10^{-5}M$/HISTAMINE

FIG. 3. Dose-response curves to histamine in the absence and presence of metiamide. Control (•), 3×10^{-5} M metiamide (▲). Each point is the mean of seven observations. Vertical bars show the S.E. of mean. Analysis of variance showed that there was no significant difference in the slope of the two lines and metiamide caused a significant displacement of the dose-response curve from the line obtained with histamine alone.

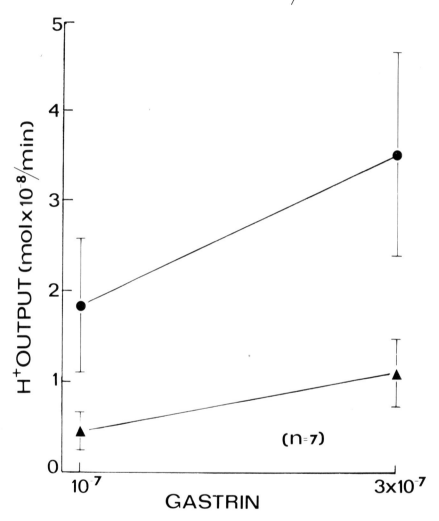

FIG. 4.   Dose-response curves to gastrin in the absence and presence of metiamide. Control (•),
3×10^{-5} M metiamide (▲). Each point is the mean of seven observations. Vertical bars show the
S.E. of mean. Analysis of variance showed that there was no significant difference in the slope of
the two lines and metiamide caused a significant displacement of dose-response curve from the
line obtained with gastrin alone.

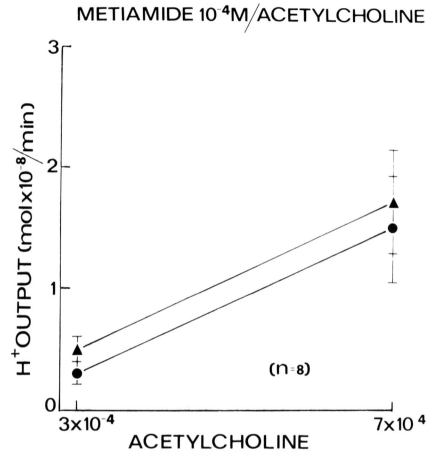

FIG. 5.   Dose-response curves to acetylcholine in the absence and presence of metiamide. Control (●), 10^{-4} M metiamide (▲). Each point is the mean of eight observations. Vertical bars show the S.E. of mean. Analysis of variance showed that there was no significant difference in the slope of the two lines and metiamide did not cause a significant displacement of the dose-response curve from the line obtained with acetylcholine alone.

Acetylcholine

The dose-response curve to acetylcholine was linear over the range 3×10^{-4}–10^{-3} M. A higher concentration of 3×10^{-3} M not only failed to stimulate acid output but also diminished the basal rate of H^+ secretion. Metiamide at concentrations of 10^{-4} M (Fig. 5) and 10^{-3} M failed to produce a shift of the dose-response curve to the right.

dbcAMP

The threshold level for stimulation with dbcAMP was 5×10^{-6} M and the dose-response curve was linear over the range 5×10^{-5}–1.5×10^{-4} M. Metiamide at concentrations up to 10^{-3} M (Fig. 6) did not inhibit dbcAMP-stimulated secretion in this preparation.

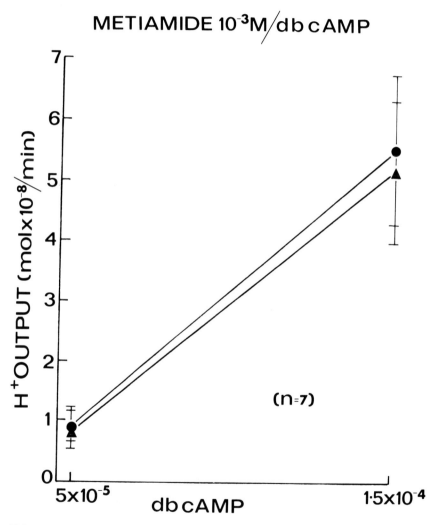

FIG. 6.   Dose-response curves to dbcAMP in the absence and presence of metiamide. Control (●), 10^{-3} M metiamide (▲). Each point is the mean of seven observations. Vertical bars show the S.E. of mean. Analysis of variance showed that there was no significant difference in the slope of the two lines and metiamide did not cause a significant displacement of the dose-response curve from the line obtained with dbcAMP alone.

I.C.I. 63,197

As noted above, repeated administration of this phosphodiesterase inhibitor led to marked tachyphylaxis of the response. Therefore only a single dose of the compound was administered to each preparation. Under control conditions in the absence of metiamide I.C.I. 63,197 at a dose of 7×10^{-7} M gave a mean secretory response above basal of 3.95 ± 0.58 (mean $\pm$ S.E.M.) H^+ mol $\times 10^{-8}$ minute^{-1} (n = 11). In the presence of 10^{-3} M metiamide, the mean response was 6.12 ± 1.28 H^+ mol $\times 10^{-8}$ minute^{-1} (n = 11). Clearly, although there is a marked between preparation variation in the secretory response to I.C.I. 63,197, metiamide tended to increase the response (although this was not statistically significant) rather than causing an inhibition.

DISCUSSION

The experiments described in the present paper clearly establish that the isolated perfused whole rat stomach preparation is a valuable tool for the study of the control of gastric acid secretion. It allows repeated doses of stimulants to be given to a single preparation and responds in a dose-related manner to a variety of gastric secretagogues. The origin of the basal secretion in the preparation is not clear. The failure of high concentrations of metiamide to have an inhibitory action indicates that endogenous histamine is unlikely to be the stimulant. Although atropine did inhibit this secretion, it only did so at concentrations some 100 times higher than those effective against acetylcholine-stimulated secretion (Bunce and Parsons, unpublished observations), which also argues against the involvement of endogenous acetylcholine. The concentrations of atropine are those effective against gastrin-stimulated secretion (Bunce and Parsons, unpublished observations), which may indicate that the basal secretion is controlled by endogenous gastrin release. This idea is supported by the fact that stomachs from fed animals have a higher basal secretion than those from starved animals. However the stability of the basal secretion over extended periods is difficult to explain and if endogenous gastrin is involved, the studies with metiamide against exogenously applied gastrin suggest that the histamine H_2-receptor antagonist should be effective against basal secretion. The origin of the basal secretion may be species-dependent since in amphibia an H_2-antagonist abolishes the spontaneous secretion (Shoemaker *et al.* 1974).

No explanation can be provided for the tachphylaxis associated with repeated pentagastrin stimulation but the same phenomenon has been found by other workers, *in vitro* (Kaskebar, 1972) and *in vivo* (Emas, 1960). The fact that the stomach responds normally to histamine and other secretagogues when the stomach has exhibited almost complete tachyphylaxis to pentagastrin indicates that it is not a toxic phenomenon and suggests that an essential intermediary for pentagastrin's action may have been depleted.

Equally difficult to explain is the fade seen in the response to all the stimulants when a constant bath concentration is maintained by infusion of the agonist. Other workers have maintained a plateau of secretion from an *in vitro* stomach provided the agonist is still present in the serosal solution (Spencer, 1974).

The studies with metiamide against histamine-stimulated secretion confirm that the compound is an effective inhibitor *in vitro* as well as *in vivo* . The calculated pA_2 value of 5.91 agrees closely with values reported for the other nongastric tissues containing histamine H_2 receptors, the guinea-pig atrium, and the rat uterus (Parsons, 1973). Although the slope of the regression of log (DR-1) on log [B] is incompatible with competitive antagonism, other factors may be operating which obscure the underlying competitive nature of the antagonism (Bunce and Parsons, 1976). The results provide evidence for homogeneity between histamine H_2 receptors in the gastric mucosa and those in other nongastric tissues.

The results with gastrin provide further evidence that the acid secretory responses to this agonist are mediated at least in part through a histaminergic pathway. The reduction of the maximal response to gastrin in the presence of metiamide could be interpreted as indicating a noncompetitive type of antagonism and is similar to results obtained *in vivo* using pentagastrin in the Heidenhain pouch rat (Lundell, 1975) and in the Heidenhain pouch dog (Black, 1973). An alternative explanation involving an inhibitory receptor for pentagastrin has been put forward (Black, 1973).

The ineffectiveness of metiamide against acetylcholine-stimulated secretion indicates that acetylcholine stimulates secretion through a direct cholinergic pathway and not via mobilisation of mucosal histamine. The inhibition of cholinergically evoked secretion by H_2-antagonists *in vivo* may be explained by the ability of the cholinergic agents to release endogenous gastrin, the secretory effect of which would be blocked by the H_2 antagonists.

Exogenous histamine increases the activity of gastric mucosal adenylate cyclase and elevates the level of cyclic AMP in the rat gastric mucosa and these changes can be prevented by H_2-antagonists (McNeill and Verma, 1974; Ruoff and Sewing, 1975). The latter experiments show that cAMP operates at a position distal to histamine in the stimulation of acid secretion. This conclusion is supported by the results obtained in the present study in which metiamide failed to inhibit secretion stimulated by exogenously applied dbcAMP. The I.C.I. phosphodiesterase inhibitor is assumed to stimulate secretion by an elevation of endogenous cyclic AMP levels and again the failure of metiamide to inhibit the response is the expected result. The elevation of cyclic AMP concentrations in dog gastric mucosal preparations caused by this compound has been found to be insensitive to H_2-receptor antagonists (Scholes *et al.* 1976).

In conclusion therefore, there appear to be both histamine H_2 and acetylcholine receptors on the rat gastric mucosa, whereas gastrin acts, at least in part, through a release of histamine. The failure of high concentrations of metiamide to inhibit exogenous or endogenous cyclic AMP stimulated secretion provides further evidence that cAMP operates at a point distal to histamine.

REFERENCES

Black, J.W. (1973). Speculation about the nature of the antagonism between metiamide and pentagastrin, in International Symposium on Histamine H_2-receptor Antagonists, C.J. Wood and M.A. Simkins, eds.,pp. 219-224. Research and Development Division, Smith Kline and French Laboratories Ltd., Welwyn Garden City.

Bunce, K.T., and Parsons, M.E. (1976). A quantitative study of metiamide, a histamine H_2 antagonist, on the isolated whole rat stomach. *J. Physiol.* **258**, 453-465.

Bunce, K.T., Parsons, M.E., and Rollings, N.A. (1976). The effect of metiamide on acid secretion stimulated by gastrin, acetylcholine and dibutyryl cyclic adenosine 3', 5'-monophosphate in the isolated whole stomach of the rat. *Br. J. Pharmac.* **58**, 149-156.

Emås, S. (1960). Gastric secretory responses to repeated intravenous infusions of histamine and gastrin in non-anaesthetised and anaesthetised gastric fistula cats. *Gastroenterology* **39**, 771-782.

Kasbekar, D.K. (1972). Secretagogue-induced tachyphylaxis of gastric H^+ secretion and its reversal. *Am. J. Physiol.* **223**, 294-299.

Lundell, L. (1975). Displacement by metiamide of the dose-response curves to pentagastrin and methacholine in the conscious rat. *Br. J. Pharmac.* **54**, 507-509.

McNeill, J.H., and Verma, S.C. (1974). Stimulation of rat gastric adenylate cyclase by histamine and histamine analogues and blockade by burimamide. *Br. J. Pharmac.* **52**, 104-106.

Parsons, M.E. (1973). The evidence that inhibition of histamine-stimulated gastric secretion is a result of the blockade of Histamine H_2-receptors, in International Symposium on Histamine H_2-receptor Antagonists, C.J. Wood and M.A. Simkins eds., pp. 207-217. Research and Development Division, Smith Kline and French Laboratories Ltd., Welwyn Garden City.

Ruoff, H.J., and Sewing, K.-Fr. (1975). Influence of atropine, metiamide and vagotomy on cAMP of resting and stimulated gastric mucosa. *Eur. J. Pharmac.* **32**, 227-232.

Shoemaker, R.L., Buckner, E., Spenny, J.G., and Sachs, G. (1974). Action of burimamide, a histamine antagonist, on acid secretion *in vitro*. *Am. J. Physiol.* **226**, 898-902.

Scholes, P., Cooper, A., Jones, D., Major, J., Walters, M., and Wilde, C. (1976). Characterisation of an adenylate cyclase system sensitive to histamine H_2-receptor excitation in cells from dog gastric mucosa. *Agents and Actions* **6**, 677-682.

Spencer, J. (1974). Gastric secretion in the isolated stomach of the guinea-pig. *J. Physiol.* **237**, 1-3P.

5

Esophageal Histamine Receptors

**Sidney Cohen, John J. Kravitz, and
William J. Snape, Jr.**
Gastrointestinal Section
Hospital of the University of Pennsylvania
Philadelphia, Pennsylvania

INTRODUCTION

The esophagus is similar to other organ systems in that it also responds to histamine. The histamine response varies in different species. The role of endogenous histamine release in the physiological control of esophageal function is not known. The purpose of this presentation is to discuss histamine receptors in esophageal smooth muscle and to evaluate possible physiological and clinical implications of these receptor mechanisms.

The esophagus both controls the propulsion of food from mouth to stomach and prevents the reflux of gastric contents from the stomach into the esophagus. Propulsive function occurs through the mechanism of peristalsis in the body of the esophagus, whereas the antireflux function resides in the intrinsic competence of the physiological lower esophageal sphincter (LES). The distal esophagus and the LES in man and in other species to be discussed here is composed of smooth muscle. LES function has therefore become a convenient area to evaluate the effect of histamine and its receptor antagonists. The LES is manifest as a zone of high pressure which can be regulated by histamine and other hormones or drugs. The changes in pressure are easily quantified in terms of dose-response curves. Thus, the LES provides an accessible and measureable area of pure smooth muscle where the pressure is generated totally by the intrinsic sphincter itself. Additionally, and perhaps most significantly, the LES is an important area in terms of its direct clinical association with several esophageal diseases in man.

METHODS

Animal Studies

Studies were performed in the opossum species, *Didelphis virginiana,* and in man. Animal studies were done both *in vivo* and *in vitro.* Male and female animals, weighing between 2.4 and 5.4 kg were anesthetized with 2.0% chloralose (3.0 cm^3/kg) and supplemented once with pentobarbital, (10.0 mg) during surgery and tube insertion. After successful anesthesia, a heparin-treated cannula was inserted into the femoral vein. All drugs were administered as a constant intravenous infusion in 0.9% saline.

Intraluminal pressures were measured through water-filled polyvinyl catheters (1.4 mm inside diameter) connected to external transducers (Statham P23 series). Recording tubes were arranged as a fixed unit with three side orifices, 1.2 mm in diameter, spaced 5 cm apart over the distal segment of the tube. Each recording tube was constantly perfused with distilled water by a Harvard infusion pump (Harvard Apparatus Co., Inc., Millis, Mass.) at 1.2 cm^3/minute. After insertion into the animal's stomach the entire recording assembly was withdrawn at 0.5-cm intervals, with measurements being recorded at each level for 1 minute. For changes in LES pressure in response to drugs, the middle recording orifice was positioned in the sphincter with the proximal lumen in the esophagus and the distal pressure orifice in the stomach. The middle orifice was maintained at the zone of maximal LES pressure by the evaluation of a complete pull-through at each 5-minute inteval. To evacuate the stomach, gastric aspiration was done through the distal orifice approximately every 30 minutes. All intraluminal pressures were graphed on a Beckman rectilinear, ink-writing recorder (Beckman Instruments, Inc., Fullerton, Calif.).

LES pressure was recorded as millimeters of mercury with gastric fundal pressure used as a zero reference. The values were obtained as the midrespiratory value during a 1-minute interval from the portion of the sphincter demonstrating the highest pressure. Mean LES pressure was obtained by determining the stable pressure at a minimum of four points during a 1-minute period.

Gastric secretion was obtained by continuous suction through a collecting tube with perforations 4 to 8 cm below the distal pressure recording site. The recording and collecting apparatus consisted of three polyvinyl tubes as described above. Specimens were collected over 10-minute intervals. Each specimen was titrated to pH 7.0 using an automatic titrator (Beckman Instruments, Inc.). Acid secretion was expressed as milliequivalents of acid output per 10-minute period.

Control values of LES pressure were obtained after insertion of the intravenous cannula and before the instillation of drugs or hormones. A period of 1 hour for stabilization to baseline levels was observed after administration of each agent. Studies *in vivo* were performed using gastrin I (residue 2–17; hexadecapeptide amide, (Imperial Chemical Industries Ltd., Alderley Park, Cheshire, England) or metiamide (Smith Kline & French Laboratories, Philadelphia, Pa.). All studies were performed utilizing the continuous intravenous infusion of gastrin or metiamide over a 1-hour period. Doses of metiamide or gastrin were given in random order. Statistical analysis was performed using the student's t-test.

Circular smooth muscle of the distal esophagus at the region of the LES was obtained through techniques previously described in detail (Lipshutz and Cohen, 1971; Lipshutz and Cohen, 1972). In brief, adult opossums were anesthetized and underwent esophageal manometric evaluation as described above. The LES was identified by manometry and each animal was killed with intravenous Nembutal. The LES, as determined by manometry, was identified and marked. The esophagus and stomach were removed intact, washed in Krebs–Ringer solution with the composition in millimoles per liter: Na^+ 138.6; K^+ 4.6; Ca^{2+} 2.5; Mg^{2+} 1.2; Cl^- 126.2; HCO_3^- 21.9; PO_4^{3-} 1.2; glucose 49.6 at 37–38°C, and transferred to an organ bath of Krebs–Ringer solution bubbled with 95% O_2 and 5% CO_2. The mucosa from the esophagus was removed to the level of the submucosa. A single, circular smooth muscle strip, 0.5 cm wide and 1.0 cm long, was obtained from the distal esophagus at the region identified as the LES high pressure zone. This strip was designed the LES circular muscle, but it represented the circular smooth muscle of the distal esophagus obtained at the region of the LES.

Each muscle was mounted in a 20-ml bath of Krebs–Ringer solution, bubbled with 95% O_2 and 5% CO_2, and kept at 37–38° C. Muscle strips were arranged to record the isometric tension of the circular smooth muscle of each region. One end of the muscle was attached to an inflexible wire which was hooked to an external force transducer (Grass Ft 03C). The other end was attached to a metal rod which could be raised and lowered by adjustment of a screw micrometer. The outputs of the transducers were graphed on a Beckman rectilinear recorder.

After a 30-minute equilibration period, length-tension curves were constructed as previously described (Lipshutz and Cohen, 1971; Lipshutz and Cohen, 1972). All muscles were then set at their respective length of maximum tension development, L_0, for the remainder of the experiment. Dose-response curves were constructed on each muscle strip at L_0. At L_0 the peak muscle response or active tension, P_0, to a given stimulus was quantified. Initially, each agent was studied separately with doses being given in random order. Cumulative dose-response curves were not preformed. In studies using a combination of metiamide with either gastrin or histamine, the metiamide was given prior to the other agent. In drug combination studies, each muscle served as its own control. Each agent was solubilized in Krebs–Ringer solution and 1-ml volumes were added to a 20-ml bath to obtain the final molar concentration as noted. The response to each drug or combination of agents was evaluated for 30 minutes. Responses occurred within the initial 10-minute period and the peak tension recorded at each dose was used to construct the dose-response curves. LES muscle showed no spontaneous activity. Studies were performed using gastrin I (hexadecapaetide amide), histamine diphosphate, and metiamide.

In additional isometric studies, muscle responses were evaluated during depolarization with 60 mM KCl. In these studies, the muscle was contracted submaximally with KCl and then was tested with either histamine or gastrin at the concentration shown to give the maximal active tension. This response to gastrin or histamine on KCl-depolarized muscle was next tested in the presence of either atropine sulfate or diphenhydramine, respectively. The inhibitory responses to gastrin or histamine in this setting were next evaluated for antagonism by metiamide.

Specificity of the metiamide antagonism of this inhibitory response to histamine or gastrin was evaluated using isoproterenol or electrical stimulation. The inhibition to isoproterenol or electrical stimulation (60 v, 10 Hz, 1.0 msecond duration) was tested against metiamide (Tuch and Cohen, 1973).

Human Studies

Studies in man were performed using methods similar to those used in the live opossum. LES pressure was recorded continuously with complete pull-through of the recording orifices each 5-minute period. Subjects were studied in the supine position. Drugs were given as continuous intravenous infusions through an antecubital vein. Solutions were delivered by a constant infusion pump (Harvard Apparatus Co., Inc.). The following compounds are used: Histamine phosphate (Eli Lilly and Co.); diphenhydramine (Benadryl, Parke-Davis & Co.); cimetidine (Tagamet, Smith Kline & French Laboratories). Cimetidine was given either orally or by intravenous infusion.

Gastric secretion was obtained by continuous aspiration through a collecting tube with perforations at 4 to 8 cm below the distal pressure recording orifice. Specimens were collected over 15-min periods and titrated as described above.

All records were evaluated by two investigators without knowledge of the drug being administered.

RESULTS

In Fig. 1 are shown the dose-response curves of histamine with metiamide or diphenhydramine in LES smooth muscle. Diphenhydramine, an H_1 antagonist, was selected at a concentration known to block the maximal

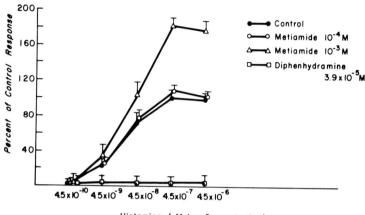

FIG. 1.   Lower esophageal sphincter circular muscle dose-response curves to histamine alone and in combination with diphenhydramine or metiamide. All values are expressed as a percent of the control histamine response. Diphenhydramine was selected at a dose which abolished the maximal histamine response on the muscle. Metiamide ($10^{-3}M$) augmented the maximal histamine responses of the muscle without altering the threshold response. Metiamide ($10^{-4}M$) had no effect at any portion of the histamine dose-response curve. Each value represents the mean + SEM for experiments obtained on a minimum of eight muscle strips. (Reproduced with permission of *Gastroenterology* **69**, 911–919, 1975).

excitatory muscle response to histamine. Metiamide at $10^{-4}M$ had no effect on the histamine dose-response curve. Metiamide at $10^{-3}M$ increased the maximal histamine responses without altering the threshold value. Thus, the excitatory response on LES smooth muscle seemed to be an H_1 effect while H_2 antagonism augmented the maximal contractile response to histamine. These data suggested that the H_2 receptor at the LES was inhibitory. Since a large concentration of metiamide was required to elicit this effect, it is possible that metiamide had a very low affinity for the LES H_2 receptor as compared to histamine, itself.

The LES muscle H_2 inhibitory receptor hypothesis was next tested directly. In Fig. 2 is shown the response of a single strip of LES circular muscle contracted by KCl depolarization. During KCl depolarization, histamine gave only a slightly further increase in active tension. When diphenhydramine was administered at a concentration previously shown to antagonize the histamine excitatory response, histamine caused inhibition of the KCl-contracted muscle. The inhibition elicited by histamine was blocked by metiamide. Thus, H_1 antagonism allowed the H_2 mediated inhibitory

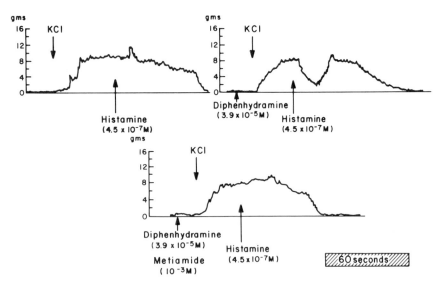

FIG. 2.   Lower esophageal sphincter circular muscle responses to KCl depolarization in combination with histamine and diphenhydramine. histamine minimally altered the maximal response to KCl depolarization. Following diphenhydramine, histamine gave an inhibitory response on the muscle. Inhibition to histamine could be antagonized by metiamide. (Reproduced with permission of *Gastroenterology* **69**, 911–919, 1975.)

response to be recorded. Metiamide did not block the inhibitory responses to isoproterenol or electrical stimulation.

Since the effect of gastrin on gastric acid secretion is blocked by H_2 antagonists, the interaction of gastrin I and metiamide was next studied on the opposum LES smooth muscle. In Fig. 3, the LES dose-response curves of LES circular muscle to gastrin I and metiamide at two concentrations are shown. Metiamide at $10^{-4} M$ concentration attenuated the prominent phase of autoinhibition beyond the maximal response. Other portions of the dose-response were unchanged. Metiamide at $10^{-3} M$ concentration increased the maximal response without changing the threshold response. The phase of autoinhibition was again attenuated in the presence of metiamide. Metiamide, alone, at either concentration gave no change in muscle tension.

Studies in the opposum, *in vivo*, showed a similar interaction of metiamide with gastrin. metiamide at 2.0 mg/kg-hour augmented the maximal LES response to gastrin I. This augmentation was seen at doses of metiamide that completely blocked the maximal acid secretory response to gastrin I. Augmentation fo the gastrin I response by metiamide is seen only with the continuous infusion of gastrin I. Bolus injections of gastrin gave considerably greater changes in LES pressure and this response seemed to be truly maximal.

In Table I are shown the LES pressure changes in response to continuous infusions of histamine phosphate in human subjects. There was a dose-related increase in pressure with a maximal response of 37.7 ±4.6 mm Hg at 20 μg/kg-hour. Higher doses of histamine gave less marked increases in LES pressure. The maximum LES response to histamine was achieved at lower doses than required for maximal acid secretion in man.

The receptor mediating this histamine effect on human LES pressure was next evaluated. In Fig. 4 is shown the maximal LES response to histamine phosphate during either cimetidine or diphenhydramine administration. Data are shown as the maximal responses during saline, diphenhydramine, and cimetidine. Diphenhydramine did not alter the maximal LES response to histamine, while cimetidine completely abolished the response. The cimetidine effect was achieved with oral administration (300 mg, 1 hour prior to histamine infusion) and intravenous infusion at 300 mg. These studies indicate that LES pressure changes in response to histamine are H_2 mediated. The H_1 receptor in man has no demonstrable effect.

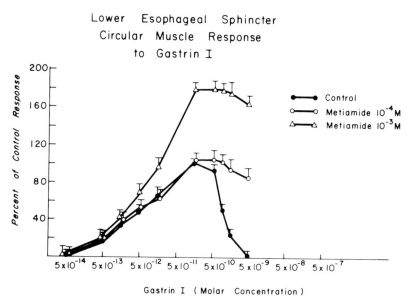

FIG. 3.   Lower esophageal sphincter circular muscle dose-response curves to gastrin I, alone and in combination with metiamide. All values are expressed as a percent of the control gastrin I response. Metiamide ($10^{-4}M$)selectively attenuated the prominent phase of autoinhibition of the gastrin dose-response curve. Metiamide ($10^{-3}M$) augmented the maximal lower esophageal sphincter muscle response to gastrin I and had a similar effect on the phase of autoinhibition. Neither concentration of metiamide altered the threshold value for gastrin I. Each value represents the mean + SEM for experiments performed on a minimum of eight muscle strips. (Reproduced with permission of *Gastroenterology* **69**, 911–919, 1975).

Table I
Effect of Histamine on Human Lower Esophageal Sphincter Pressure[a, b]

Histamine Phosphate (μg/kg–hr)	
5	27.8 ± 3.2
10	37.0 ± 4.1
20	37.7 ± 4.6
30	30.9 ± 4.9
40	27.5 ± 4.1

[a]Values are expressed in mm Hg.
[b]Control, 20.5 ± 2.3

DISCUSSION

In Table II the action of histamine on the LES pressure in several species tested to date is summarized. In all model systems, the LES is composed entirely of smooth muscle. Despite general uniformity in the LES response to

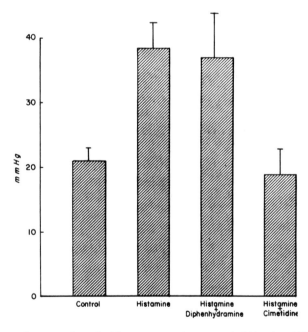

FIG. 4.   Human lower esophageal sphincter pressure in response to histamine at 20 μg/kg-hour, alone and in combination with diphenhydramine or cimetidine. Cimetidine completely abolished the response to histamine.

a wide variety of other neurohumoral substances or drugs, the LES response to histamine varies greatly in many species. Additionally, the receptor type mediating the effect in each animal also varies considerably. The lack of any consistency in the predominant LES response to histamine and the receptor producing this response is unexplained. No clear evolutionary trend is seen. However, it is apparent that in a variety of mammalian species the LES does respond to histamine (Cohen and Snape, 1975; De Carle *et al.*, 1976; De Carle and Glover, 1974; Brown and Castell, 1976; Kravitz *et al.*, 1976.

The physiological significance of histamine receptors in the LES smooth muscle is unclear. In man, histamine blockers (H_1 or H_2) fail to alter basal LES pressure, suggesting that histamine has no role in basal LES pressure (Kravitz *et al.*, 1976). However, in the opossum (North American), H_2 antagonists do increase LES pressure (Cohen and Snape, 1975). Before attributing this effect to the antagonism of endogenous histamine, it must be emphasized that metiamide also augmented the LES response to gastrin I. Thus, the physiological role of histamine in basal sphincter tone, even in the opossum, is unknown.

Although histamine cannot be shown to have a direct role in the control of basal tone, endogenous histamine release does alter LES pressure. Compound 48/80, a drug known to release histamine from mast cells contracts LES muscle *in vitro* (De Carle *et al.*, 1976). The endogenous release of histamine under physiological conditions may therefore play some role during digestive processes where histamine is released. Unfortunately, the factors causing the release of histamine under physiological conditions are not known.

Table II
Lower Esophaeal Sphincter Histamine Receptors

Species	Types of histamine receptor	Major response[a] *in vivo*
Opossum (N.A.)		
Didelphis virginiana	H_1, H_2	Excitatory (H_1)[b,c]
Opposum (Australian)		
Trichosurus vulpecula	H_2	Inhibitory[d]
Monkey (*Macaca nemestrinas*)	H_2	Inhibitory[d]
Baboon	H_1	Excitatory[e]
Man	H_2	Excitatory[f]

[a]Response to exogenous histamine in the absence of any antagonists.
[b]Cohen, S., and Snape, W.J., Jr. (1975).
[c]De Carle, D.J. *et al.* (1976).
[d]De Carle, D.J., and Glover, W.E. (1974).
[e]Brown, F.D., and Castell, D.O. (1976).
[f]Kravitz, J.J. *et al.* (1976).

The LES studies using histamine were of further significance in several important areas. First, studies in the opossum indicate that H_1 and H_2 receptors mediate opposite responses in the gastrointestinal tract. Second, either an H_1 or H_2 receptor may be demonstrable without the apparent presence of the other receptor type. Third, the H_2 receptor in gastrointestinal smooth muscle may be excitatory. These general observations regarding the LES most likely apply to all gastrointestinal smooth muscle and indicate that gut muscle is very similar to other smooth muscle organs where histamine receptors have been described (Ash and Schild, 1966; Ambach et al., 1973; Wood and Simkins, 1973).

The interaction of gastrin with H_2 antagonist drugs is reminiscent of that seen in the stomach. Gastric acid secretion in response to histamine or gastrin is blocked by H_2 antagonists (Wood and Simkins, 1973). In the opossum esophagus, H_2 antagonists blocked the inhibitory H_2 receptor leading to augmented responses to histamine and gastrin. This observation suggested that gastrin may act at the H_2 receptor in esophageal muscle. However, the high concentration of metiamide required to produce augmentation of the gastrin response may indicate a nonspecific effect.

REFERENCES

Ambache, N., Killick, S.W., and Zar, M. Aboo (1973). Antagonism by burimamide of inhibitions induced by histamine in plexus-containing longitudinal muscle preparations from guinea-pig ileum. Br. J. Pharmacol. **48**, 362.

Ash, A.S.F., and Schild, H.O. (1966). Receptors mediating some actions of histamine. Br. J. Pharmac. Chemother. **27**, 427–439.

Brown, F.C., and Castell, D.O. (1976). Histamine receptors on primate lower esophageal sphincter (LES) smooth muscle. Clin. Res. **24**(4), 533A.

Cohen, S., and Snape, W.J., Jr. (1975). Action of metiamide on the lower esophageal sphincter. Gastroenterology **69**, 911–919.

De Carle, D.J., Brody, M.J., and Christensen, J. (1976). Histamine receptors in esophageal smooth muscle of the opossum. Gastroenterology **70**, 1071–1075.

De Carle, D.J., and Glover, W.E. (1974). Independence of gastrin and histamine receptors in the lower esophageal sphincter of the monkey and possum. J. Physiol. (London) **245**, 78P–79P.

Kravitz, J.J., Snape, W.J., Jr., and Cohen, S. (1976). Role of histamine receptors in the control of human lower esophageal sphincter (LES) function. Clin. Res. **24**(5), 628A.

Lipshutz, W.H., and Cohen, S. (1971). Physiological determinants of lower esophageal sphincter function. Gastroenterology **61**, 16–24.

Lipshutz, W.H., and Cohen, S. (1972). Interaction of gastrin I and secretin on gastrointestinal circular muscle. Am. J. Physiol. **222**, 775–781.

Tuch, A., and Cohen, S. (1973). Lower esophageal sphincter relaxation: studies on the neurogenic inhibitory mechanism. J. Clin. Invest. **52**, 14–20.

Wood, C.J., and Simkins, M.A. (eds.) (1973). International symposium on histamine H_2-receptor anatagonists. Smith Kline & French, Ltd., London.

6

Imidazoline Stimulants of Gastric Secretion

T.O. Yellin and S.H. Buck
Biomedical Research Department
Pharmaceuticals R & D
ICI Americas Inc.
Wilmington, Delaware

E.M. Johnson, Jr.
Department of Pharmacology
Medical College of Pennsylvania
Philadelphia, Pennsylvania

INTRODUCTION

The discovery of histamine H_2-receptor blockers and the simultaneous description of gastric, cardiac, and vascular H_2 receptors by Black and his co-workers (Black et al., 1972) has recently led to the appreciation that some of the pharmacologic activity of several adrenergic imidazolines may be due to activation of H_2 receptors. Thus, Karppanen and Westermann (1973) showed that burimamide, an H_2-receptor blocker, antagonized the increases in acid secretion and gastric mucosal cAMP levels produced by clonidine [2-(2, 6-dichloroanilino)-2-imidazoline] in the rat. Stimulation of rat brain adenylate cyclase by clonidine was also antagonized by the H_2-receptor blocker, metiamide (Audigier et al., 1976) and the positive inotropic effect of clonidine in isolated guinea pig hearts was competitively antagonized by burimamide (Csongrady and Kobinger, 1974). Sanders et al. (1975) found that the positive chronotropic effect of tolazoline and tetrahydrozoline (structures shown in Fig. 1) in isolated guinea pig atria was inhibited by metiamide, and they concluded that these compounds activate H_2 receptors.

Our interest has centered on tolazoline, an α-adrenergic blocking agent with a number of pharmacologic effects that resemble those of histamine (Ahlquist et al., 1947; Nickerson, 1949). These include peripheral vasodilatation which underlies its clinical use in the treatment of peripheral vascular disease, cardiac stimulation, and, of greatest interest to us, tolazoline's ability to provoke copious acid secretion in a variety of species including man (Nasio, 1944; Grossman et al., 1952). It is interesting to note that N-

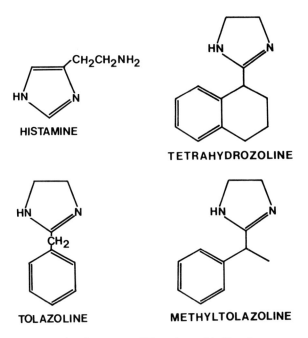

FIG. 1. Structures of histamine and imidazolines.

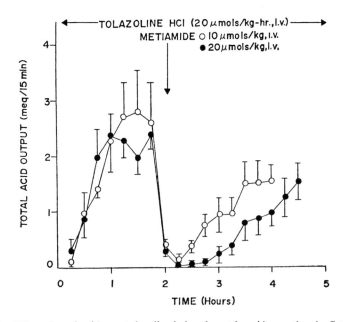

FIG. 2. Effect of metiamide on tolazoline-induced gastric acid secretion in fistula dogs. Experimental procedure was as described in Methods. Mean ± s.e.m. (N = 4 each curve).

TABLE I
Inhibitor Dissociation Constants

	Agonist	
Antagonist	Histamine[a,b]	Tolazoline[c]
Burimamide	7.8×10^{-6} M	3.2×10^{-6} M
Metiamide	9.2×10^{-7} M	8.5×10^{-7} M

[a]Black *et al.* (1972).
[b]Parsons (1973).
[c]Yellin *et al.* (1975a).

methylation of tolazoline abolishes its histamine-like activity (Gowdey, 1948), similar to ring N-methylation of histamine.

The new availability of H_2 blockers made it possible to test an old question, namely, is tolazoline a histaminergic agonist. In earlier work (Yellin *et al.*, 1975a), we showed that the gastric secretagogue activity of tolazoline in gastric fistula dogs could be blocked by small doses of metiamide as shown in Fig. 2. Also, using isolated guinea pig atria as a model system of H_2 receptors, we demonstrated that metiamide and burimamide were competitive inhibitors of the positive chronotropic action of tolazoline whereas propranolol, a β-adrenergic receptor blocker, or H_1-receptor antagonists, such as diphenhydramine, did not antagonize tolazoline. Inhibitor constants calculated from our data with the use of Schild plots were in close agreement with those obtained by Black *et al.* (1972) and Parsons (1973) using histamine (Table I). Here we describe a further characterization of the histaminergic actions of imidazolines.

METHODS

In Vitro Experiments

Spontaneously beating guinea pig right atria

Male Hartley guinea pigs (500–700 gm) were stunned by a blow to the head and killed by exsanguination. The heart was removed immediately and placed in oxygenated (95% O_2: 5% CO_2) Krebs–Henseleit buffer (pH 7.4). The right atrium was dissected rapidly and suspended at 1 gm tension in a thermostatically controlled (30° C) 25-ml tissue bath of the same oxygenated buffer. Tissues were allowed to stabilize, with repeated washing, for 1–2 hours. Individual contractions were recorded with a force-displacement transducer through a strain gage coupler, and instantaneous rates were obtained with a cardiotachometer. Cumulative dose-response curves were constructed after sequential additions of drug as a concentrated solution in saline so that total added volume was less than 1% of bath volume. Heart rate was allowed to stabilize before addition of each subsequent dose. The positive chronotropic response was defined as the increase over baseline rate just before addition of agonist. Fresh atria were used for each agonist studied.

Isolated guinea pig gastric mucosa

A modification of the method of Holton and Spencer (1976) was used. Male Hartley guinea pigs (240–300 gm) were fed only lettuce for 2 days and then fasted for 2 days with water *ad lib*. The animals were stunned by a blow to the head and the stomach was excised quickly. The stomach was cut open along the lesser curvature and rinsed with chilled mucosal solution. The cleaned organ was stretched over the end of a glass cylinder (3 cm diameter), fundic mucosa facing inward, and held in place with a rubber O-ring. Excess tissue was trimmed away and the cylinder was mounted upright in a 50-ml bath containing serosal solution bubbled with 95% O_2:5% CO_2 and maintained at 34° C. Fifteen milliliters of mucosal solution was added to the cylinder and bubbled with 100% O_2. The mucosal solution was maintained at pH 5.6 by automatic titration with 0.01 N NaOH using a pH-stat system (Radiometer) to provide a continuous record of acid secretion. The unbuffered mucosal solution contained NaCl 136 mM, KCl 5 mM, MgSO$_4$ 1.3 mM, CaCl$_2$ 3.6 mM, and glucose 16.7 mM. The buffered serosal solution contained NaCl 110 mM, KCl 5 mM, MgSO$_4$ 1.3 mM, CaCl$_2$ 3.6 mM, glucose 16.7 mM, and NaHCO$_3$ 26 mM. After equilibration of the tissue for 1–2 hours, a cumulative dose-response curve was obtained by adding drug to the serosal solution. Each dose was added when the response to the previous one had plateaued. Fresh tissues were used for each agonist studied.

In Vivo Experiments

Gastric fistula dogs

Female, chronic gastric fistula beagles (9–12 kg) were fasted overnight with water allowed *ad lib*. During experiments the dogs were lightly restrained in a standing position. After ascertaining the absence of basal secretion, continuous intravenous infusion of secretagogue was begun in 0.9% saline. Gastric acid samples were collected every 15 minutes and for each sample the volume of secretion was measured and then a 1-ml aliquot was titrated to neutrality with 0.1 N NaOH to determine acid concentration. In the constant-dose experiments with tetrahydrozoline, phentolamine (10 mg/kg) was injected subcutaneously 1 hour before the infusion to reduce the α-adrenergic side effects of tetrahydrozoline. Phentolamine at several dose levels and by several methods of administration had no effect on acid secretion in fistula dogs. In the dose-response gastric secretion studies, successive doses of secretagogue were each infused for a 1-hour period and the total acid secreted during the last 30 minutes of each period was determined.

Anesthetized gastric fistula cats

Cats of either sex (2–4 kg) were fasted overnight with water *ad lib*. The animals were anesthetized with methoxyflurane by inhalation followed by α-chloralose 80 mg/kg, i.v. The femoral veins were cannulated for intravenous administrations, and a femoral or carotid artery was cannulated and connected to a Statham blood pressure transducer. A tracheal cannula was inserted and connected to a Statham respiration transducer. Both transducers were monitored through strain gage couplers and a cardiotachometer wired into the blood pressure coupler allowed instantaneous heart rate to be recorded as well. After occlusion of the pylorus, an acute gastric fistula was sutured into the stomach at the oxyntopyloric junction and exteriorized through an abdomnal wall incision. Drugs were administered in 0.9% saline. Gastric acid samples were collected every 15 minutes by gravity and the total acid output in each was determined as described above.

Anesthetized rabbits

New Zealand rabbits of either sex (2–4 kg) were anesthetized with Dial-Urethane 0.7 ml/kg, i.v., and provided with a tracheal cannula. A femoral vein was cannulated for drug administration and a carotid artery was cannulated to measure blood pressure. Blood pressure and heart rate were monitored as described above.

Guanethidine-sympathectomized rats

Sprague–Dawley neonatal rats were sympathectomized with guanethidine as previously described (Johnson *et al.*, 1976). The procedure resulted in complete functional denervation of peripheral structures including the vascular system (Johnson *et al.*, 1975, 1977).

RESULTS AND DISCUSSION

Studies with Tolazoline

Experiments on rabbits

In preliminary experiments (Yellin *et al.*, 1975b), we observed that tolazoline produced pressor effects in some anesthetized rabbits and

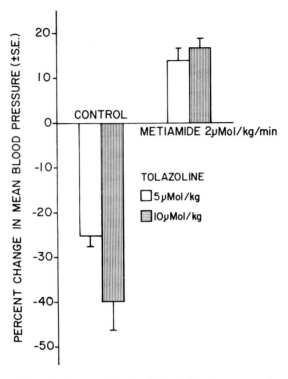

FIG. 3. Effect of metiamide on tolazoline-induced blood pressure changes in rabbits. Experimental procedure as described in Methods. Mean ± s.e.m. (N = 4 each dose).

depressor responses in others, thus, resembling histamine in its action on rabbit blood pressure. The hypotensive effect of tolazoline in anesthetized rabbits is unequivocally H_2-histaminergic. Figure 3 summarizes the results from a series of four rabbits responding to tolazoline with falls in blood pressure. Bolus injections of 5 and 10 μmol/kg tolazoline produced an average decrease in mean blood pressure of 25% and 40%, respectively. One hour after the effect of tolazoline had disappeared the injections were repeated during an infusion of metiamide at the rate of 2 μmol/kg/minute. It can be seen that metiamide completely abolished the depressor effect of tolazoline unmasking the pressor component of its action. In the dose used, metiamide had little or no effect on blood pressure. Since the hypotensive effect of tolazoline was completely blocked by metiamide, it could not have been due to the drug's well-known α-adrenergic blocking action, a conclusion which is in accord with previous investigators who have noted a direct vasodilative action of tolazoline (cf. Nickerson, 1949; Nickerson and Hollenberg, 1967).

In rabbits giving pressor responses to tolazoline, the injection of an H_1 antagonist (pyrilamine, 10 μmol/kg, i.v.) reversed the effect of succeeding doses of tolazoline unmasking a depressor action which could then be eliminated by an H_2 antagonist (metiamide). These results seemed to indicate that the vascular effects of tolazoline are mediated, at least in part, by both H_1 and H_2 receptors (Yellin *et al.,* 1975b). However, in subsequent experiments using guinea pig ileum, we were unable to demonstrate specific antagonism by antihistamines of the spasmogenic effect of tolazoline which was, in any case, quite different from histamine in its characteristics (cf. Ahlquist *et al.,* 1947). Furthermore, when tolazoline was administered to guinea pigs, which are exquisitely sensitive to the H_1 effects of histamine, it produced no evidence of histamine-like activity in intraperitoneal doses from 5 up to a lethal dose of 1500 μmol/kg. Death was not by asphyxiation and on autopsy the lungs were normal in appearance as were the intestines and other viscera. The stomach, however, was greatly distended by a large quantity of acid juice. It is unlikely, therefore, that tolazoline possesses a high degree of H_1 activity or that its histaminergic actions can be attributed exclusively to histamine release. In consequence of the foregoing, we are unclear at present about the possible H_1 effects of tolazoline on blood pressure and plan to investigate this question more carefully in the future with special attention to the α-agonist activity of tolazoline (Benfey and Varma, 1964) as an alternative explanation for our earlier observations.

Experiments on sympathectomized rats

Evidence that the relaxant effect of tolazoline on vascular smooth muscle is due not only to α-adrenergic blockade but also to a direct action had already been demonstrated in surgically denervated patients (Lindqvist, 1943; Grimson *et al.,* 1948). We have reinvestigated this question by testing the effects of tolazoline on systemic blood pressure using chemically sympathectomized rats. Johnson *et al.* (1975) have described the remarkably complete and permanent sympathectomy that can be achieved by treating newborn rats with guanethidine sulfate daily (50 mg/kg) for the first 3 weeks of life. Figure 4 shows typical evidence of functional vascular sympathectomy in such a rat which had been atropinized, curarized, and pithed. Electrical stimulation of the spinal cord in the control rat, shown at the top of Fig. 4, resulted in graded hypertensive responses. In sharp contrast, vasomotor outflow was completely absent in the treated animal, which also showed the expected supersensitivity to exogenous norepinephrine.

Both histamine and tolazoline invariably produced hypotensive responses in normal rats. However, in sympathectomized rats histamine frequently produced sharp pressor effects whereas tolazoline continued to give only

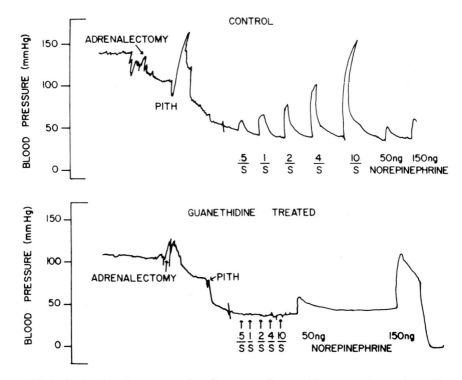

FIG. 4.   Typical blood pressure tracing of responses of a control (upper panel) rat and a rat 12 weeks old (lower panel) treated as a newborn with guanethidine (100 mg/kg/day, s.c., for 20 days) to adrenalectomy, pithing, stimulation of the vasomotor outflow, and exogenous norepinephrine. From Johnson *et al.*, 1975; reprinted with permission of *J. Pharmacol. and Exper. Ther.*

depressor effects (Yellin and Johnson, unpublished observations). This difference, which may have been due to the well-known ability of histamine to liberate epinephrine from the adrenals coupled with the adrenergic supersensitivity of sympathectomized rats, was not investigated further. Yet, if tolazoline were also capable of discharging epinephrine from the adrenals, either directly or by histamine release, its action in this regard could be masked by concomitant α-adrenergic blockade. Bearing on this question and the larger one of whether tolazoline is a direct-acting histaminergic agent, a careful comparison was made of tolazoline and compound 48/80, a known histamine releaser, using suspensions of rat peritoneal mast cells. The study showed that tolazoline (10^{-6}–10^{-2} M) did not release histamine whereas 48/80 produced typical concentration-response curves (Fertel and Yellin, unpublished observations).

Figure 5 illustrates the dose-related hypotensive activity of tolazoline in a series of four sympathectomized rats. The decreases in blood pressure which were produced by tolazoline were antagonized by metiamide, an H_2-receptor blocker. Since the heart and vasculature of guanethidine-sympathectomized rats are devoid of sympathetic innervation as judged by functional, histologic, and biochemical criteria (Johnson et al., 1975), α-adrenergic blockade is ruled out as a mechanism. Thus, these experiments clearly dissociate the antiadrenergic activity of tolazoline from its direct action on vascular smooth muscle. It is concluded that an H_2-histaminergic action underlies the fall in blood pressure due to tolazoline.

Furthermore, we can show that H_2-receptor blockade antagonizes the hypotensive activity of infused tolazoline without affecting its α-blocking action. Figure 6 is a photograph of a portion of the actual blood pressure tracing from a typical experiment using cats. It may be observed that a small dose of the H_2 blocker, cimetidine, 10 μmol/kg, i.v., counteracted the depressor effect of tolazoline without eliminating the α-blockade which was made evident by norepinephrine reversal.

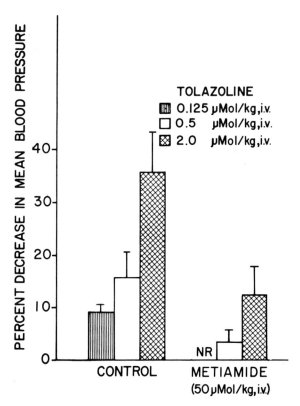

FIG. 5.   Effect of metiamide on tolazoline-induced blood pressure changes in guanethidine-sympathectomized rats. Experimental procedure was as described in Fig. 4. Mean ± s.e.m. (N = 4 each dose). NR = no response.

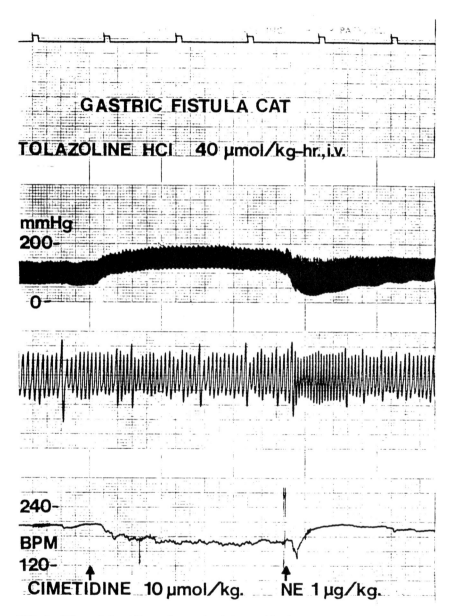

FIG. 6. Effect of cimetidine and norepinephrine on blood pressure and heart rate during tolazoline infusion in fistula cat. Experimental procedure was as described in Methods. Photograph of actual tracing from one animal. BPM = beats per minute.

Experiments on cats

The anesthetized gastric fistula cat is a very convenient preparation for simultaneously observing the primary actions of tolazoline *in vivo*. Figure 7 shows that tolazoline stimulates acid secretion and lowers blood pressure in the gastric fistula cat. Furthermore, it is seen that the injection of 5 μmol/kg metiamide sharply reduced secretion and simultaneously raised the blood pressure. As the action of the antagonist wore off, there was a gradual fall in blood pressure which was mirrored by a gradual rise in acid secretion following a similar time course toward plateau. A second injection of metiamide at a dose of 10 μmol/kg again demonstrated that the inverse relationship between blood pressure and secretion was maintained before as well as after H_2-blockade. These results suggest the involvement of a common

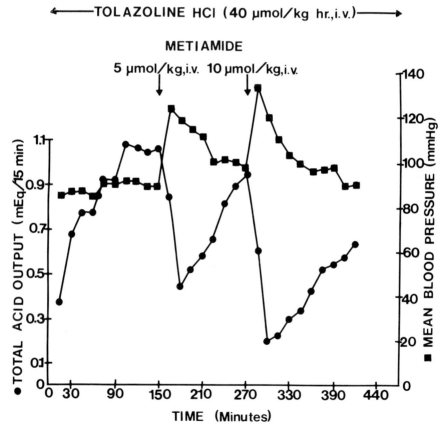

FIG. 7.   Effect of metiamide on tolazoline-induced blood pressure changes and gastric acid secretion in fistula cats. Experimental procedure was as described in Methods. (N = 3).

mechanism in the vasodilatory and secretagogue activities of tolazoline, namely, activation of H_2 receptors.

In order to strengthen the argument that tolazoline is an H_2 agonist we determined the depressor response to graded doses of tolazoline (2.5–40 μmol/kg, i.v.) in the anesthetized cat before and after H_2-blockade with metiamide. The results in Fig. 8 show that metiamide (5 μmol/kg, i.v.) produced a parallel shift to the right of the dose-response curve. This finding is consistent with the hypothesis that tolazoline and metiamide compete at H_2 receptors.

It is known that in cats and dogs H_2-receptor blockers do not antagonize the vasodepressor responses of small to moderate doses of histamine except if H_1 receptors have been blocked also (e.g., Black et al., 1975; Powell and Brody, 1976). We have repeatedly confirmed this in experiments using histamine and tolazoline in a wide range of doses producing comparable falls in blood pressure (although the duration of action of tolazoline is longer). Whereas the hypotensive effect of histamine was insensitive to H_2 blockers, that of tolazoline could be completely eliminated by metiamide or cimetidine. Such results argue that tolazoline is not acting by releasing histamine.

Our results provide strong evidence for the classification of tolazoline as an H_2 agonist. Along with the drug's well-known adrenergic properties, this conclusion helps to explain many of the diverse actions of tolazoline. Thus,

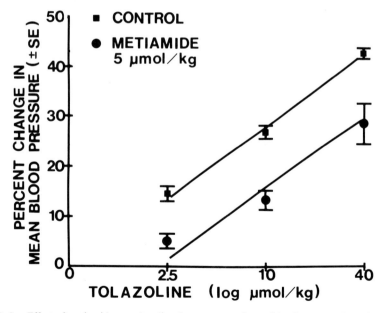

FIG. 8.   Effect of metiamide on tolazoline dose-response for cat blood pressure. Experimental procedure as described in Methods. Mean ± s.e.m. (N = 16 control; N = 7 metiamide).

the therapetuic utility and many of the clinical side-effects of tolazoline are probably due to activation of histamine H_2 receptors by the drug.

Studies with Tetrahydrozoline

Sanders *et al.* (1975) discovered that, in addition to tolazoline, the potent α-adrenergic agonist tetrahydrozoline (Fig. 1), produced concentration-dependent increases in the rate of spontaneously beating isolated guinea pig atria *in vitro,* an effect which was blocked by metiamide. Two closely related sympathomimetic imidazolines, naphazoline and oxymetazoline, were inactive. These results interested us because tolazoline and tetrahydrozoline have opposite effects at adrenergic receptors but appeared similar in their action on H_2 receptors. This made it possible to rule out possible adrenergic or vascular mechanisms in explaining the gastric secretagogue activity of tolazoline (cf. Holton, 1973). More importantly, we envisioned that a wider study of related imidazolines would yield structural clues helpful to an understanding of histamine receptors. An added interest lay in the fact that tetrahydrozoline has an asymmetric center and it could be hoped that its resolution might result in complete separation of adrenergic and histaminergic activity. To the same end, Dr. David Gilman of ICI kindly provided us with the congeneric methyltolazoline which we hope can also be resolved into its optical isomers and then studied in greater detail than in the present study (see below).

We proceeded by testing the effect of tetrahydrozoline on acid secretion using total gastric fistula beagles. In preliminary experiments we found that, given alone, tetrahydrozoline stimulated gastric secretion as well as tolazoline. However, the drug caused the dogs obvious discomfort which was considerably reduced by treatment with phentolamine. Therefore, we have used phentolamine in all subsequent experiments to reduce the marked adrenergic effects of tetrahydrozoline. In separate experiments we determined that phentolamine neither stimulates acid secretion nor reduces the secretagogue activity of tetrahydrozoline. As may be seen in Fig. 9, continuous intravenous infusions of tetrahydrozoline (12 μmol/kg/hour) provoked a brisk and steady output of acid secretion which was nicely blocked by cimetidine. In the course of doing these experiments, we noticed that tetrahydrozoline was more potent and produced a greater maximal acid output than tolazoline. Since this was in contrast to the results gotten by Sanders *et al.* (1975) in guinea pig atria, we investigated further the possible tissue specificities of the histaminergic imidazolines at our disposal. Figure 10 summarizes experiments comparing the H_2-agonist activity of several imidazolines and histamine in isolated right atria from guinea pigs. The order of increasing efficacy in this preparation was tetrahydrozoline, tolazoline, methyltolazoline, and histamine. Thus, the imidazolines appear to be partial

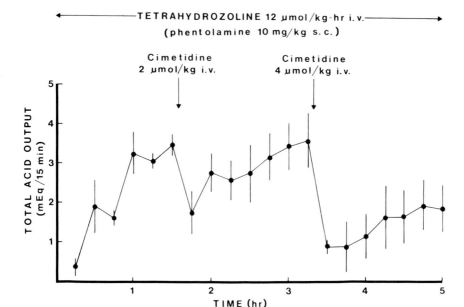

FIG. 9. Effect of cimetidine on tetrahydrozoline-induced gastric acid secretion in fistula dogs. Experimental procedure was as described in Methods. Mean ± s.e.m. (N = 3).

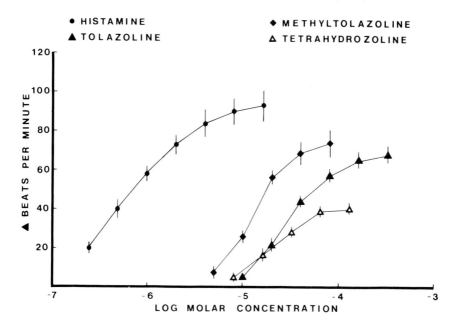

FIG. 10. Dose-response curves for positive chronotropic action of histamine and imidazolines in isolated guinea pig atria. Experimental procedure was as described in Methods. Mean ± s.e.m. (N = 4 each curve).

agonists. 2-Methyl-2-imidazoline (not shown) was inactive in concentrations up to $10^{-2}M$.

We also compared the compounds as gastric secretagogues *in vivo*. The results are shown in Fig. 11. These are step-dose experiments done in five gastric fistula bitches on successive weeks taking the drugs in random order, one experiment per week. Each dose of secretagogue was infused intravenously for 1 hour followed by the next dose and so forth. The values indicated on the graph represent the second half-hour at each dose. In experiments where it was used, phentolamine was administered at the rate of 1 mg/kg/hour, i.v. throughout.

It is apparent from Figs. 10 and 11 that the relative efficacies of tolazoline and methyltolazoline bear the same relationship in gastric fistula dogs as in guinea pig atria *in vitro*. However, the potencies and relative efficacies of tolazoline and tetrahydrozoline are reversed in the two preparations. Several possible explanations may account for this difference, namely, species differences, differences in the tissue distributions of the two agonists, or, more interesting, subtle differences between gastric and cardiac H_2 receptors.

To rule out the first possibility, we tested the secretagogue activity of tolazoline and tetrahydrozoline in isolated guinea pig gastric mucosa (see Methods) and found that, as in the dog, tetrahydrozoline was more potent and more efficacious than tolazoline (Fig. 12), opposite to the ranking

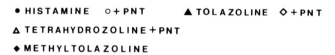

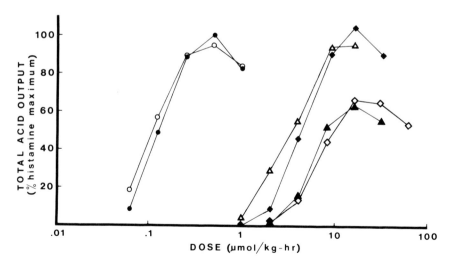

FIG. 11.   Dose-response curves for secretagogue action of histamine and imidazolines in fistula dogs. Experimental procedure was as described in Methods. Mean (N = 3 histamine + PNT; N = 5 all other curves). PNT = phentolamine.

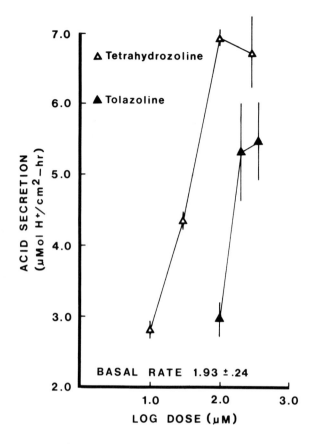

FIG. 12.   Dose-response curves for secretagoguge action of tetrahydrozoline and tolazoline in isolated guinea pig gastric mucosa. Experimental procedure was as described in Methods.   Mean ± s.e.m. (N = 3 tetrahydrozoline; N = 4 tolazoline; N = 7 basal rate).

observed in guinea pig atria (Fig. 10). Using oxyntic cell suspensions from dog gastric mucosa such as he describes in this volume, Peter Scholes found that tetrahydrozoline was also more potent than tolazoline in stimulating histamine-sensitive adenylate cyclase (Scholes, personal communication), consistent with our *in vivo* data. On the whole, therefore, it seems unlikely that species differences or differences in the tissue distributions of these drugs can account for our observations.

We are led to suspect the existence of histamine H_2 isoreceptors and to hope that useful tissue specific agonists and antagonists may be possible in the future, as has been the case in the β-adrenergic receptor area. Our results are, however, largely circumstantial in nature and further study is needed to bring more direct evidence to bear on this question

Speculation

If, as our data indicate, the imidazolines discussed here are direct-acting histaminergic agents, it is of interest to speculate on how they could bind to and activate the histamine receptor. So we would like to try to imagine how tolazoline might fit the receptor such that at least some of the differences in structure between it and histamine are reconciled.

It is generally agreed that there are at least two sites in the active center of the histamine receptor, namely, a ring binding site, and a side-chain nitrogen binding site. Fig. 13 schematically depicts several alternative ways that tolazoline could bind at the receptor. The first (a) would be to suppose that the aromatic ring of tolazoline binds at the imidazole site with the imidazoline ring taking the place of the ethylamine side-chain in histamine. This is very unappealing because it is difficult to imagine the hydrophobic benzene ring substituting for the hydrophilic, albeit aromatic, imidazole ring. Furthermore, there is overwhelming evidence available that at least one ring-nitrogen is required for activity at histamine receptors (Barlow, 1968; see also Ganellin, and Green *et al.,* this volume). In the following choices, therefore, we have

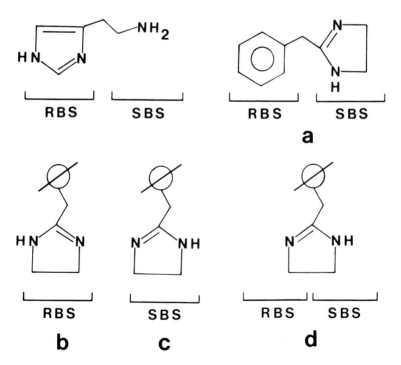

FIG. 13.   Speculative nature of binding of histamine and tolazoline to H_2-receptors. RBS = ring binding site. SBS = side-chain binding site.

drawn the aromatic ring in a way to indicate that it hasn't anything to do with receptor activation. We propose that it contributes nothing to intrinsic activity, only to binding affinity. Thus, we can now imagine the imidazoline ring either taking the place of imidazole in histamine and activating the receptor without benefit of a side-chain nitrogen (b) or we can take the opposite situation at the side-chain binding site (c). But here again there is simply too much evidence that an interaction with both sites is needed for receptor activation to seriously contemplate these possibilities. We are left with the last choice (d) in which we speculate that sites R and S are close, only a bond length or so apart, and that the imidazoline ring overlaps the imino nitrogen and side-chain amino binding sites of histamine. At physiological pH, tolazoline, which is a strong base, pKa 10.3, will be in protonated form as depicted in Fig. 14. The two nitrogens then become equivalent until subject to the influence of the receptor, which may possibly be anionic at site S. In this proposal, tautomerism, which has been proposed to be important in receptor activation by histamine (Weinstein *et al.*, 1976), could occur between the R and S binding sites.

To make the foregoing speculation more plausible, we require more evidence that the histaminergic imidazolines act directly on the receptor and

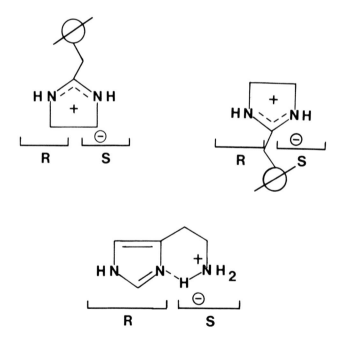

FIG. 14.   Speculative ionic nature of binding of histamine and tolazoline to H_2-receptors. R = ring site. S = side-chain site.

that histamine activates the receptor in an analogous way, i.e., in the folded conformation (Fig. 14) as suggested by Niemann and Hays (1942) for histamine at H_1 receptors. If tolazoline and other imidazolines are H_2 agonists then any theory about how histamine binds to and activates the H_2 receptor would have to deal with these structures if it is to be complete or completely believable.

ACKNOWLEDGMENTS

We thank J. G. Francis and R. A. Macia for technical assistance.

REFERENCES

Ahlquist, R.P., Huggins, R.A., and Woodbury, R.A. (1947). The pharmacology of benzyl-imidazoline (priscol). *J. Pharmacol. Exp. Ther.* **89**, 271–288.

Audigier, Y., Virion, A., and Schwartz, J.C. (1976). Stimulation of cerebral histamine H_2-receptors by clonidine. *Nature (London),* **262**, 307–308.

Barlow, R.B. (1968). Direct actions on tissues: drugs affecting histamine receptors, in "Introduction to Chemical Pharmacology." 2nd ed. pp. 344–377. Methuen, U.K.

Benfey, B.G., and Varma, D.R. (1964). Vasoconstrictor action of tolazoline. *Brit. J. Pharmacol.* **22**, 66–71.

Black, J.W., Duncan, W.A.M., Durant, C.J., Ganellin, C.R., and Parsons, M.E. (1972). Definition and antagonism of histamine H_2-receptors. *Nature (London)* **236**, 385–390.

Black, J.W., Owen, D.A.A., and Parsons, M.E. (1975). An analysis of the depressor responses to histamine in the cat and dog: involvement of both H_1- and H_2-receptors. *Brit. J. Pharmacol.* **54**, 319–324.

Csongrady, A., and Kobinger, W. (1974). Investigations into the positive inotropic effect of clonidine in isolated hearts. *Naunyn-Schmied. Arch. Pharmacol.* **282**, 123–128.

Gowdey, C.W. (1948). The change in pharmacological action produced by the introduction of a methyl group into Priscol. *Brit. J. Pharmacol.* **3**, 254–262.

Grimson, K.S., Reardon, M.J., Marzoni, F.A., and Hendrix, J.P. (1948). The effects of Priscol (2-benzyl-4, 5-imidazoline HCl) on peripheral vascular diseases, hypertension, and circulation in patients. *Ann. Sug.* **127**, 968–991.

Grossman, M.I., Robertson, C., and Rosiere, C.E. (1952). The effect of some compounds related to histamine on gastric acid secretion. *J. Pharmacol. Exp. Ther.* **104**, 277–283.

Holton, P. (1973). Catecholamines and gastric secretion, in "International Encyclopedia of Pharmacology and Therapeutics," vol. 1, Section 39A, *Pharmacology of Gastrointestinal Motility and Secretion.* (G. Peters, ed.) pp. 287–315. Pergamon Press, New York.

Holton, P., and Spencer, J. (1976). Acid secretion by guinea-pig isolated stomach. *J. Physiol. (London)* **255**, 465–479.

Johnson, E.M., Jr., Cantor, E., and Douglas, J.R., Jr. (1975). Biochemical and functional evaluation of the sympathectomy produced by the administration of guanethidine to newborn rats. *J. Pharmacol. Exp. Ther.* **193**, 503–512.

Johnson, E.M. Jr., O'Brien, F., and Werbitt, R. (1976). Modification and characterization of the permanent sympathectomy produced by the administration of guanethidine to newborn rats. *Eur. J. Pharmacol.* **37**, 45–54.

Johnson, E.M., Jr., Macia, R.A., and Yellin, T.O. (1977). Marked difference in the susceptibility of several species to guanethidine induced chemical sympathectomy. *Life Sci.* **20**, 107–112.

Karppanen, H.O., and Westermann, E. (1973). Increased production of cyclic AMP in gastric tissue by stimulation of histamine H_2-receptors. *Naunyn-Schmied. Arch. Pharmacol.* **279**, 83–87.

Lindqvist, T. (1943). Die Behandlung der Raynaudschen Krankheit mit 2-Benzyl-4, 5-Imidazolin (Priscol, Ciba). *Acta Med. Scan.* **113**, 83–108.

Nasio, J. (1944). A new test for gastric function. *Amer. J. Dig. Dis.* **11**, 227–229.

Nickerson, M. (1949). The pharmacology of adrenergic blockade. *Pharmacol. Rev.* **1**, 27–101.

Nickerson, M., and Hollenberg, N.K. (1967). Blockade of α-adrenergic receptors, in "Physiological Pharmacology," vol. 4, *The Nervous System—Part D: Autonomic Nervous System Drugs.* (W.S. Root, and F.G. Hofman, eds.), pp. 243–305. Academic Press, New York.

Nieman, C., and Hays, J.T. (1942) The relation between structure and histamine-like activity. *J. Amer. Chem. Soc.* **64**, 2288–2289.

Parsons, M.E. (1973). The evidence that inhibition of histamine-stimulated gastric secretion is a result of the blockade of histamine H_2-receptors, in "International Symposium on Histamine H_2-Receptor Antagonists. (C.J. Wood and M.S. Simkins, eds.), pp. 207–216. SK&F Labs, Welwyn Garden City, U.K.

Powell, J.R., and Brody, M.J. (1976). Identification and specific blockade of two receptors for histamine in the cardiovascular system. *J. Pharmacol. Exp. Ther.* **196**, 1–14.

Sanders, J., Miller, D.D., and Patil, P.N. (1975). Adrenergic and histaminergic effects of tolazoline-like imidazolines. *J. Pharmacol. Exp. Ther.* **195**, 362–371.

Weinstein, H., Chou, D., Johnson, C.L., Kang, S., and Green, J.P. (1976). Tautomerism and the receptor action of histamine: a mechanistic model. *Mol. Pharmacol.* **12**, 738–745.

Yellin, T.O., Sperow, J.W., and Buck, S.H. (1975a). Antagonism of tolazoline by histamine H_2-receptor blockers. *Nature (London)* **253**, 561–563.

Yellin, T.O., Sperow, J.W., Buck, S.H., and Johnson, E.M., Jr. (1975b). H_2-histaminergic activity of tolzaoline. *Fed. Proc.* **34**, 717.

PART II
CARDIOVASCULAR HISTAMINE RECEPTORS

7

Histamine–Drug–Disease Interactions and Cardiac Function*

Roberto Levi, James H. Zavecz,† Chi-Ho Lee, and Geoffrey Allan‡**
Department of Pharmacology
Cornell University Medical College
New York, N. Y.

The cardiac stimulant effect of histamine was first noted by Dale and Laidlaw (1910). Although independent of sympathetic activation (Trendelenburg, 1960; Levi and Gershon, 1970), this effect appeared to be refractory to classic antihistamines (Trendelenburg, 1960; Bartlet, 1963; Flacke et al., 1967). Consequently, the characterization of specific cardiac histamine receptors was left unresolved until a second type of histamine receptor (H_2 receptor) was defined (Black et al., 1972). With the availability of selective histamine H_1- and H_2-receptor agonists and antagonists (Black et al., 1972; Durant et al., 1975) the characterization of cardiac histamine receptors became possible (Levi et al., 1976).

Pertinent to our interests is the fact that histamine is stored in large amounts in cardiac tissues (Vugman and Rocha e Silva, 1966), particularly in the regions of the right atrium which comprise the sinoatrial and atrioventricular nodes (Conrad, 1974). Although a physiological role for cardiac histamine is not known at present, histamine could be of pathophysiological importance when one considers that mobilization of histamine from its storage sites can be provoked by a variety of stimuli, e.g., drugs (Douglas, 1975), immunological mechanisms (McIntire, 1973), and various surgical and diagnostic procedures (Lorenz, 1975). Furthermore, it is conceivable that the cardiac effects of histamine may be potentiated by commonly used drugs, e.g., digitalis (Levi and Capurro, 1975) and by disease states, e.g., hyperthyroidism

---
*Supported by USPHS, grant no. RO1 GM 20091.
†Recipient of the USPHS Research Fellowship no. F32 HL 05013.
**Recipient of the USPHS Research Fellowship no. F32 HL 05536.
‡Graduate student in pharmacology.

(Lee and Levi, 1977). Thus, an understanding of the cardiac effects of histamine, and of the receptor mechanisms involved, will allow the development of selective pharmacological means to antagonize the potential cardiac dysfunctions caused by histamine, released at any site by any means.

CARDIAC EFFECTS OF HISTAMINE
IN THE GUINEA PIG

In the guinea pig histamine, whether exogenous or endogenously released by immunologic mechanisms, enhances the force of ventricular contraction (positive inotropic effect), increases the sinus rate (positive chronotropic effect), impairs atrioventricular conduction (negative dromotropic effect), and induces ventricular arrhythmias (Levi, 1972; Capurro and Levi, 1975; Levi et al., 1976; Zavecz and Levi, 1977a). Classical histamine antagonists (H_1-receptor antagonists, e.g., diphenhydramine, promethazine, cyclizine, chlorpheniramine, and tripelennamine) fail to inhibit the histamine-induced stimulation of cardiac rate and contractility in the guinea pig; however, all inhibit in a concentration-dependent fashion the negative dromotropic effect of histamine (Levi and Kuye, 1974; Fig. 1). It is therefore apparent that the negative dromotropic effect of histamine is mediated by H_1 receptors, whereas different receptors mediate the positive inotropic and chronotropic effects of histamine (Table I). Burimamide (an H_2-receptor blocker) antagonizes the positive chronotropic and ventricular inotropic effects of

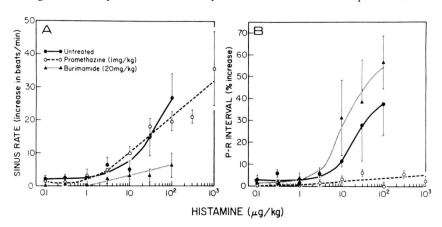

FIG. 1.   Effects of histamine (i.v.) on sinus rate (A) and atrioventricular conduction (B) in guinea pigs anesthetized with sodium pentobarbital (35–50 mg/kg, i.p.) and artificially ventilated. The guinea pigs were untreated (n = 6) or treated with either promethazine (1 mg/kg, s.c.; n = 5) or burimamide (20 mg/kg, s.c.; n = 5). Points (means ±S.E.) represent maximum changes from values immediately preceding each histamine injection. Modified from Levi et al., 1975a with permission.

Table I
Receptors Mediating the Cardiac Effects of Histamine

Parameter	Effect	Receptor
Sinus rate	increase	H_2
A-V conduction time	increase	H_1
Ventricular automaticity	increase	H_2
Ventricular contractility	increase	H_2
	decrease	H_1

histamine in the guinea pig heart. The negative dromotropic effect of histamine is not antagonized by burimamide at concentrations that clearly inhibit the increase in sinus rate (Levi et al., 1975a; Fig. 1). Thus, by the use of selective antagonists it appears that the cardiac effects of histamine are mediated by two types of receptors, H_2, mediating the increase in sinus rate and ventricular contraction, and H_1, mediating the impairment of atrioventricular (A–V) conduction (Table I).

Cardiac histamine receptor differentiation has also been aided by the use of selective agonists. As a function of dose 4-methylhistamine (4-MeH), a histamine H_2-receptor agonist (Black et al., 1972), selectively causes positive chronotropic and ventricular inotropic effects. Conversely, histamine H_1-receptor agonists 2-methylhistamine, 2-(2-pyridyl)ethylamine (PEA), and 2-(2-thiazolyl)-ethylamine (ThEA) (Durant et al., 1975) selectively impair A–V conduction (Levi et al., 1975a,b; Levi et al., 1976).

Recent experiments in our laboratory have suggested that histamine H_1 receptors are present in the ventricular myocardium, and mediate a negative inotropic effect (Table I). Indeed the inotropic effect of histamine in the isolated guinea pig heart is biphasic, and the initial increase in contractility is followed by a depression (Fig. 2a). This negative inotropic effect of histamine is unmasked when the positive inotropic effect is eliminated by H_2-receptor blockade (Fig. 2b). Furthermore, this negative inotropic effect is abolished by H_1-receptor antagonists (Fig. 2c). Confirmative studies have been carried out with the H_1 agonist ThEA, which selectively produces a negative inotropic effect (Fig. 2d). Conversely, the H_2 agonist 4-MeH selectively produces a positive inotropic effect which is not followed by a depression in contractility (Fig. 2e; Zavecz and Levi, 1977b).

Although histamine causes changes in inotropism and chronotropism, by far the most distinctive effect of histamine is its ability to cause severe arrhythmias which result from a direct effect on the A–V node and the specialized conductive tissue of the ventricles. Histamine indirectly impairs A–V conduction as a consequence of the enhanced decremental conduction that occurs during tachycardia. However, a direct effect of histamine at the A–V node is also evident since the increase in P–R interval during histamine induced tachycardia is far larger than during a similar tachycardia attained by

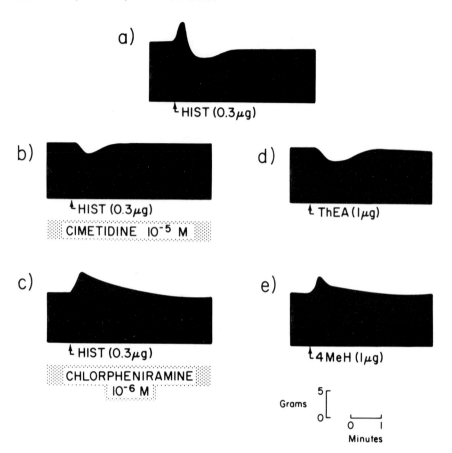

FIG. 2.   Effects of histamine (HIST), 2-(2-thiazolyl)ethylamine (ThEA), and 4-methyl-histamine (4-MeH) on the isometric ventricular contraction amplitude of isolated guinea pig hearts. A qualitative comparison. (b) The heart was continuously perfused with cimetidine; (c) with chlorpheniramine.

electrical pacing of the right atrium (Levi, 1972). This negative dromotropic effect of histamine, as previously mentioned, is mediated by H_1 receptors (Table I). We have recently investigated the ability of histamine to enhance ventricular automaticity and to cause idioventricular arrhythmias. For this purpose, we have studied the effects of histamine in the isolated guinea pig heart with surgically induced permanent atrioventricular dissociation (Zavecz and Levi, 1976a). In this preparation, the atria and ventricles beat independently. It is therefore an ideal model for studying the effects of drugs on ventricular automaticity without the influence of atrial pacemakers. As a function of dose, histamine enhances idioventricular rates, either by increasing the rate of firing of the dominant pacemaker or by enhancing the automaticity of latent pacemakers causing a shift in pacemaker site. Although this effect of histamine is similar to that of norepinephrine, it is not modified by beta blockade (Zavecz and Levi, 1976a), whereas it is susceptible to antagonism by cimetidine, an H_2-receptor antagonist, but not by chlorpheniramine, an H_1-receptor antagonist (Fig. 3). It thus appears the H_2 receptors mediate histamine-induced idioventricular tachyarrhythmias (Table I). This view is substantiated by preliminary data obtained with agonists which are selective for H_1- or H_2-histamine receptors. Although both 4-MeH (H_2 agonist) and ThEA (H_1 agonist) increase idioventricular rates, 4-MeH is one-hundred times more potent in this respect (Zavecz and Levi, unpublished). The discovery that histamine can cause idioventricular tachyarrhythmias and the characterization of the receptor involved, may well have important implications for the treatment of ventricular arrhythmias caused by histamine release.

CARDIAC EFFECTS OF HISTAMINE IN PRIMATES

In order to appreciate the clinical important of cardiac histamine release it was germane to our interest to determine how histamine will affect cardiac function in primates. Using the positive chronotropic effect as an index of cardiac histamine sensitivity, we have quantitatively compared the cardiac effects of hsitamine in the squirrel monkey with those observed in the guinea

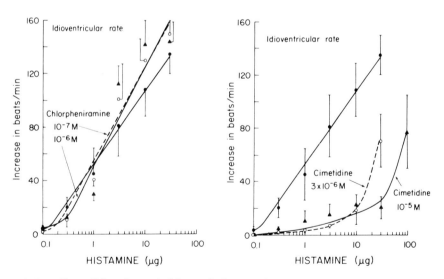

FIG. 3.   Effects of histamine on the idioventricular rate of isolated guinea pig hearts. Permanent atrioventricular block was obtained by ligature of the His bundle. Points (means $\pm$S.E., n = 5–6) represent maximum changes from values immediately preceding each histamine injection.

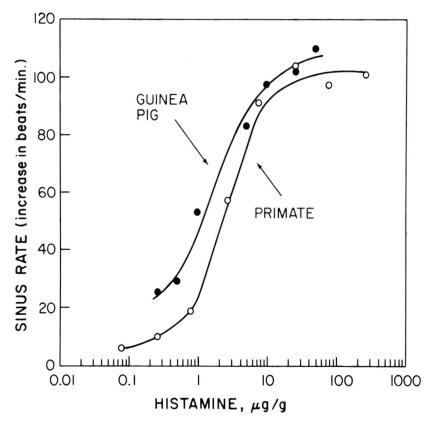

FIG. 4.   Effects of histamine on the sinus rate of the isolated heart of the guinea pig and squirrel monkey. Points (means, $n = 11$ for the guinea pig, and $n = 2$ for the primate) represent the maximum changes from values immediately preceding each histamine injection.

pig. The results obtained demonstrate that the positive chronotropic response to histamine is similar in both species (Fig. 4).

Spontaneously firing human right-atrial cells respond to histamine with an increase in the rate of phase 4 depolarization, which leads to an increased rate of firing (Fig. 5). Similar effects, at similar histamine concentrations, are observed in the sinoatrial preparation of the guinea pig (Fig. 6).

These findings demonstrate that histamine can indeed modify human cardiac function and suggest that a possible cardiac histamine release by drugs, immunological mechanisms, or surgical procedures should be recognized as a clinical entity. Furthermore, the results of these experiments emphasize the validity of the guinea pig model for the study of the cardiac effects of histamine.

HUMAN RIGHT ATRIUM

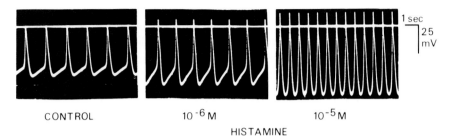

CONTROL $10^{-6}M$ $10^{-5}M$

HISTAMINE

FIG. 5.   Effect of histamine on the electrical activity of a spontaneously firing cell from a human right atrial specimen obtained during cardiac surgery. Voltage and calibration apply to all 3 records; zero potential is indicated by horizontal lines. (Levi, and Rosen, unpublished observations).

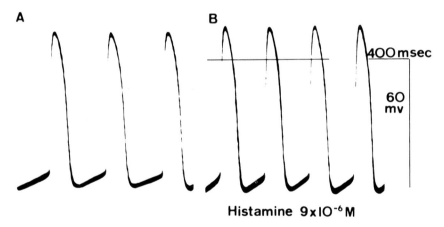

Histamine $9 \times 10^{-6}M$

FIG. 6.   Effect of histamine on the electrical activity of a pacemaker cell from the sinus node of the guinea pig heart. Voltage and calibration apply to both records; zero potential indicated by horizontal line in B; A, control. B, 30 seconds after addition of $9 \times 10^{-6}M$ histamine. (Levi and Pappano, unpublished observations).

HISTAMINE–DRUG–DISEASE INTERACTIONS

Histamine-Digitalis Interaction

Some of the cardiac effects of histamine resemble those of digitalis, in particular, atrioventricular conduction block and increase in ventricular automaticity. This prompted us to investigate a possible cardiac histamine–digitalis interaction. Ouabain, at concentrations which do not affect parameters of cardiac function, selectively potentiates the arrhythmogenic effects of histamine in the isolated guinea pig heart (Levi and Capurro, 1975). Ouabain shifts to the left the dose-response curve describing the prolongation of the P–R interval by histamine (fig. 7a). The larger the concentration of ouabain, the greater the potentiation. This leads to an increase in the incidence of atrioventricular block. Ventricular automaticity is also increased and re-entrant arrhythmias occur more frequently (Fig. 8). However, over the same concentration range ouabain does not modify the positive inotropic and chronotropic effects of histamine (Fig. 7b and c; Levi and Capurro, 1975). The histamine-induced increase in ventricular automaticity, as expressed by the number of ventricular ectopic beats, is potentiated by ouabain (Fig. 8).

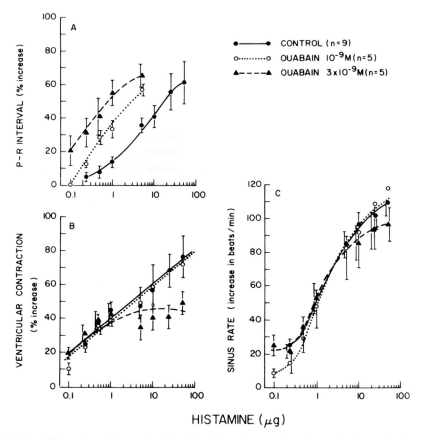

FIG. 7.   Effects of ouabain on the histamine-induced increase in atrioventricular conduction time, ventricular contraction, and sinus rate in the isolated guinea pig heart. Points (means ±S.E., n = 6–11) represent maximum changes in P–R interval (A), ventricular contractile force (B), and sinus rate (C) from values immediately preceding each histamine injection. (Reprinted from Levi and Capurro, 1975, with permission).

VENTRICULAR
ECTOPIC BEATS

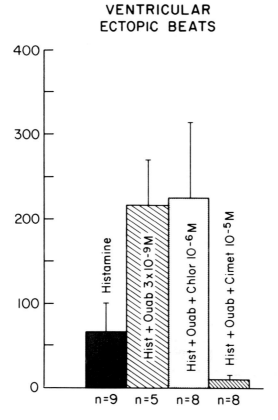

FIG. 8. Effects of ouabain on histamine-induced ventricular arrhythmias and their modifications by chlorpheniramine or cimetidine in isolated guinea pig hearts. Ventricular ectopic beats were measured over a 2 minute period following a 50 μg dose of histamine (means ±S.E.).

Whereas chlorpheniramine (an H_1 antagonist) fails to modify the potentiation by ouabain of the arrhythmogenic effects of histamine, cimetidine (an H_2 antagonist) abolishes the increase in ventricular automaticity (Fig. 8). This suggests that H_2 receptors are involved in the idioventricular arrhythmias generated by the histamine–digitalis interaction (Zavecz and Levi, 1976b).

We have also demonstrated that digitalis interacts with immunologically released histamine. Hearts excised from sensitized guinea pigs respond to antigenic challenge with histamine release, which causes sinus tachycardia, atrioventricular conduction block, and increase in ventricular automaticity. During anaphylaxis in the presence of ouabain, 10^{-9} and $3 \times 10^{-9} M$, although there is no change in either the amounts of histamine released or the intensity of sinus tachycardia, the duration of atrioventricular block is greatly increased (Fig. 9) as is the incidence of ventricular automaticity (Levi and Capurro, 1975). These results clearly demonstrate that ouabain, at concentrations that do not modify any parameter of cardiac function, selectively potentiates the arrhythmogenic properties of immunologically released histamine.

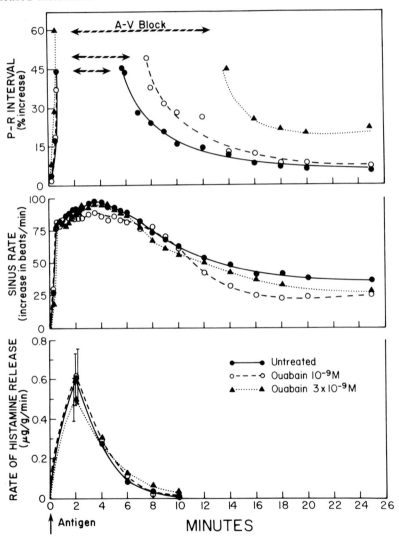

FIG. 9.   Effects of ouabain on the time-courses of histamine release, increase in sinus rate, and prolongation of P–R interval during anaphylaxis to penicillin antigens in isolated guinea pig hearts. (Reproduced from Levi and Capurro, 1975, with permission).

The ouabain–histamine interaction could have definite clinical implications since digitalis is widely used and histamine release, either immunologically or directly by drugs, is a common phenomenon. Since ventricular arrhythmias and conduction disturbances are known to occur during anaphylaxis in humans (Bernreiter, 1959; Booth and Patterson, 1970; Criep and Woehler, 1971), it is conceivable that digitalis could enhance cardiac manifestations of allergic reactions.

Digitalis cardiotoxicity cannot be explained solely on the basis of digitalis serum levels. One particular case of interest is that of patients who, after cardiopulmonary bypass, exhibit arrhythmias compatible with digitalis toxicity at relatively low digitalis serum levels (Morrison and Killip, 1973; Rose *et al.*, 1975). Since histamine is released during extracorporeal circulation (Hollenberg *et al.*, 1963; Meyer-Burgdorff *et al.*, 1973), it might be implicated in what was assumed to be an "increased myocardial sensitivity to digitalis" after cardiopulmonary bypass. Moreover, ouabain-induced cardiotoxicity, as expressed by the onset of ventricular tachycardia and fibrillation, is significantly delayed in the presence of metiamide, a histamine H_2-receptor antagonist (Somberg *et al.*, 1975). This suggests that histamine may participate in digitalis-induced arrhythmia. Thus, on the basis of our findings, an interaction between released histamine and digitalis could explain some instances of digitalis toxicity that are presently simply accepted as digitalis adversity *per se*.

Histamine–Angiotensin Interaction

"High renin" patients, who represent 20% of the total hypertensive population, will probably have raised levels of angiotensin II. Some of the cardiac effects of angiotensin II, particularly the impairment of atrioventricular conduction (Bonnardeaux and Regoli, 1974), are analogous to the cardiac effects of histamine. Furthermore, there is evidence of increased histamine synthesis in the aortic wall of rats with surgically induced short-term hypertension (Yarnal and Hollis, 1976). These considerations have recently led us to investigate the possibility of cardiac histamine-angiotensin interaction. In the isolated guinea pig heart perfused with $8.3 \times 10^{-9} M$ angiotensin II, the dose-response curve describing the histamine-induced prolongation of the P–R interval is displaced to the left (Fig. 10). Furthermore, at this concentration of angiotensin, histamine-induced atrioventricular conduction block occurs more frequently and ventricular ectopic activity is enhanced. Thus, it is possible that in high renin hypertensive patients atrioventricular block due to released histamine will occur more frequently. Furthermore, there may be an increased incidence and severity of ventricualr tachyarrhythmias.

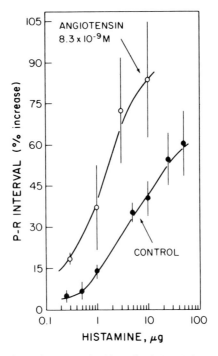

FIG. 10.   Effect of angiotensin II on the histamine-induced increase in atrioventricular conduction time in isolated guinea pig hearts. Points (means ±S.E., *n* = 5–11) represent maximum changes in P–R interval from values immediately preceding each histamine injection.

Cardiac Effects of Histamine in Hyperthyroidism

Cardiac excitability and automaticity are enhanced in the thyrotoxic state (Sobel and Braunwald, 1971). We have recently studied the cardiac effects of histamine in isolated hearts excised from hyperthyroid guinea pigs in order to determine whether thyroid hormone might sensitize the myocardium to the arrhythmogenic effects of histamine. The positive chronotropic and inotropic effects of histamine are not modified in the hyperthyroid state (Lee and Levi, 1977). However, as a function of the severity of the thyrotoxic state, the arrhythmogenic effects of histamine are potentiated, as evidenced by the increased incidence and duration of ventricular arrhythmias (Fig. 11). Histamine-induced conduction arrhythmias are also potentiated in the hyperthyroid state (Lee and Levi, 1977). These results demonstrate that hyperthyroidism selectively enhances the arrhythmogenic properties of histamine and suggest that cardiac dysfunctions caused by histamine release may be exacerbated in the hyperthyroid state.

VENTRICULAR ARRHYTHMIAS

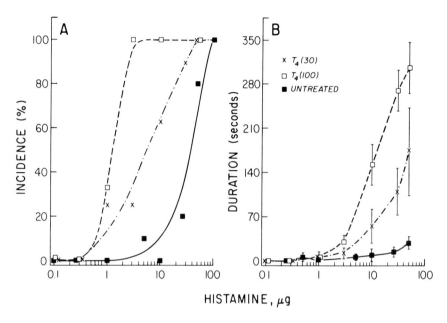

FIG. 11.   Arrhythmogenic effects of histamine and their potentiation in the hyperthyroid state. Guinea pigs were either untreated or treated with thyroxine (T₄ at 30 or 100 μg/day/300 g animal for 8 consecutive days) and their excised hearts were perfused *in vitro* (Langendorff preparation). In A, points represent the percent incidence (n = 8–9), and in B, the duration of ventricular arrhythmias (multifocal ventricular ectopic beats, junctional rhythms or ventricular tachycardia; means ±S.E.; n = 8–9) following each dose of histamine.

SUMMARY

The major points to have emerged from our studies are:

(1) Histamine affects many parameters of cardiac function. In the guinea pig, it causes tachycardia, an increase–decrease in ventricular contraction, impairment of atrioventricular conduction, and severe ventricular arrhythmias.

(2) In the guinea pig heart both types of histamine receptors coexist. The selective activation of these receptors is required for the expression of the various cardiac effects of histamine.

(3) The sensitivity of the sinoatrial node to histamine in the monkey and in humans is similar to that of the guinea pig.

(4) The arrhythmogenic effects of histamine can be potentiated by certain drugs and disease states.

REFERENCES

Bartlet, L.A. (1963). The action of histamine on the isolated heart. *Br. J. Pharmacol.* **21**, 450–461.

Bernreiter, M. (1959). Electrocardiogram of patient in anaphylactic shock. *J. A. M. A.* **170**, 1628–1630.

Black, J.W., Duncan, W.A.M., Durant, G.J., Ganellin, C.R., and Parsons, M.E. (1972). Definition and antagonism of histamine H_2-receptors. *Nature (London)* **236**, 385–390.

Bonnardeaux, J.L., and Regoli, D. (1974). Action of angiotensin and analogues on the heart. *Can. J. Physiol. Pharmacol.* **52**, 50–60.

Booth, B.H., and Patterson, R. (1970). Electrocardiographic changes during human anaphylaxis. *J. A. M. A.* **211**, 627–631.

Capurro, N., and Levi, R. (1975). The heart as a target organ in systemic allergic reactions: comparison of cardiac anaphylaxis *in vivo* and *in vitro*. *Circ. Res.* **36**, 520–528.

Conrad, M.J. (1974). A systems analysis of atrial and oviductal anaphylaxis. Ph.D. Thesis, Stanford University, California.

Criep, L.H., and Woehler, T.R. (1971). The heart in human anaphylaxis. *Ann. Allergy* **29**, 399–409.

Dale, H.H., and Laidlaw, P.P. (1910). The physiological action of β-iminazolylethylamine. *J. Physiol. (London)* **41**, 318–344.

Douglas, W.W. (1975). Histamine and antihistamines; 5-hydroxytryptamine and antagonists, in "The Pharmacological Basis of Therapeutics." (L.S. Goodman and A. Gilman, eds.) pp. 590–629. Macmillan, New York.

Durant, G.J., Ganellin, C.R., and Parsons, M.E. (1975). Chemical differentiation of histamine H_1- and H_2-receptor agonists. *J. Med. Chem.* **18**, 905–909.

Flacke, W., Atanackovic, D., Gillis, R.A., and Alper, M.H. (1967). The actions of histamine on the mammalian heart. *J. Pharmacol. Exp. Ther.* **155**, 271–278.

Hollenberg, M., Pruett, R., and Thal, A. (1963). Vasoactive substances liberated by prolonged bubble oxygenation. *J. Thorac. Cardiov. Surg.* **45**, 402–411.

Lee, C.-H. and Levi, R. (1977). Arrhythmogenic effects of histamine and their potentiation in hyperthyroidism. *Fed. Proc.* **36**, 1043.

Levi, R. (1972). Effects of exogenous and immunologically released histamine on the isolated heart: a quantitative comparison. *J. Pharmacol. Exp. Ther.* **182**, 227–238.

Levi, R., Allan, G., and Zavecz, J.H. (1976). Cardiac histamine receptors. *Fed. Proc.* **35**, 1942–1947.

Levi, R., and Capurro, N. (1975). Cardiac histamine–ouabain interaction: potentiation by ouabain of the arrhythmogenic effects of histamine. *J. Pharmacol. Exp. Ther.* **192**, 113–119.

Levi, R., Capurro, N., and Lee, C.-H. (1975a). Pharmacological characterization of cardiac histamine receptors: sensitivity to H_1- and H_2-receptor agonists and antagonists. *Eur. J. Pharmacol.* **30**, 328–335.

Levi, R., Ganellin, C.R., Allan, G., and Willens, H.J. (1975b) Selective impairment of atrioventricular conduction by 2-(2-pyridyl)-ethylamine and 2-(2-thiazolyl)ethylamine, two histamine H_1-receptor agonists. *Eur. J. Pharmacol.* **34**, 237–240.

Levi, R., and Gershon, M.D. (1970). Chemical sympathectomy and cardiac action of histamine. *Fed. Proc.* **29**, 612.

Levi, R., and Kuye, J.O. (1974). Pharmacological characterization of cardiac histamine receptors: sensitivity to H_1-receptor antagonists. *Eur. J. Pharmacol.* **27**, 330–338.

Levi, R., and Pappano, A.J. (1978). Modifications of the effects of histamine and norepinephrine on the sinoatrial node pacemaker by potassium and calcium. *J. Pharmacol. Exper. Ther.* **204**, 625–633.

Lorenz, W. (1975). Histamine release in man. *Agent. Action* **5**, 402–416.

McIntire, F. C. (1973). Histamine release by antigen-antibody reactions, in "International Encyclopedia of Pharmacology and Therapeutics," (M. Schachter, sec. ed.) Vol. 1, Section 74, Histamine and Antihistamines, pp. 45–99. Pergamon Press, Oxford.

Meyer-Burgdorff, C., Seidel, G., and Schlütter, F. J. (1973). Freisetzung von Histamin und Serotonin bei extrakorporaler Zirkulation. *Anesthesist* **22**, 212–216.

Morrison, J., and Killip, T. (1973). Serum digitalis and arrythmia in patients undergoing cardiopulmonary bypass. *Circulation* **47**, 341–352.

Rose, M.R., Glassman, E., and Spencer, F.C. (1975). Arrhythmias following cardiac surgery: relation to serum digoxin levels. *Am. Heart J.* **89**, 288–294.

Sobel, B.E., and Braunwald, E. (1971). Cardiovascular system, in "The Thyroid," (S.C. Werner and S.H. Ingbar, eds.) Third Ed., pp. 551–560. Harper and Row, New York.

Somberg, J., Cagin, N.A., Kleid, J., Bounous, H., Levitt, B., and Levi, R. (1975). The influence of metiamide on ouabain cardiotoxicity. *Eur. J. Pharmacol.* **34**, 233–236.

Trendelenburg, U. (1960). The action of histamine and 5-hydroxytryptamine on isolated mammalian atria. *J. Pharmacol. Exp. Ther.* **130**, 450–460.

Vugman, I., and Rocha e Silva, M. (1966). Biological determiantion of histamine in living tissues and body fluids, in "Handbook of Experimental Pharmacology," Vol. 18, Part 1, Histamine. (M. Rocha e Silva, ed.), pp. 81–115. Springer-Verlag, New York.

Yarnal, J.R., and Hollis, T.M. (1976). Rat aortic histamine synthesis during short-term hypertension. *Blood Vessels* **13**, 70–77.

Zavecz, J.H. and Levi, R. (1976a). Pharmacological characterization of the receptors mediating histamine-induced idioventricular tachyarrhythmias. *Fed. Proc.* **35**, 645.

Zavecz, J.H., and Levi, R. (1976b). Histamine–digitalis interaction: modification by histamine H_1- and H_2-receptor antagonists. *Pharmacologist* **18**, 168.

Zavecz, J.H., and Levi, R. (1977a). Separation of primary and secondary cardiovascular events in systemic anaphylaxis. *Circ. Res.* **40**, 15–19.

Zavecz, J.H., and Levi, R. (1977b). Negative inotropic effect of histamine: an H_1-response. *Pharmacologist* **19**, 187.

8

Histamine Receptors in Vascular Smooth Muscle: Mechanisms of Vasodilatation[1]

Michael J. Brody, Mark Kneupfer, M. R. Strait, and Richard A. Shaffer
Department of Pharmacology and
the Cardiovascular Center
College of Medicine
The University of Iowa
Iowa City, Iowa

INTRODUCTION

The development of a new class of histamine-receptor antagonists (Black *et al.*, 1972) has provided a tool for studying the receptor mechanisms involved in the cardiovascular responses to histamine. Since the earliest experiments of Dale it has been known that histamine is an extremely potent vasoactive material. In most species the substance lowers arterial pressure through a complex set of interactions between cardiac and vascular effects. In several species such as the rabbit and frog histamine produces an elevation in arterial pressures. Since most of the species known to respond to histamine do so with a fall in blood pressure this review will focus on the receptor mechanisms involved in producing histamine-mediated vasodilatation.

The traditional antihistamines, hereafter referred to as H_1-receptor blockers, do not abolish the vasodepressor or vasodilator actions of histamine. When Black and co-workers developed the new H_2-receptor antagonists burimamide and metiamide it became possible to test the hypothesis that the residual response to histamine involved a second type of histamine receptor. Our laboratory and others were able to demonstrate that the vascular actions of histamine in fact involved interactions with H_1 and H_2 receptors; however, these studies documented that the interactions of histamine with its receptors were quite complex.

---

[1]This study was supported in part by USPHS Grants HLB-14388 and GM 00141.

The following is a summary of some of our studies which have helped identify the mechanisms of histamine interaction with receptors in vascular smooth muscle (Powell and Brody, 1973, 1976a,b).

Initial studies were performed on the gracilis muscle of the dog perfused under conditions of constant blood flow. Intra-arterial injection of graded doses of histamine produced dose related vasodilator responses. The administration of the H_2-receptor antagonists burimamide or metiamide failed to affect the response to histamine even when given in enormous concentrations. However when the preparation was first treated with mepyramine a significant shift of the histamine dose-response curve was produced and the subsequent administration of an H_2-receptor antagonist abolished the response to histamine. These data demonstrated that there may not be an important physiological role for H_2 receptors in promoting vasodilatation since their activation can be demonstrated only when H_1 receptors are blocked. Using relatively specific H_1- and H_2-receptor agonists, namely 2-(2-pyridyl) ethylamine (PEA) and 4-methyl histamine, it was possible to demonstrate that H_2 receptors could be activated in the absence of H_1-receptor blockade. PEA produced vasodilatation which was essentially blocked by mepyramine while 4-methyl histamine produced vasodilatation which was large attenuated by metiamide. Thus, H_2 receptors are available for interaction with a specific agonist; however, histamine appears to preferentially bind to H_1 receptors.

The chemical form of an agonist may be the factor that determines its preference for either H_1 or H_2 receptors. It appears that those compounds possessing a high affinity for H_2 receptors, like 4-methyl histamine, display 1, 3-protrophic tautomerism while PEA exists primarily in a nontautomeric hydrogen bonded form (Durant *et al.*, 1974).

There have now been a substantial number of papers published which support the concept that histamine has the potential to interact with H_1 and H_2 receptors in producing its depressor or vasodilator effects. These studies have been detailed in a recent review (Chand and Eyre, 1975) and will be only briefly summarized here. In addition to the dog, in which both H_1 and H_2 receptors mediate vasodilatation, it appears that the cat, chicken, guinea pig, and rat possess similar histamine receptor mechanisms. Recent papers have suggested that H_1 and H_2 receptors are also involved in mediating vasodilator responses in monkey (Doyle and Stike, 1976) and man (Chipman and Glover, 1976). Vasoconstrictor responses induced by H_1-receptor activation are seen in the guinea pig, calf, rabbit, and horse. In the rabbit especially, administration of H_1-receptor antagonists unmasks depressor responses mediated by H_2 receptors. Vasoconstrictor effects of histamine are not limited to species exhibiting pressor activity. For example, pulmonary vessels and cranial vessesl in species such as cat and dog exhibit vasoconstriction mediated by H_1 receptors.

The physiological functions of histamine as a mediator of vasodilatation have been examined (Powell and Brody, 1976b). Histamine has been proposed to be involved in mediating reflex vasodilatation induced by activation of baroreceptors, an analog of baroreceptor-mediated vasodilatation, i.e., the vasodilator response which follows termination of sympathetic nerve stimulation, reactive hyperemia, the vasodilatation associated with exercise, sustained vasodilatation seen primarily in the cutaneous circulation, and finally vasodilatation mediated by release of histamine from mast cells. Evidence was found for the involvement of H_2 as well as H_1 receptors in baroreceptor-mediated reflex vasodilatation and in poststimulation vasodilatation. No evidence for the role of histamine release in reactive hyperemia or exercise-induced hyperemia could be obtained. An unexpected observation was the demonstration that compound 48/80 produced vasodilatation which unlike that of histamine could be blocked only when H_2-receptor antagonists were present.

The present studies were undertaken to examine further the relationships between histamine receptors in vascular smooth muscle and the effects of histamine release from endogenous storage sites. At least two such sites are known to exist, a mast cell and nonmast cell storage pool. With respect to vascular smooth muscle, histamine is localized exclusively in a nonmast cell pool in most species (El-Ackad and Brody, 1975). The release of this nonmast cell pool appears to be involved in mediating baroreceptor-induced reflex vasodilatation. Such vasodilatation develops when adrenergic vasoconstrictor tone is inhibited by the reflex arc. Thus, there appears to be a close functional relationship between adrenergic innervation to vascular smooth muscle and responses involving release of nonmast cell histamine. Furthermore, the release of mast cell histamine appears to selectively involve activation of H_2 receptors. These considerations led to an examination of the influence of removal of adrenergic innervation on the responsiveness of vascular smooth muscle to histamine as well as an examination of the reflex vasodilator mechanisms involving histamine in the cat.

METHODS

The gracilis muscle of dogs was treated with 6-hydroxydopamine to destroy adrenergic nerve terminals. The animals were treated 1 week before experimentation. Six-hydroxdopamine was administered directly into the gracilis artery in a dose of 2.5 mg. To accomplish this the dogs were anesthetized with sodium pentobarbital, 30 mg/kg, and the gracilis artery was exposed in each limb under sterile conditions. An injection of 6-hydroxydopamine was made into one limb while the contralateral muscle received the injection vehicle (saline bubbled with nitrogen). The skin incisions were closed and the animals allowed to recover.

The experiments were performed using bilateral, constant flow perfusion of the isolated gracilis muscles in dogs anesthetized with sodium pentobarbital, 30 mg/kg. The animals were tracheotomized and the brachial artery was cannulated for blood pressure measurement. The jugular vein was cannulated for intravenous administration. The muscles were perfused using Sigmamotor pumps after preparation according to the method described in detail by Dorr and Brody (1965). Flow was adjusted so that perfusion pressure in each muscle approximated systemic blood pressure. Two Sigmamotor pumps were precalibrated so that the flows were equal to the two muscles.

All drugs were administered into the tubing leading to the gracilis artery. Tests for destruction of sympathetic innervation included loss of reflex vasoconstriction produced by bilateral carotid artery occulsion, supersensitivity to norepinephrine injected intra-arterially, and the absence of vasodilatation following sectioning of the gracilis nerve.

Histamine-mediated vascular responses were studied in the perfused hindquarters of cats. The animals were anesthetized with an injection of chloralose, 60 mg/kg, administered intravenously. The hindquarters were isolated as described by Beck (1965) and perfused with a Sigmamotor pump at constant flow. Drugs were administered intra-arterially through the tubing leading to the hindquarters or intravenously through a jugular venous catheter. Reflex vasodilatation was produced by intravenous administration of several doses of norepinephrine. The contribution of neurogenic vasoconstrictor tone to vasodilator responses was evaluated by sectioning the lumbar sympathetic chains bilaterally at the termination of each experiment.

Drugs used in these experiments included norepinephrine bitartrate, histamine hydrochloride, nitroglycerin, compound 48/80 (obtained as a gift from Burroughs–Wellcome, Inc., Research Triangle Park, North Carolina), mepyramine maleate (Pfaltz and Bauer, Inc., Flushing, New York), metiamide (obtained as a gift from Smith Kline and French, Philadelphia, Pennnsylvania), and 6-hydroxydopamine hydrobromide (Regis Chemical). Data were analyzed by means of paired t-tests (Steele and Torrie, 1960) or by parallel line bioassay (Finney, 1952).

RESULTS AND DISCUSSION

Histamine-Mediated Vasodilatation in Cat

The possibility that histamine mediates active reflex vasodilatation has been examined in both dogs and cats. There is substantial agreement about the existence of active vasodilatation in dogs and its mediation by histamine (Heitz and Brody, 1975). The situation is more complicated in cats. For example, several papers have failed to demonstrate the existence of anything other than sympatho-inhibition as a reflex vasodilator mechanism (Zimmerman, 1971; Zimmerman and Liao, 1973), while others have suggested that an antihistamine-sensitive vasodilator system exists (Tuttle, 1966, 1967; Weaver and Gebber, 1974). Since there have been no reports of the use of combined H_1- and H_2-receptor blockade on reflex vasodilatation in cats the current study was undertaken.

Results are summarized in Table I. Two doses of norepinephrine were used to induce reflex vasodilatation. Responses to graded doses of histamine and nitroglycerin, both given itnra-arterially, were also tested. Following the administration of mepyramine the responses to histamine were abolished while the responses produced by nitroglycerin and the reflex vasodilator responses produced by norepinephrine were unaffected. Subsequent administration of metiamide (10 mg given over a 10-minute period) had no effect on reflex vasodilatation or the vasodilator effects produce by nitroglycerin. When the lumbar sympathetic chains were sectioned at the termination of the experiment the fall in perfusion pressure was as great as that produced by the large dose of norepinephrine (ratio equals 0.28 ± 0.08).

Table I

The Influence in the Cat of Antihistamines on Reflex
Vasodilatation and Vasodilatation Produced by Histamine

Treatment	Change in Hindquarter Perfusion Pressure (Ratio)*	
	Control	Mepyramine†
Histamine (IA)		
50 ng	0.21 ± 0.02	—
200 ng	0.53 ± 0.08	—
Reflex vasodilatation via norepinephrine		
0.3 μg/kg	0.16 ± 0.03	0.16 ± 0.06
1.0 μg/kg	0.29 ± 0.02	0.30 ± 0.04
Nitroglycerin		
3 μg	0.21 ± 0.06	0.18 ± 0.04
9 μg	0.43 ± 0.08	0.47 ± 0.08

*Ratio determined by dividing change in perfusion pressure by the initial pressure.

†5 mg infused directly into the hindquarters over a 10-minute period. Blood flow to the hindquarters averaged 16.4 ml/minute in 10 preparations used to compile data in this table. After metiamide (10 mg IA) reflex vasodilatation averaged 0.18 ± 0.02 and 0.36 ± 0.05 for the low and high doses of norepinephrine.

These data demonstrate that reflex vasodilatation induced by elevation of arterial pressure in cats does not involve activation of a histaminergic system. A possible explanation for the discrepancy between this finding and that of other investigators who have demonstrated histaminergic vasodilatation in cats is the nature of the stimulus. In this study and those by Zimmerman (Zimmerman, 1971; Zimmerman and Liao, 1973) arterial pressure was raised by norepinephrine. In other studies demonstrating histaminergic vasodilatation the stimuli have been electrical stimulation in brain stem (Tuttle, 1966, 1967; Weaver and Gebber, 1974) or stimulation of the afferent end of the sectioned vagus nerve (Weaver and Gebber, 1974). Thus, histaminergic vasodilatation in the cat appears to involve activation of central pathways which may to be functionally distinct from the baroreceptor pathway.

It is also of interest to note that we were unable to demonstrate the existence of two types of histamine receptors in the hindlimb of the cat. This was an unexpected finding since previous studies from this laboratory have demonstrated that the systemic arterial pressure effects of histamine involve two types of histamine receptor (Powell and Brody, 1973) and because others have found that vasodilatation produced in the hindquarters of cats involves both H_1- and H_2-receptor mechanisms (Flynn and Owen, 1975). This latter paper is of special interest because the experimental conditions are almost identical to those in the present paper. There are several differences, however. Flynn and Owen anesthetized their animals with pentobarbital while we used chloralose. In their experiments the antihistamines were administered by the intravenous route while we gave the agents intra-arterially. In computing the relationship between doses of histamine and antihistamine in the two papers it appears that the sensitivity of the hindquarters to histamine in the experimental preparations of Flynn and Owen was much less than those described in the present paper. We achieved equivalent percent changes in perfusion pressure (20%) by the intra-arterial injection of 50 ng histamine, while Flynn and Owen appeared to require approximately 400 ng. It is difficult to compare the concentrations of mepyramine. However, if it is assumed that instantaneous concentrations are maintained, Flynn and Owen would have had approximately 33 μg/ml of mepyramine in blood while our concentration was approximately 13 μg/ml blood in the hindlimb. Thus, the concentrations of antihistamines were roughly comparable while the absolute sensitivity of the hindquarter vessels to histamine was much greater in our findings. These comparisons, while pointing out differences between the experimental preparations, do not help explain the discrepancy. It is interesting to note that in an older study performed on chloralose anesthetized cats, the vasodilator effects of histamine in the hindquarters were abolished by the antihistamine benadryl (Folkow et al., 1948). The concentrations of histamine producing such effects were similar to those used in the present study. It is conceivable that the nature of histamine receptors in

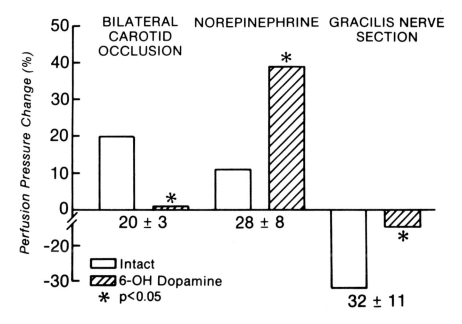

FIG. 1. Tests for completeness of pharmacological denervation induced by 6-hydroxydopamine-treated muscles. Bilateral carotid occlusion was performed for 45 seconds. Responses to norepinephrine are shown for the dose of 0.3 μg injected intraarterially. Values underneath each pair of bars represent the mean difference ± standard error of the mean for the paired comparison t-test.

the cat might be altered by anesthesia, but this hypothesis needs much more investigation.

Histamine Receptors in Denervated Vessels

The effectiveness and selectivity of 6-hydroxydopamine is confirmed by the data summarized in Fig. 1. Bilateral carotid artery occlusion produced reflex vasoconstriction in the intact muscle and produced essentially no response in the muscle treated with 6-hydroxydopamine. Supersensitivity to norepinephrine, injected intra-arterially, was observed in the treated muscles. Although response to only a single dose of norepinephrine (0.3 μg) is illustrated, a larger dose (1.0 μg) also produced a significantly greater response in the treated muscle. Finally, at the termination of the experiment, section of the gracilis nerve produced a large fall in perfusion pressure in the intact muscle, i.e., a vasodilatation due to interruption of adrenergic vasoconstrictor tone, whereas a very small fall in perfusion pressure was seen in the treated muscles. It may be concluded that the intra-arterial injection of 6-hydroxydopamine

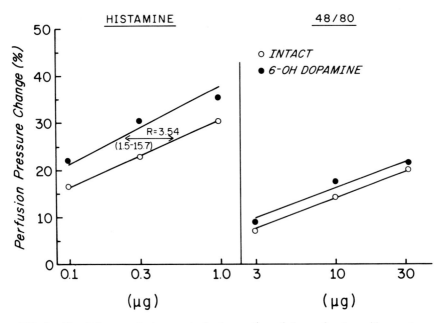

FIG. 2. The influence of pharmacologic denervation of the perfused gracilis muscle on vasodilator responses to histamine and compound 48/80. The significant potency ratio including its confidence interval is shown for histamine. No significant difference in responses to compound 48/80 was observed.

into a single muscle effectively destroys the vascular innervation to that muscle without affecting innervation in the contralateral limb.

The influence of 6-hydroxydopamine treatment on responses of the gracilis muscle to histamine and to compound 48/80 was determined in five dogs. Dose-response curves were determined for histamine, using doses ranging from 0.01 to 3 μg, and for 48/80, using doses ranging from 1 to 30 μg. The steep portions of these curves were used to analyze the data depicted in Fig. 2. The muscles treated with 6-hydroxydopamine were more sensitive to histamine than the control muscles. The potency ratio of 3.54 means that the muscles treated with 6-hydroxydopamine responded as if they were receiving three to four times more histamine than the control muscles. No such difference was observed in the case of compound 48/80. Since flows were the same in the two muscles the amount of drug being delivered to each was equivalent. In addition, perfusion pressures between the two muscles were not significantly different. Thus, the change in response of the gracilis muscle vessels to histamine appears to be due to a true increase in sensitivity. As a test for the capacity of the vessels to dilate, the response to a nonspecific vasodilator, nitroglycerin, was tested. There was no significant difference in the response of the control and 6-hydroxydopamine-treated muscles to nitroglycerin. Furthermore, the direct vasodilator effect of the antihistamine mepyramine was also unchanged in the two muscles. These data are summarized in Fig. 3.

The difference between the increased sensitivity seen with histamine and the failure to see such a change in the case of compound 48/80 provides further evidence that these substances produce effects which are mediated by a different histamine receptor. In an earlier study from this laboratory it was found that compound 48/80, which is thought to act by liberating mast cell histamine stores, produced vasodilator effects which were unaltered by the H_1-receptor blocker, mepyramine (Powell and Brody, 1976c). In contrast the response to histamine was reduced significantly by mepyramine. Thus, it appears that the histamine liberated by compound 48/80 does not gain access to the H_1 receptors which are available to histamine injected via the blood stream. H_2-receptor blockade attenuated the response to compound 48/80 (Powell and Brody, 1976c), but this was accomplished only after H_1-receptor blockade was established. It was postulated that there might well be a spatial orientation of type H_1 and H_2 receptors which could explain the selective effect of H_2-receptor blockade on the vasodilator response produced by compound 48/80. Specifically, H_2 receptors might be more heavily concentrated on the outside of the vessel wall whereas there might be a higher

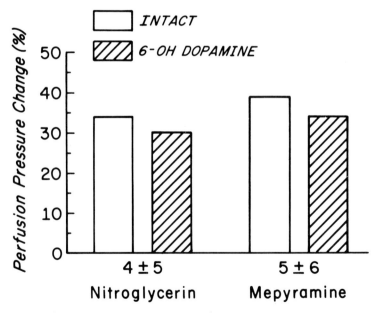

FIG. 3.   Vasodilator responses produced in intact and 6-hydroxydopamine-treated gracilis muscles by nitroglycerin and mepyramine. The dose of nitroglycerin was 3 μg while that for mepyramine was 50 mg. infused over a 20-minute period. The peak response to mepyramine is plotted. Values under each pair of bars represent the mean difference ± standard error. No significant differences exist between the values.

concentration of H_1 receptors on the luminal side. Since mast cells are never found within the vessel wall in species such as dog and cat (El-Ackad and Brody, 1975) but rather are found outside the wall proper, histamine liberated by compound 48/80 could be anticipated to act preferentially on the H_2 receptors proposed to lie on the outer side of the vessel wall. Although this hypothesis about histamine-receptor location is not supported directly by the present experiments concerning increased sensitivity to histamine in pharmacologically denervated vessels, they do suggest that blood-borne histamine and histamine liberated by compound 48/80 either have access to different receptor sites or work through different mechanisms.

An attempt was made to determine if the increased sensitivity observed with histamine was associated with activation of a specific histamine receptor. Mepyramine (50 mg infused over a 20-minute period) was given simultaneously to the control and 6-hydroxydopamine treated muscles. As described above (Fig. 3) mepyramine produced a direct vasodilator action which was not significantly different between the two muscles. Responses to histamine were tested when perfusion pressure had returned to its control values in each muscle. As summarized in Fig. 4 there was an approximately equivalent shift of the dose response curve to histamine in both muscles. In fact histamine retained a significantly greater potency in sympathectomized ($R = 2.41$) after H_1-receptor blockade. The subsequent administration of metiamide (50 mg

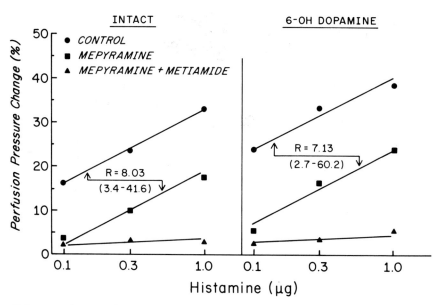

FIG. 4. Influence of H_1- and H_2-receptor blockade on responses of intact and 6-hydroxydopamine-treated gracilis muscles to histamine. The potency ratios (R) were not significantly different between the intact and 6-hydroxydopamine treated muscles.

infused over a 20-minute period) essentially abolished the vasodilator effects of histamine in both the control and 6-hydroxydopamine treated muscles. Responses to the nonspecific vasodilator nitroglycerin were not affected significantly by either antihistamine. These data suggest that the increase in sensitivity to histamine may be associated with a specific alteration in type H_2 receptor mechanisms. This conclusion is based upon the fact that the difference in sensitivity between the two muscles was unaffected by H_1-receptor blockade leaving the residual histamine response mediated solely by activation of type H_2 receptors.

What is the mechanism by which degeneration of adrenergic nerve terminals induces an increase in sensitivity of vascular smooth muscle to histamine, apparently through a change in the nature of histamine's interaction with H_2 receptors? A schematized version of the mechanisms by which histamine produces vasodilatation is shown in Fig. 5. On the left-hand side of the figure is an adrenergic nerve terminal which liberates norepinephrine which in turn activates an alpha-adrenergic receptor on the vascular smooth muscle wall. The function of this receptor is to activate vasoconstriction. It has recently been demonstrated that histamine interferes with vasoconstriction induced by neurogenic release of norepinephrine by inhibiting the release of transmitter (McGrath and Shepherd, 1976). This effect of histamine was blocked specifically by H_2-receptor blockade, but not H_1-receptor antagonism. H_2 blockade also specifically decreases the uptake of histamine by the vascular smooth muscle (Goodman et al., 1975). Although the study by Goodman et al., did not determine whether the histamine uptake was associated with binding to a neurogenic store, the studies by McGrath and Shepherd (1976) suggest that this may well be the case. The diagram in Fig. 5 illustrates an H_2 receptor associated with the adrenergic nerve terminal. If histamine binds to nerve terminal receptors as well as to the receptors on vascular smooth muscle associated with its vasodilator action, it could be predicted that the destruction of nerve terminal binding sites might be associated with an enhanced effect of histamine due to greater availability of histamine at vascular receptors. The fact that increased sensitivity to histamine appeared to be associated with the H_2-receptor mechanism suggests tha the histamine ordinarily bound to nerve terminals has the capacity to find preference for those receptors proposed to be on the outside of the vessel wall, i.e., in closer association with nerve terminals which usually innervate only to the level of the adventitial-medial border.

The remainder of the schematic concerns the mechanisms by which endogenous histamine stores are involved in vasodilatation. The nerve terminal depicted ont he right-hand side of Fig. 5 does not play a vasoconstrictor role. The existence of such a special type of adrenergic innervation was identified functionally by experiments demonstrating that histamine-mediated vasodilatation was produced at the termination of nerve

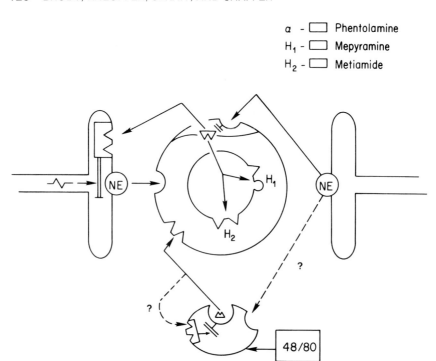

FIG. 5.   Schematic depiction of interactions between histamine and its receptors on vascular smooth muscle, adrenergic nerve terminals, and mast cells.

stimulation when release of norepinephrine and vasoconstriction had been prevented (for details see Heitz and Brody, 1975; Powell and Brody, 1976c). This nerve terminal is thought to regulate the release of histamine from its non-mast cell storage pool (Ryan and Brody, 1972; Heitz and Brody, 1975; El-Ackad and Brody, 1975). The release of non-mast cell histamine appears to be involved in the histamine mediated component of reflex vasodilatation produced by activation of barorecptors (Beck and Brody, 1961; Beck, 1965; Brody, 1966). Non-mast cell histamine release appears to involve activation of both H_1 and H_2 receptors (Powell and Brody, 1976c). Figure 5 suggests that a second mechanism by which non-mast cell histamine, released during inhibition of adrenergic nerve activity, might produce vasodilatation is by inhibiting the nerve terminal release of norepinephrine involved in vasoconstriction.

    The final portion of the schematic concerns the release of histamine from its mast cell storage site. Compound 48/80 liberates histamine which appears to interact preferentially with H_2 receptors. The regulation of histamine from the mast cell by systems depicted in Fig. 5 is not well understood.

Norepinephrine is not particularly potent in its action on the mast cell and its effect appears to be to activate the release of histamine (Beavan, 1976a, b; Goth and Johnson, 1975). It is conceivable that neurogenically liberated norepinephrine may have access to the mast cell and help promote this release (Rothschild and Oliveria, 1973). Histamine itself, via activation of an H_2 receptor and subsequent formation of cyclic AMP, appears to inhibit histamine release from the mast cell (Lichtenstein *et al.,* 1973; Beavan, 1976a, b). Beta-adrenergic receptor activation, also acting through the cyclic nucleotide mechanism, possesses the capacity to inhibit histamine release from mast cells (Goth and Johnson, 1975).

In conclusion, the vasodilator effects of histamine are not restricted to simple interaction with vascular smooth muscle receptors. Although histamine has the capacity to interact with H_1 and H_2 receptors it is difficult to demonstrate H_2-receptor mechanisms unless H_1 receptors are blocked. Under physiological conditions histamine appears to produce vasodilatation not only by reacting with vascular receptors but by inhibiting vasoconstriction induced by neurogenic release of norepinephrine from adrenergic nerve terminals. This effect is mediated by H_2 receptors. Two sources of endogenous histamine are involved in promoting histamine-mediated vasodilatation. The non-neurogenic, non-mast cell pool of histamine mediates reflex vasodilatation. The release of histamine from this pool is inhibited by physiological discharge of norepinephrine from special nonvasoconstrictor nerves. Non-mast cell histamine interacts with H_1 and H_2 receptors. Mast cell histamine appears to act selectively on H_2 receptors. Physiologic stimuli for release of this histamine pool have not been identified but it may well be that the release of histamine from mast cells is regulated by histamine itself acting on H_2 receptors and by antagonistic releasing and inhibitory effects of alpha- and beta-adrenergic receptors, respectively.

ACKNOWLEDGMENTS

The authors are indebted to Drs. C. R. Ganellin and P. Ridley of Smith Kline and French for generous gifts of metiamide and to Dr. R.A. Maxwell of Burroughs–Wellcome for graciously providing us with samples of compound 48/80.

REFERENCES

Beaven, M.A. (1976a). Histamine. *N. Eng. J. Med.* **294**, 30-36.
Beaven, M.A. (1976b). Histamine. *N. Eng. J. Med.* **294**, 320-325.
Beck, L., and Brody, M.J. (1961). The physiology of vasodilatation. *Angiology* **12**, 202-221.

Beck, L. (1965). Histamine as the potential mediator of active reflex vasodilatation. *Fed. Proc.* **24,** 1298-1310.

Black, J.W., Duncan, W.A.M., Durant, C.J., Ganellin, C.R., and Parsons, E.M. (1972). Definition and antagonism of histamine H₂-receptors. *Nature (London)* **236,** 385-390.

Bogaert, M.G., De Schaepdryver, A.F., and Willems, J.L. (1977). Dopamine-induced neurogenic vasodilatation in the intact hindleg of the dog. *Br. J. Pharmac.* **59,** 283-292.

Brody, M.J. (1966). Neurohumoral mediation of active reflex vasodilatation. *Fed. Proc.* **25,** 1583-1592.

Carroll, P.R., and Glover, W.E. (1977). Modification of cardiovascular responses to histamine by dithiothreitol. *Br. J. Pharmac.* **59,** 333-341.

Chand, N., and Eyre, P. (1975). Classification and biological distribution of histamine receptor sub-types. *Agents and Actions* **5,** 277-295.

Chipman, P., and Glover, W.E. (1976). Histamine H₂-receptors in the human peripheral circulation. *Br. J. Pharmac.* **56,** 494-496.

Dale, M.M., Evinc, A., and Vine, P. (1976). The denervated cremaster muscle of the guinea-pig as a pharmacological preparation. *Br. J. Pharmac.* **58,** 229-237.

Dorr, L.D., and Brody, M.J. (1965). Functional separation of adrenergic and cholinergic fibers to skeletal muscle vessels. *Am. J. Physiol.* **208,** 417-424.

Doyle, T.F., and Strike, T.A. (1976). Histamine-induced hypotension modified by H₁ and H₂ antagonists in the monkey (macaca mulatta). *Experientia* **32,** 1428-1430.

Durant, C.J., Ganellin, C.R., and Parsons, M.E. (1974). Chemical differentiation of histamine H₁-and H₂-receptor antagonists, *Pro. 168th Am. Chem. Soc. Nat. Meet. MEDI* **29.**

El-Ackad, T.M., and Brody, M.J. (1975). Evidence for non-mast cell histamine in the vascular wall. *Blood Vessels* **12,** 181-191.

Finney, D.J. (1952). "Statistical Methods in Biological Assay," Charles Griffin, London.

Flynn, S.B., and Owen, D.A.A. (1975). Histamine receptors in peripheral vascular beds in the cat. *Br. J. Pharmac.* **55,** 181-188.

Folkow, B., Haeger, K., and Kahlson, G. (1948). Observations on reactive hyperaemia as related to histamine, on drugs antagonizing vasodilatation induced by histamine and on vasodilator properties of adenosinetriphosphate. *Acta Physiol. (Scandinavia).* **15,** 264-278.

Goodman, F.R., Debbas, G., and Weiss, G.B. (1975). Effects of metiamide on distribution of ¹⁴C-histamine in aortic smooth muscle. *Arch. Int. Pharmacodyn.* **218,** 212-220.

Goth, A., and Johnson, A.R. (1975). Current concepts on the secretory function of mast cells. *Life Sci.* **16,** 1201-1214.

Heitz, D.C., and Brody, M.J. (1975). Possible mechanism of histamine release during active vasodilatation. *Am. J. Physiol.* **228,** 1351-1357.

Lichtenstein, L.M., Plaut, M., Henney, C., and Gillespie, E. (1973). The role of H₂-receptors on the cells involved in hypersensitivity reactions, in "International Symposium on Histamine H₂-Receptor Antagonists" (C.J. Wood and M.A. Simkins, eds.) pp. 187-198. Smith Kline & French Laboratories Limited, Welwyn Garden City.

McGrath, M.A., and Shepherd, J.T. (1976). Inhibition of adrenergic neurotransmission in canine vascular smooth muscle by histamine. Mediation by H₂-receptors. *Circ. Res.* **39,** 566-573.

Powell, J.R., and Brody, M.J. (1973). Identification of two vascular histamine receptors in the dog, in "International Symposium on Histamine H₂-Recptor Antagonists" (C.J. Wood and M.A. Simkins, eds.) pp. 137-146. Smith Kline & French Laboratories Limited. Welwyn Garden City.

Powell, J.R., and Brody, M.J. (1976a). Identification and specific blockade of two receptors for histamine in the cardiovascular system. *J. Pharmacol. Exper. Ther.* **196,** 1-14.

Powell, J.R., and Brody M.J. (1976b). Identification and blockade of vascular H₂ receptors. *Fed. Proc.* **35,** 1935-1941.

Powell, J.R., and Brody, M.J. (1976c). Participation of H₁ and H₂ histamine receptors in physiological vasodilator responses. *Am. J. Physiol.* **231**, 1002-1009.

Rothschild, A.M. and Oliveira, M.P. (1973). "Histamine release and mast cell degranulation by sympathetic stimuli in the rat, in Histamine" (C. Maslinski, ed.) Dowden, Hutchinson & Ross, Inc. pp. 81-90. Stroudsburg, Pennsylvania.

Ryan, M.J. and Brody, M.J. (1972). Neurogenic and vascular stores of histamine in the dog. *J. Pharmacol. Exper. Ther.* **181**, 83-91.

Steele, R.G.D., and Torrie, J.H. (1960). "Principles and Procedures of Statistics with special reference to Biological Sciences," McGraw-Hill, New York.

Tuttle, R.S. (1966). Evidence for histaminergic nerves in the pyramidal cat. *Am. J. Physiol.* **211**, 903-910.

Tuttle, R.S. (1967). Physiological release of histamine-^{14}C in the pyramidal cat. *Am. J. Physiol.* **213**, 620-624.

Weaver, L.C., and Gebber, G.L. (1974). Electrophysiological analysis of neural events accompanying active dilatation. *Am. J. Physiol.* **226**, 84-89.

Zimmerman, B.G. (1971). Comparison of reflex vasodilator responses in hindlimb of dog and cat. *Am. J. Physiol.* **221**, 1171-1177.

Zimmerman, B.G., and Liao, J.C. (1973). Reflex vasodilatation in the cat and dog anesthetized with ketamine. *Proc. Soc. Exper. Biol. Med.* **144**, 268-272.

9

H₁- and H₂-Histamine Receptors in the Gastric Microcirculation

Paul H. Guth and Esther Smith
Medical and Research Services
VA Wadsworth Hospital Center
Los Angeles, California

University of California at Los Angeles
School of Medicine
Los Angeles, California

INTRODUCTION

The Gastric Microcirculation

The specialized epithelial cells of the gastric mucosa are responsible for its secretory, protective, and absorptive functions. In order to provide these cells with energy sources sufficient to meet their metabolic needs and to provide for removal of metabolic wastes, there must be an intimate relation between the epithelial cells and the mucosal microcirculation. This relationship has been recognized for some time. In spite of numerous studies over the past half century, there is still debate over such basic issues as the anatomical organization and physiological control of the gastric microcirculation.

In 1951, Barlow *et al.*, using a double-injection technic, described submucosal arteriovenous anastomoses in the human stomach. On the basis of glass microsphere injection studies, Walder (1952) concluded that these shunts play a major role in the control of gastric mucosal blood flow. Normally, shunt resistance is higher than mucosal arteriolar resistance and most of the blood flows throught the mucosa. In the presence of agents or stimuli which constrict the arterioles, mucosal arteriolar resistance increases and more blood then passes through the shunts. However, the existence of shunts has been seriously questioned by recent investigations with improved accurately sized microspheres with radioactive labels. These permit quantitative estimates of shunt flow. Delaney and Grim (1964) injected microspheres into the left gastric artery of the living dog. No 35-μm spheres and at the most 5.2% of 12-μm spheres were recovered in the venous effluent. In similar

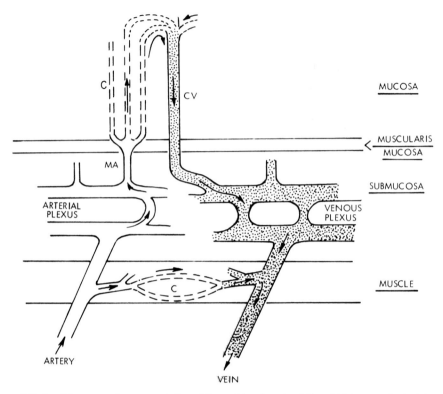

FIG. 1.   Diagrammatic representation of the gastric microcirculation. MA =mucosal arteriole, C= capillary, C.V. = collecting vein. The microvasculature of the muscle layer is in parallel with that of the mucosa, while the microvasculature of the submucosa is in series with that of the mucosa. There are no arteriovenous anastomoses.

studies Shoemaker and Powers (1966) and Archibald *et al.* (1974) recovered no spheres in the venous outflow.

We have used a different approach, *in vivo* microscopy (Guth and Rosenberg, 1972) to study this problem. A fasted rat or cat was anesthetized, the abdomen opened, and the stomach exteriorized. The gastric wall was then transilluminated and the gastric microvasculature directly visualized microscopically. With apprropriate modifications, the external muscle layer, submucosa, or mucosa, could be studied. Details of the techniques for visualizing the submucosal vaculature and the image-splitting procedure for measuring changes in arteriolar diameter are presented in the Methods section of this paper. Careful study of the submucosal plexuses revealed completely separate arterial and venous plexuses. No shunts were seen. The organization of the microcirculation of the stomach as seen by *in vivo* microscopy is diagrammatically depicted in Fig. 1.

Physiological studies employing nerve stimulation and the close intra-arterial injection or topical superfusion of various humoral agents were then performed (Guth and Smith, 1975b and 1976b). On the basis of these studies we concluded that the submucosal arterioles are the major resistance vessels in the gastric microcirculatory bed. Constriction of these vessels results in an increase in resistance and a decrease in mucosal blood flow, while dilatation of these vessels decreases resistance and increases mucosal flow. These vessels are under both nervous and humoral control. The parasympathetic nerves, the vagi, dilate while the sympathetic nerves, the splanchnics, constrict them. Under humoral control, both biogenic amines and hormones appear to play a role. Histamine dilates while norepinephrine constricts these vessels. Of the gastrointestinal hormones, only cholecystokinen may have a role in the physiological control of mucosal blood flow.

Histamine and Histamine Receptors

Histamine plays a major role in the regulation of blood flow throughout the body. Histamine exerts its actions via two types of receptors, mepyramine-sensitive receptors (e.g., those mediating bronchial constriction), termed H_1 (Ash and Schild, 1966), and mepyramine-insensitive receptors (e.g., those mediating gastric secretion) termed H_2 (Black et al., 1972). The latter are subject to blockade by a new class of antihistamines, the H_2 antagonists (Black et al., 1972). The development of these two types of histamine receptor antagonists has permitted study of the distribution and function of histamine receptors in different vascular beds. In arterial segment studies H_1-receptors subserving vasoconstriction and H_2 receptors subserving vasodilation were present in the rabbit ear artery (Parsons and Owen, 1973); Glover et al., 1973), while only H_2 receptors subserving vasodilatation were present in the human temporal artery (Glover et al., 1973). Both H_1 and H_2 receptors subserving vasodilatation have been observed in the general circulation (i.e., depression of systemic arterial blood pressure) of the dog (Powell and Brody, 1973, 1976) and cat (Parsons and Owen, 1973), in the skeletal muscle of the dog (Powell and Brody, 1973, 1976), and in the intestinal circulation of the cat (Guth and Smith, 1976). When, as in the last-mentioned studies, both receptors subserve vasodilatation, the H_1-receptor effects predominate, i.e., an H_2 effect cannot be demonstrated unless the H_1 receptor is blocked.

The purpose of the present investigation was to ascertain the types and functions of histamine receptors in the submucosal arterioles of the corpus and antrum of the stomach of the cat and rat.

METHODS

Cats weighing between 2 and 4 kg and male Sprague–Dawley rats weighing between 150 and 200 gm were used throughout this study. The animals were fasted but allowed free access to water for 24 hours prior to study. An *in vivo* microscopy technique was employed to study gastric submucosal arteriolar responses (Guth and Rosenberg, 1972). The animals were anesthetized with sodium pentobarbital, 35 mg/kg, i.p., the abdomen opened, and the stomach exteriorized. For visualization of the antrum a clad fiberglass rod was passed into the stomach through a small incision in the duodenum. For visualization of the corpus, the rod was passed into the stomach through a small incision high in the fundus of the cat stomach or in the rumen of the rat stomach. The gastric wall was then transilluminated by passing light from a high intensity light source through this rod. Using a compound microscope with long working distance objectives, the microvascular bed was visualized. For optimum visualization of the submucosal vascular network, it was necessary to carefully remove serosal and muscle layers from a small area of either the corpus or antrum, thus exposing the submucosal plexi to direct viewing. The flow of blood through the submucosal arteriolar arcades to the mucosal arterioles and the capillary bed at the base of the mucosa and then back from the mucosa through collecting venules and into the submucosal

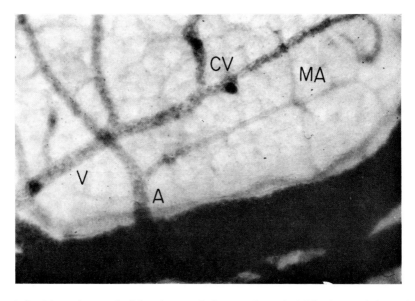

FIG. 2.   Photomicrograph of the submucosal microvasculature (rat). The characteristic arterial (A) and venous (V) plexuses are seen. The venous network can be distinguished by the larger diameter of its vessels and the presence of collecting veins (CV), seen in cross-section, which drain into the venous anastomotic network. An arterial arcade gives rise to a mucosal arteriole (MA) which divides and enters the capillary network. This mucosal arteriole appears to be entering a vein, but in actuality it goes beneath the vein to enter the mucosa. The honeycomb-like appearance of the capillary bed is barely visible. (×100).

venular network could clearly be seen (Fig. 2). The area under study was continuously superfused with a Krebs solution at 38° C. Body temperature was monitored and maintained between 37 and 38° C by a heating pad.

The responses of one of the smaller branches of the submucosal arterial plexus to superfusion of the various agents were studied. Vessel diameter was measured by the image-splitting technique via a microscope recording system (Baez, 1966). This method provides permanent graphic recordings of the amount of shearing of the microscopic image of the small blood vessels and permits quantitation of diameter changes with accuracy (standard deviation expressed as coefficient variation of 1.8% in our experience, Guth and Smith, 1975a). As the dial on the image splitter is turned, the vessel image is split in two. When the two images lie side by side, just touching, the vessel has been split exactly one diameter. Turning the dial alters the resistance in a potentiometer and the current flowing to the recorder. The recorder needle is deflected proportionately. By rapidly splitting the image exactly in two and then returning to one image several times, several measurements of diameter size are made. During the course of a study, numerous measurements are easily recorded and the tracings are analyzed after the study by reference to a standard calibration recording.

For study of histamine and histamine antagonists, the compounds were added to the superfusing fluid so that the submucosal vascular network was continuously bathed with solutions of known molarity. The concentrations employed were: histamine, $10^{-4} M$, mepyramine, an H_1 antagonist, $10^{-5} M$, and metiamide, an H_2 antagonist, $10^{-4} M$. Previous studies revealed that these were the optimally effective concentrations of mepyramine and metiamide. Higher concentrations of these agents by themselves inhibited norepinephrine vasoconstriction. While histamine produced readily measureable marked dilatation of the rat corpus submucosal arterioles, the dilatation of cat and rat antral arterioles and cat corpus arterioles was relatively small. In order to amplify this effect so that the antagonists could be more readily studied, the antral submucosal bed in the cat and rat and the corpus bed in the cat were superfused with norephinephrine, $10^{-5}-10^{-7}$ M, to partially constrict the arterioles. Subsequent superfusions with histamine with and without the antagonists contained norepinephrine. Six to ten minutes were allowed between superfusion episodes to permit effects of the previously superfused agents to wear off. During these intervals, superfusion with the Krebs solution alone was maintained. Repeat superfusions with histamine (rat corpus studies) or with norepinephrine alone and with histamine (antrum and cat corpus studies) were performed at the end of each series of studies to be certain the histamine response had not changed. To ascertain whether the H_1- and H_2-antagonist effects were specific for histamine, similar studies were performed with another vasodilator, papaverine $10^{-3} M$.

RESULTS

Corpus

Results of the microcirculatory studies in the corpus of 7 cats are presented in Table I. The size of the arterioles studied was similar in all cats, averaging 36.0 ± 2.9 μm (mean ± SE, prior to norepinephrine constriction). Histamine caused dilatation in all animals, averaging 72.8 ± 8.9% above control diameter. Both the H_1 antagonist and the H_2 antagonist partially inhibited this response in all animals. The average diameters were 31.2 ± 8.1 and 44.2 ± 7.3% above control with the H_1 and H_2 antagonists, respectively. These were significantly less than the histamine dilated diameter. When the antagonists were given together, there was complete inhibition of the histamine effect, the diameter being 5.6 ± 7.4% above control (not significantly different from 0). The effects of the antagonists were nearly perfectly additive: 31.2% dilatation due to H_2 effect + 44.2% dilatation due to H_1 effect = 75.8% dilatation together (and histamine alone yielded 72.8 8.9% dilatation).

Results of the microcirculatory studies in the corpus of 7 rats are presented in Table II. Vessels of similar size to those in the cat, 32.9 ±2.6 μm, were studied. Again dilatation occurred in all rats, the arteriolar diameter increasing to 36.1 ± 5.1% above control, on the average. Both H_1 and H_2 antagonists inhibited the histamine dilatation in all animals studied. Interestingly, H_2-receptor antagonism alone nearly completely inhibited the response, the diameter being only 6.2 ± 3.6% above control. However, the H_1

Table I
Percent Increase in Cat Corpus Submucosal Arteriolar Diameter in Response to Histamine and the Histamine Antagonists[a]

Cat No.	H	H + H_1A	H + H_2A	H + H_1A + H_2A
		Δ Diameter (%)		
1	80.7	29.8	43.3	2.9
2	86.4	57.2	57.2	28.0
3	63.8	59.4	52.7	34.0
4	116.9	31.0	63.1	-5.9
5	54.1	22.6	43.2	9.5
6	51.5	20.4	46.2	-11.5
7	56.2	-1.7	4.0	-17.7
Mean ± SE	72.8 ± 8.9	31.2 ± 8.1	44.2 ± 7.3	5.6 ± 7.4

[a]Δ Diameter = % above control; control = diameter of norepinephrine-constricted arteriole (or resting arteriole in rat corpus studies); H = histamine; H_1A = H_1-receptor antagonist, mepyramine; H_2A = H_2-receptor antagonist, metiamide.

Table II
Percent Increase in Rat Corpus Submucosal Arteriolar Diameter in
Response to Histamine and the Histamine Antagonists[a]

Rat No.	Δ Diameter (%)			
	H	H + H$_1$A	H + H$_2$A	H + H$_1$A + H$_2$A
1	57.9	28.2	−7.2	2.4
2	24.7	12.1	2.1	13.0
3	15.9	3.4	4.3	
4	45.6	7.9	12.2	6.3
5	34.0	11.1	1.1	−8.4
6	38.1	10.1	7.3	−2.9
7	36.6	3.2	23.3	4.2
Mean ± SE	36.1 ± 5.1	10.9 ± 3.2	6.2 ± 3.6	2.4 ± 3.0

[a] Δ Diameter = % above control; control = diameter of norepinephrine-constricted arteriole (or resting arteriole in rat corpus studies); H = histamine; H$_1$A = H$_1$-receptor antagonist, mepyramine; H$_2$A = H$_2$-receptor antagonist, metiamide.

antagonist alone also markedly inhibited the histamine effect, the average diameter being 10.8 ± 3.2% above control. The two antagonists together also completely inhibited the effect of histamine. The more marked effect of the H$_1$ and H$_2$ antagonists alone, seen in the rat study, might be due to the smaller histamine effect seen in the rat without norepinephrine constriction (36.1% dilatation) than in a cat with norepinephrine constriction (72.8% dilatation).

Antrum

Results of microcirculatory studies in 6 cats are presented in Table III. The arterioles studied averaged 54.6 ± 7.8 μm in diameter. Histamine produced arteriolar dilatation in all animals 46.3 ± 11.8% above control). The H$_1$ antagonist partially inhibited this response in all animals, the dilatation now averaging only 17.3 ± 10.6% above control. The H$_2$ antagonist alone had no effect on the histamine response in any cat, but when it was administered with the H$_1$ antagonist, there was complete inhibition of the histamine effect.

Results obtained in the rat are presented in Table IV. The arterioles studies averaged 32.7 ± 2 μm in diameter. Histamine produced arteriolar dilatation in all 7 rats studied, 48.1 ± 11.4% above control. The H$_1$ antagonist markedly inhibited this response, dilatation now averaging 12.7 ± 10.1% above control. The H$_2$ antagonist alone had no effect, and when administered with the H$_1$ antagonist it did not significantly increase the inhibition obtained with the H$_1$ antagonist alone.

Table III

Percent Increase in Cat Antrum Submucosal Arteriolar Diameter in
Response to Histamine and the Histamine Antagonists[a]

	Δ Diameter (%)			
Cat No.	H	H + H_1A	H + H_2A	H + H_1A + H_2A
8	78.0	48.1	104	33.0
9	85.9	49.3	81.4	−19.0
10	30.4	10.6	26.7	−26.4
11	12.9	−16.2	21.1	−26.0
12	34.0	4.8	35.7	−3.0
13	37.0	7.1	50.8	−26.4
Mean ± SE	46.3±11.8	17.3 ± 10.6	53.3 ± 13.4	−11.3 ± 9.6

[a]Δ Diameter = % above control; control = diameter of norepinephrine-constricted arteriole (or resting arteriole in rat corpus studies); H = histamine; H_1A = H_1-receptor antagonist, mepyramine; H_2A = H_2-receptor antagonist, metiamide.

Specificity of the Histamine Antagonists

The effect of the histamine antagonists on papaverine induced dilatation of corpus submucosal arterioles was studied in 5 cats. Results are presented in Table V. Papaverine produced a 45.2 ± 7.5% dilatation of the norepinephrine-constricted arterioles. The H_1 and H_2 antagonists, separately or together, had

Table IV

Percent Increase in Rat Antrum Submucosal Arteriolar Diameter in
Response to Histamine and the Histamine Antagonists[a]

	Δ Diameter (%)			
Rat No.	H	H + H_1A	H + H_2A	H + H_1A + H_2A
8	78.8	38.6	80.0	13.3
9	12.6	−28.4	16.5	−12.8
10	15.4	7.7	18.1	2.2
11	44.5		34.3	4.9
12	34.1	13.8	32.8	10.3
13	61.5	37.6	63.3	15.7
14	90.1	7.0	86.1	18.4
Mean ± SE	48.1±11.4	12.7 ± 10.1	47.3 ± 10.9	7.4 ± 4.0

[a]Δ Diameter = % above control; control = diameter of norepinephrine-constricted arteriole (or resting arteriole in rat corpus studies); H = histamine; H_1A = H_1-receptor antagonist, mepyramine; H_2A = H_2-receptor antagonist, metiamide.

Table V
Specificity of the Histamine Antagonists; Percent Increase in Cat
Corpus Submucosal Arterioles in Response to Papaverine (P) and the
Histamine Antagonists[a]

Cat No.	Δ Diameter (%)			
	P	P + H_1A	P + H_2A	P + H_1A + H_2A
14	61.0	44.0	64.1	54.8
15	47.1	29.7	36.3	33.6
16	23.7	58.0	26.1	27.3
17	61.3	84.0	76.1	106.6
18	32.8	30.4	38.2	39.5
Mean $\pm$ SE	45.2 $\pm$ 7.5	49.2 $\pm$ 10.1	48.2 $\pm$ 9.4	52.4 $\pm$ 14.3

[a]Δ Diameter = % above control; control = diameter of norepinephrine-constricted arteriole (or resting arteriole in rat corpus studies); H = histamine; H_1A = H_1-receptor antagonist, mepyramine; H_2A = H_2-receptor antagonist, metiamide.

no effect on the papaverine induced dilatation. This finding is consistent with mepyramine and metiamide being specific histamine antagonists.

DISCUSSION

The results of the present investigation indicate a distinct difference in the behavior of histamine receptors on the submucosal arterioles of the antrum and corpus. In both regions the H_1 and H_2 receptors subserve vasodilatation. However, in the antrum the receptors behave in a fashion similar to that found in the small intestine submucosal arterioles (Guth and Smith, 1976). The H_1 receptor antagonist partially inhibited histamine dilatation and the effect of the H_2 antagonist could not be demonstrated unless the H_1 receptor was blocked. This was clear in the cat antrum but not in the rat antrum studies, where, because of the marked H_1 antagonist effect, an H_2 effect was not demonstrable. The predominance of H_1 receptors when both receptors subserve vasodilation has also been found in skeletal muscle and the general circulation when the depressor effect of histamine was studied. (Powell and Brody, 1973, 1976; Parsons and Owen, 1973). In the corpus, on the other hand, independent H_1 and H_2 receptor effects subserved vasodilation. In the cat studies, these effects were additive. In the rat studies, the inhibition by either antagonist was so marked that interpretation of the effect of the two antagonists administered together was difficult.

The corpus and antrum perform different functions. The secretion of acid is a major function of the corpus where histamine is an important stimulant of acid secretion. H_2 receptors on the parietal cell are responsible for this function of histamine. While an increase in mucosal blood flow will not stimulate acid secretion, an increase in flow is essential to meet the increased metabolic needs of the actively secreting parietal cell and conversely, marked inhibition of mucosal blood flow will diminish acid secretion (Jacobson *et al.*, 1966). Direct histamine effect on submucosal arterioles therefore might be expected. It is of interest that H_1 and H_2 receptors independently subserving vasodilation were demonstrated on these arterioles.

Since all stimuli of acid secretion increase mucosal blood flow (probably via vasoactive catabolites from the parietal cell), it is difficult to separate gastric secretory and primary blood flow effects using standard flow measurement techniques. For example, Jacobson and Chang (1969) found that both histamine and gastrin increased gastric mucosal blood flow, as determined by aminopyrine clearance, in the dog. However, the ratio of gastric mucosal blood flow to acid secretory rate was greater for histamine than for gastrin. This suggested, but did not prove, that the increased flow due to histamine represented both a direct pharmacological vasodilating effect and an indirect metabolic effect secondary to secretion. In previous studies we have shown that the gastric submucosal arterioles are the major resistance vessels regulating blood flow to the gastric mucosa (Guth, and Smith, 1975); when they constrict, mucosal flow decreases, when they dilate, flow increases. Thus, the effect of histamine on H_2 receptors on the parietal cell, to increase acid secretion, would simultaneously call forth an increase in blood flow to these cells via the dilating effect of H_2, as well as H_1, receptors on the corpus submucosal arterioles.

SUMMARY

The types and functions of histamine receptors in the submucosal arterioles of the corpus and antrum of the cat and rat stomach were studied using an *in vivo* microscopy technique. Change in arteriolar diameter in response to superfusion of histamine with and without antagonists was measured by an image-splitting technic. H_1- and H_2-histamine receptors subserving vasodilatation were demonstrated in both the antral and corpus submucosal arterioles of the cat and rat. However the H_1 effect was predominant in the antrum (the H_2 antagonist inhibited histamine dilatation only in the presence of the H_1 antagonist) while H_1 and H_2 effects were approximately equal and independent in the corpus.

ACKNOWLEDGMENTS

This work was supported by NIAMDD Grant 17328 to CURE (Center for Ulcer Research and Education) and V.A. Medical Research Funds.

The metiamide used in this study was kindly supplied by Mr. J. G. Paul of the Smith, Kline & French Laboratories, Philadelphia.

REFERENCES

Archibald, L.H., Moody, F.G., and Simons, M. (1974). Effect of isoproterenol on canine gastric acid secretion and blood flow. *Surg. Forum* **25**, 409.

Ash, A.S.F., and Schild, H.O. (1966). Receptors mediating some actions of histamine. *Br. J. Pharmacol.* **27**, 427-439.

Baez, S. (1966). Recording of microvascular dimensions with an image-splitter television microscope. *J. Appl. Physiol.* **21**, 299-301.

Barlow, T.E., Bently, F.H., and Walder, D.N. (1951). Arteries, veins,and arteriovenous anastomoses in the human stomach. *Surg. Gyne. and Obst.* **93**, 657-671.

Black, J.W., Duncan, W.A.M., Durant, C.V., Ganellin, C.L., and Parsons, M.E. (1972). Definition and antagonism of histamine H_2-receptors. *Nature (London)* **236**, 385-390.

Delaney, J.P., and Grim, E. (1964). Canine gastric blood flow and its distribution. *Am. J. Physiol.* **207**, 1195-1202.

Glover, W.E., Carroll, P.R., and Latt, N. (1973). Histamine receptors in human temporal and rabbit ear arteries, in "International Symposium on Histamine H_2-Receptor Antagonists" (C.J. Wood and M.A. Simkins, eds.), pp. 169-174. Smith, Kline and French Laboratories Ltd., London.

Guth, P.H., and Rosenberg, A. (1972). *In vivo* microscopy of the gastric microcirculation. *Am. J. Dig. Dis.* **17**, 391-398.

Guth, P.H., and Smith, E. (1975a). Escape from vasoconstriction in the gastric microcirculation. *Am. J. Physiol.* **228**, 1893-1895.

Guth, P.H., and Smith, E. (1975b). Neural control of gastric mucosal blood flow in the rat. *Gastroenterology* **69**, 935-940.

Guth, P.H., and Smith, E. (1976a). H_1 and H_2 receptors in the cat mesenteric circulation. *Microvasc. Res.* **11**, 119.

Guth, P.H., and Smith E. (1976b). The effect of gastrointestinal hormones on the gastric microcirculation. *Gastroenterology* **71**, 435-438.

Jacobson, E.D., and Chang, A.C.K. (1969). Comparison of gastrin and histamine on gastric mucosal blood flow. *Proc. Soc. Exp. Biol. Med.* **130**, 484-486.

Jacobson, E.D., Linford, R.H., and Grossman, M.I. (1966). Gastric secretion in relation to mucosal blood flow studied by a clearance technique. *J. Clin. Invest.* **45**, 1-13.

Parsons, M.E., and Owen, D.A.A. (1973). Receptors involved in the cardiovascular responses to histamine, in "International Symposium on Histamine H_2-Receptor Atagonists"(C.J. Wood and M.A. Simkins, eds.), pp. 127-135. Smith, Kline and French Laboratories Ltd., London.

Powell, J.R., and Brody, M.J. (1973). Identification of two vascular histamine receptors in the dog, in "International Symposium on Histamine H_2-Receptor Antagonists"(C.J. Wood and M.A. Simkins, eds.), pp. 137-146. Smith, Kline & French Laboratories Ltd., London.

Powell, J.R., and Brody, M.J. (1976). Identification and specific blockade of two receptors for histamine in the cardiovascular system. *J. Pharmacol. Exper. Ther.* **196**, 1-14.

Shoemaker, C.P., Jr., and Powers, S.R., Jr. (1966). The absence of large functional arteriovenous shunts in the stomach of the anesthetized dog. *Surgery* **60**, 118-126.

Walder, D.N. (1952). Arteriovenous anastomoses of the human stomach. *Clin. Sci.* **11**, 59-71.

10

Characteristics of H_1 and H_2 Histamine Receptors Which Mediate the Chronotropic Response of Rabbit Atrial Muscle

M. J. Hughes and Ralph Lydic
Texas Tech University
School of Medicine
Department of Physiology
Lubbock, Texas

INTRODUCTION

The advent of two compounds, burimamide and metiamide, capable of blocking histamine's H_2 receptors (Black *et al.*, 1972, 1973) and evidence that promethazine, an H_1 blocker, is capable of inhibiting cardiac chronotropic activity in rabbit atria (Hughes and Coret 1972, 1974) have resulted in a number of reports concerning the nature of the cardiac receptor as well as H_2 receptor activity in other areas. Most of the research has been done using guinea pig cardiac tissue with a number of different experimental techniques.

McNeill and Verma (1974a) using a guinea pig Langendorff preparation reported that promethazine blocked the inotropic and chronotropic response and the elevation of cardiac cAMP, which resulted from histamine stimulation. Levi and Kuye (1974) also using a Langendorff guinea pig preparation tested a series of H_1 antihistaminics including promethazine. They reported that the chronotropic and inotropic responses were mediated by H_2 receptors while the atrioventricular node and coronary vessels contained H_1 receptors. Ercan *et al.*, (1974) using a similar guinea pig preparation reported that coronary dilation and increase in force and rate initiated by histamine could be blocked by metiamide. Reinhardt *et al.*, (1974) studied isolated guinea pig right and left atrial preparations and reported that burimamide blocked chronotropic activity and promethazine blocked the inotropic response to histamine. Ledda *et al.*, (1974) and Moroni *et al.*, (1974) reported that histamine had a greater inotropic effect on guinea pig ventricular muscle strips than norepinephrine and that this response could be blocked with burimamide and metiamide. Steinberg and Holland (1975) using spontaneously beating right and driven left guinea pig atria reported that the chronotropic response was mediated by H_2 receptors while the atrial inotropic response was the result of H_2 receptor stimulation. Levi et al., (1975a, b, 1976) using specific H_1 and H_2 agonists as well as antagonists reaffirmed their earlier conclusions in very careful and well planned studies and made the distinction between the ventricular (H_2) and atrial (H_1) inotropic response. Reinhardt et al., (1976), in general, confirmed the findings of Levi's group.

It would thus appear that the predominant receptor type responsible for each of the various histamine activities in guinea pigs has been worked out. There has been very little recent attention given to the character of the cardiac receptors of other species, with some exceptions. Powell and Brody (1976) did an extensive study of the action of histamine in the cardiovascular system of the dog. They concluded that histamine stimulation of the dog heart rate was mediated by the activation of H_1 receptors and that H_2 receptors were responsible for a negative inotropic response. Broadley (1975) reported results obtained with Langendorff guinea pig and rabbit preparations and concluded that the coronary receptors are of the H_1 type since both the excitatory and inhibitory responses to histamine could be blocked by mepyramine. In the spontaneous beating rabbit atrial preparation, promethazine causes a noncompetitive and long-lasting blockade of the chronotropic response to histamine (Hughes and Coret, 1972). Hughes and Coret (1974) using the same preparation reported that a number of other tricyclic compounds could also block histamine stimulation of rabbit atrial rate. Hughes and Coret (1975) studied the effects of burimamide which appears to be a competitive inhibitor at relatively low concentrations and to become noncompetitive at higher dose levels.

The behavior of rabbit atria in response to histamine and its antagonists appears to be different than that found for guinea pig atria. Therefore, more extensive studies of these receptors seems warranted.

METHODS

Ninety rabbits (average wt. 1.2 Kg) and forty-six guinea pigs (average wt. 0.5 Kg) unselected as to sex were killed by cervical fracture. The chest was opened along the midline and the whole heart removed and immersed in Tryode's solution which was gassed with 95% O_2/5% CO_2. The atrial pairs were dissected free of all extraneous tissue and a thread passed through the tip of each auricular apex.

The atria were mounted in a 50 ml tissue bath with one atrium tied to a glass hook and the other to a Statham strain gauge. The passive control tension was 0.43 (±0.02) gm for rabbit atria and 0.41 (±0.02) gm for guinea pig atria. The tissues were allowed to equilibrate for 60–90 minutes before experimental procedures were begun. Signals from the transducers (Model UL5 and G10B) were recorded on Beckman Biomedical Dynograph-411 recorders.

Drugs were injected into the tissue bath through a fine caliber, polyethylene tube which extended to the base of the bath. The gas mixture was bubbled into the tissue chamber through a sintered glass base and served as a source of oxygenation, regulation of pH, and rapid mixing of the injected drug solutions with the bathing medium. Drugs were injected in a total volume of 0.5 ml or less, followed immediately by the injection of air to clear the drug from the tubing.

Tissue baths were immersed in a large volume thermostated water bath, which maintained the temperature at 36°C±0.1°C. The bathing solution in the tissue chambers could be changed rapidly by a continuous flow from a 6 liter reservoir. The bathing medium was gravity-fed through glass coils (also in the thermostated bath) into the base of the tissue baths and the chamber volume kept constant by suction applied to the side-arm at the 50 ml level. Flow was stopped during the drug response period by clamping the reservoir tubing. At the end of a drug response period the baths were completely emptied three times by suction and refilled; retesting did not begin until the atrial rate had returned to the control values.

The Tyrode's solution had the following composition in mM/liter: Na^+ 145, K^+ 5.5, Mg^{2+} 2.1, Ca^{2+} 1.6, Cl^- 133.0, HCO_2^- 25.0 and glucose 10.0. The pH was 7.42±0.01. Drugs were dissolved in deionized water. The concentrations obtained after injection into the bath are specified in the section on results.

The drugs used (and their sources) are: histamine diphosphate (Sigma Chemical Co.), metiamide (a generous gift of Dr. J. W. Black of Smith, Kline and French), diphenhydramine HCl (a generous gift of Dr. A. M. Moore of Parke Davis and Co.), 3-(2-aminoethyl) 1,2,4 triazole 2 HCl (Eli Lilly and Co.), and 3-(2-aminoethyl) pyrazole 2 HCl (Eli Lilly and Co.).

Statistical calculations were done on a Hewlett–Packard Calculator Series 9800A, Model 20.

RESULTS

A series of experiments were done to ascertain the time course of inhibition by metiamide of that dose of histamine (4.5×10^{-6} M), which normally caused approximately a half-maximum increase in rate of rabbit atrial pairs (Coret and Hughes, 1974).

Three concentrations of metiamide were used (Fig. 1) and data were normalized for purposes of comparison in this way: the remaining increase in rate above control at each time interval was divided by the initial steady-state increase in rate to histamine alone. In all cases there was a rapid decrease in rate with a half time of approximately 5 minutes.

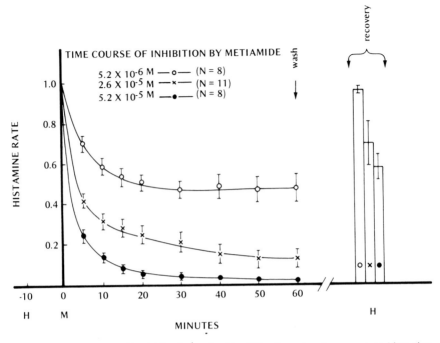

FIG. 1.   Time course of inhibition by metiamide of the chronotropic response to histamine. Histamine (H) (4.5 × 10^{-6} M), 10 minutes (at steady-state frequency) before metiamide was added to the bath. Metiamide (M) (5.2, 26, or 52 × 10^{-6} M) administered at zero time, using 27 atria. Data were normalized for comparison and each atrial pair acted as its own control. Tissues were washed, allowed to recover (> 30 minutes), and histamine repeated. Vertical axis = increase in rate to histamine (beats/minute), 1.0 for control response with decreasing frequency after metiamide as some portion of that response. Horizontal axis = time in minutes. Vertical lines = S.E.M.

The effect of metiamide (5.2 × 10^{-6} M), (the lowest dose tested) appeared to reach a maximum in approximately 30 minutes after which time a steady-state inhibition of slightly greater than 50% was maintained. At the two higher concentrations of the H_2 blocker, even after 30 minutes, there was a continued slow decline in rate. After 60 minutes, in the presence of 5.2 × 10^{-5} M (the highest dose used), inhibition of the histamine activity was virtually complete. The tissues were washed and after a recovery period retested with the same concentration of histamine to judge the reversibility of the blockade. Atrial pairs which had been treated with 5.2 × 10^{-6} M metiamide evidenced almost complete recovery (97%) after only one wash while those atria which had been treated with 5.2 × 10^{-5} M metiamide still exhibited more than a 40% inhibition after washing. The inhibitor was allowed to remain in the bath for 60 minutes before washout in all of the experiments and thus the only variable was the concentration of metiamide.

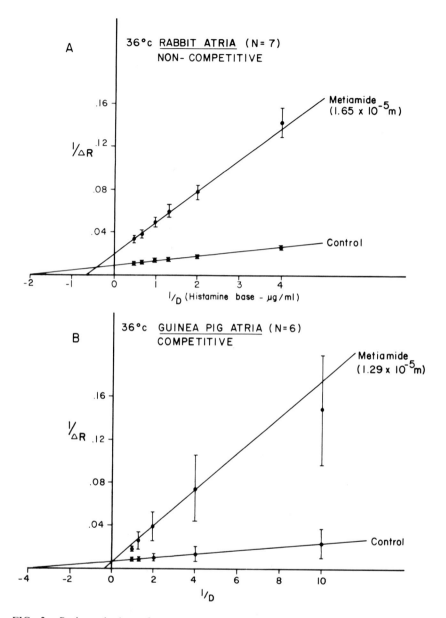

FIG. 2. Reciprocal plots of control histamine and metiamide inhibited dose response chronotropic activity (36° C). (A) Rabbit atria. (B) guinea pig atria. Vertical axis= 1/R, reciprocal of increase in rate (beats/minute). Horizontal axis=1/D, reciprocal of dose. Histamine base doses: rabbit 0.25 to 2.0 µg/ml and guinea pig 0.1 to 1.0 µg/ml of bathing solution. Vertical lines= S.E.M. (See Table I for data)

A series of experiments was then performed using rabbit atrial pairs. Atria were tested with a series of increasing histamine concentrations given at 10-minute intervals. Tissues were washed and allowed to recover; metiamide was introduced into the bath and after 30 minutes the same histamine doses were repeated. Reciprocal plots of data showed that the concentration of histamine which was necessary to cause a half-maximum increase in rate (the point at which the line intercepts the $1/D$ axis) increased after metiamide while the calculated theoretical maximum increase in rate ($1/\triangle R$ intercept) declined (Fig. 2A and Table I). Metiamide has been reported to be a competitive inhibitor of guinea pig atrial H_2 receptors, (Black *et al.*, 1973), but this did not appear to be the case for rabbit atria. Therefore, we set up experiments using guinea pig atria to compare with the rabbit data. Reciprocal plots of metiamide inhibition appeared to be competitive when guinea pig atria were used (Fig. 2B and Table I). A calculated K_1 of metiamide ($0.92 \times 10^{-6}M$ and $1.78 \times 10^{-6}M$) for the two concentrations used approximated the range of 7.4–11.5×10^{-7} M reported by others (Black *et al.*, 1973).

Experiments using two histamine analogs, 3-(2-aminoethyl) 1,2,4 triazole, reported to be intermediate in its action on H_2 receptors between 2- and 4-methyl-histamine (Black *et al.*, 1972), and 3-(2-aminoethyl) pyrazole, which is not considered to be an effective agonist at H_1 receptors, were performed with rabbit atria. The response to these compounds was very different (Table I and Fig. 3).

The dose necessary to cause a half-maximum increase in rate ($1/2$ max dose) for histamine was $4.9 \times 10^{-6}M$, for triazole $1.3 \times 10^{-4}M$, and for pyrazole $1.4 \times 10^{-3}M$, which gives ratios of $\simeq 1:27:286$ with respect to histamine. This strongly suggests that the rabbit atrial chronotropic receptors must be of both the H_1 and H_2 type. Therefore, guinea pig atrial pairs were tested to determine whether this behavior was common to atria from both kinds of animals. The results obtained in guinea pig experiments were $1.6 \times 10^{-6}M$ for histamine, $7.2 \times 10^{-6}M$ for triazole and $6.1 \times 10^{-6}M$ for pyrazole with ratios of $\simeq 1:4:4$, suggesting a much more homogenous postulation of receptors, primarily of the H_2 type. The ratio of rabbit/guinea pig (R/G) receptor activity ($1/D$ max dose) is $3:18:230$ and calculated maximum increase in rate (max rate) was less for rabbit atria with all three agonists.

Rabbit and guinea pig atrial pairs were both tested with these agonists and metiamide as the antagonist (Table III). The concentration of metiamide that had been effective in achieving a partial blockade in the rabbit atria proved to completely block the chronotropic response to lower concentrations of histamine in guinea pig atria; therefore it was necessary to reduce the amount of inhibitor administered to be able to obtain a satisfactory dose response curve. The $-1/D$ intercept ratio (I/C) for histamine is altered approximately eight fold by $5.2 \times 10^{-5}M$ metiamide when rabbit atria are used, while the same change in $-1/D$ for guinea pig atria is obtained using $6.6 \times 10^{-6}M$ metiamide($\simeq 12\%$ the concentration of the H_2 antagonist; Table I).

Table I
Histamine and Antagonists (36°C)

Molar conc	N	Control histamine responses		After metiamide/diphenhydramine			
		1/2 max dose (molar conc)[b]	max rate (beats/min)[b]	1/2 max dose (molar conc)[b]	I/C[a]	max rate (beats/min)[b]	I/C[a]
				A Rabbit			
Metiamide							
5.2×10^{-6}	5	$3.3(\pm 0.3) \times 10^{-6}$	$138(\pm 10)$	$1.7(\pm 0.3) \times 10^{-5}$	5.2	$109(\pm 9)$	0.79
2.5×10^{-5}	5	$4.8(\pm 1.0) \times 10^{-6}$	$137(\pm 21)$	$3.6(\pm 1.0) \times 10^{-5}$	7.5	$68(\pm 17)$	0.79
5.2×10^{-5}	5	$5.6(\pm 1.1) \times 10^{-6}$	$126(\pm 7)$	$4.5(\pm 1.5) \times 10^{-5}$	8.0	$51(\pm 10)$	0.44
				B Guinea Pig			
Metiamide							
6.6×10^{-6}	5	$1.4(\pm 0.3) \times 10^{-6}$	$179(\pm 10)$	$1.1(\pm 0.4) \times 10^{-5}$	7.9	$175(\pm 9)$	1.00
1.3×10^{-5}	6	$2.3(\pm 0.3) \times 10^{-6}$	$172(\pm 15)$	$1.9(\pm 0.5) \times 10^{-5}$	8.3	$175(\pm 21)$	1.00
				C Guinea Pig			
Diphenhydramine							
6.9×10^{-6}	6	$1.4(\pm 0.1) \times 10^{-6}$	$152(\pm 7)$	$2.3(\pm 0.4) \times 10^{-6}$	1.6	$133(\pm 11)$	0.88

[a]Inhibition data divided by control data.
[b]Parenthetical numbers = S.E.M.

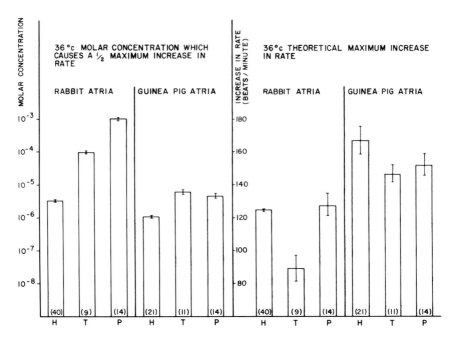

FIG. 3.   A comparison of rabbit and guinea pig atrial chronotropic response to histamine and other agonists (36° C). Vertical axis= molar concentration of the agonists which will cause a 1/2 maximum increase in rate (-1/D) and the theoretical maximum increase in rate (beats/minute) at an infinite concentration of the agonist (see Table II for detail). Horizontal axis= H_1 histamine, 4-(2-aminoethyl) imidazole; T_1 triazole, 3-(2-aminoethyl) triazole; P_1 pyrazole, 3-(2-aminoethyl) pyrazole. Vertical lines= S.E.M. Numbers in parenthesis=number of determinations.

This also proved to be true when triazole and pyrazole were used as the agonists. In rabbit atria tested with triazole, metiamide (2×10^{-5} M) caused a four-fold shift in the -1/D intercept while 17% of that concentration of metiamide (3.3×10^{-6} M) used with guinea pig atria caused a two-fold change (Table II).

When pyrazole was used as the agonist with guinea pig atria, metiamide was more (1.5 times) effective in changing the -1/D intercept as a larger dose (approximately four-fold) tested with rabbit atria (Table III).

These results suggested the possibility of a spectrum of receptor sites in rabbit atria, and to a much lesser extent in guinea pig atria as well. If both H_1 and H_2 receptors are responible for the stimulation of the chronotropic response of rabbit atria, there may also be some less specific intermediate types of receptors present, which could be affected in various degrees by both H_1 and H_2 agonist and antagonist. There have been reports (Kenakin *et al.*, 1974, Cook *et al.*, 1975) that the metabolic state of the ileum determines whether the histamine receptors appear to be of the H_1 or H_2 type. This is

Table II

Control Dose Response Curve Data (36°C)

Drug	Rabbit			Guinea pig				
	N	1/2 max dose (molar conc)[b]	max rate (beats/min)[b]	N	1/2 max dose (molar conc)[b]	R/G[a]	max rate (beats/min)[b]	R/G[a]
Histamine	40	$4.9(\pm0.1)\times10^{-6}$	125($\pm$3)	21	$1.6(\pm0.2)\times10^{-6}$	3	167($\pm$8)	0.75
Triazole	9	$1.3(\pm0.1)\times10^{-4}$	89($\pm$8)	11	$7.2(\pm0.6)\times10^{-6}$	18	147($\pm$5)	0.61
Pyrazole	14	$1.4(\pm0.1)\times10^{-3}$	128($\pm$7)	14	$6.1(\pm0.7)\times10^{-6}$	230	152($\pm$7)	0.84
Spontaneous rate before drug	63		126($\pm$4)	46			167($\pm$8)	

[a]Rabbit data divided by guinea pig data.
[b]Parenthetical numbers = S.E.M.

Table III
3-(2-Aminoethyl) 1,2,4 Triazole and 3-(2-Aminoethyl) Pyrazole with Metiamide (36° C)

Metiamide (molar conc)	N	Control response		After metiamide			
		1/2 max dose (molar conc)[b]	max rate (beats/min)[b]	1/2 max dose (molar conc)[b]	1/C[a]	max rate (beats/min)[b]	1/C[a]
				Rabbit			
		triazole			triazole		
2.6×10^{-5}	5	$1.1(\pm 0.1) \times 10^{-4}$	$103(\pm 10)$	$4.1(\pm 0.2) \times 10^{-4}$	3.7	$36(\pm 6)$	0.36
		pyrazole			pyrazole		
6.6×10^{-6}	7	$1.3(\pm 0.1) \times 10^{-3}$	$132(\pm 5)$	$2.3(\pm 0.4) \times 10^{-3}$	1.8	$76(\pm 7)$	0.58
				Guinea Pig			
		triazole			triazole		
3.3×10^{-6}	5	$6.5(\pm 0.6) \times 10^{-6}$	$157(\pm 6)$	$1.1(\pm 0.1) \times 10^{-5}$	1.7	$89(\pm 15)$	0.57
		pyrazole			pyrazole		
1.6×10^{-6}	4	$6.0(\pm 0.7) \times 10^{-6}$	$154(\pm 7)$	$1.8(\pm 0.2) \times 10^{-5}$	3.0	$154(\pm 11)$	1.00

[a] Inhibition data divided by control data.
[b] Parenthetical numbers = S.E.M.

analogous to the evidence of the interconversion of α- and β-receptors in response to temperature changes which can alter the metabolic state of the tissue. To test the possibility that the relative proportion of H_1 and H_2 receptors may be altered, a series of histamine dose response curves were done with rabbit atria at 26°, 36°, and 40°C. The temperature range that can be used for spontaneous beating atria is severely limited. This type of isolated preparation is adversely affected by high temperatures for prolonged periods of time (these experiments take at least 6 hours), and rabbit atria tend to become irregular at temperatures below 26°C. We retested some H_1 blocking agents and found that diphenhydramine (6.9×10^{-6} M; a concentration which did not decrease the spontaneous rate of rabbit atrial tissue) would cause an appreciable blockade of the histamine response.

Metiamide (1.6×10^{-5} M) and diphenhydramine (6.9×10^{-6} M) were used throughout this series of experiments (Table IV). When the ratio of inhibited to control (I/C) for -1/D intercept was calculated at the three temperatures there was a progressive decrease in degree of inhibition (3.4, 2.9, 2.0)with metiamide. However, at increasingly higher temperatures there   was a progressive increase in inhibition with diphenhydramine (1.6, 1.8, 2.6). This is graphically illustrated in Fig. 4, calculated in a different manner. The results shown in the graph were obtained by dividing the response at each dose for each atrial pair in the presence of the inhibition by its own control response ($\triangle RI/\triangle RC$). Although there is a slight decrease in the metiamide inhibition at 40°C compared to 26°C it does not appear to be statistically significant. However, the increased inhibition which occurs in the presence of diphenhydramine at 40°C does appear to be significantly different from that obtained at 26°C.

A final bit of evidence is included which involved using diphenhydramine (6.9×10^{-6} M) as the blocking agent with guinea pig atria (Table I). There is some inhibition (I/C ratio = -1.6) with diphenhydramine but it is a much smaller shift of -1/D intercept than seen with metiamide (I/C ratio = 8.0) at approximately the same molar concentration of the two inhibitors. Figure 5 shows this data calculated in the same manner for the guinea pig atria as was done with the data from rabbit atria in Fig. 4.

DISCUSSION

The population of histamine receptors responsible for the chronotropic response of rabbit atrial muscle appears to have different characteristics than those found in guinea pig atrial muscle. Previous reports from this laboratory have implicated both H_1 histamine (Hughes and Coret, 1972, 1974) and H_2 histamine (Hughes and Coret, 1975) antagonists in blockade of the chronotropic response to histamine. The blocking action of metiamide is not

Table IV

Rabbit Atria Response to Histamine at 26°, 36°, and 40° C

Temp	N	1/2 max dose (molar conc)[b]	max rate (beats/min)[b]	1/2 max dose (molar conc)[b]	I/C[a]	max rate (beats/min)[b]	I/C[a]
		Control response		After Metiamide (1.6×10^{-5} M)			
26°C	7	$4.1(\pm0.6)\times10^{-6}$	75(±2)	$1.4(\pm0.2)\times10^{-5}$	3.4	34(±6)	0.45
36°C	8	$5.0(\pm0.6)\times10^{-6}$	132(±9)	$1.4(\pm0.1)\times10^{-5}$	2.9	54(±6)	0.41
40°C	8	$4.9(\pm0.3)\times10^{-6}$	145(±10)	$1.0(\pm0.1)\times10^{-5}$	2.0	70(±6)	0.48
		Control response		After diphenhydramine (6.9×10^{-6} M)			
26°C	6	$4.4(\pm0.7)\times10^{-6}$	62(±9)	$7.1(\pm1.4)\times10^{-6}$	1.6	39(±5)	0.63
36°C	5	$4.1(\pm0.8)\times10^{-6}$	151(±7)	$7.5(\pm1.3)\times10^{-6}$	1.8	115(±9)	0.76
40°C	6	$5.3(\pm0.3)\times10^{-6}$	135(±15)	$1.4(\pm0.3)\times10^{-5}$	2.6	68(±10)	0.50
		Spontaneous rate before drugs					
26°C	40		73(±2)				
36°C	40		126(±4)				
40°C	35		153(±4)				

[a] Inhibition data divided by control data.
[b] Parenthetical numbers = S.E.M.

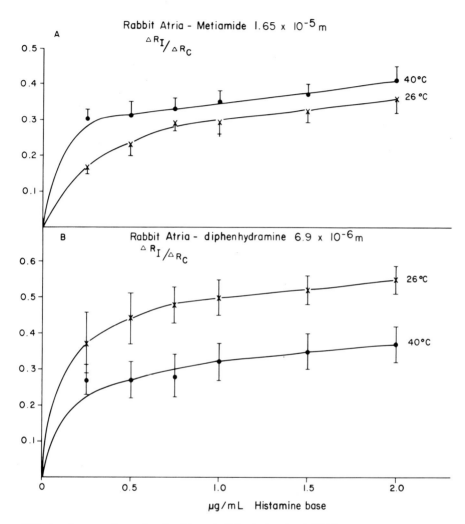

FIG. 4. A comparison of metiamide and diphenhydramine inhibition of the rabbit atrial chronotropic response to histamine at 26° *and 40°*C. (A) $\triangle R_I/\triangle R_C$, the ratio of the increase in rate (beats/minute) above control in the presence of metiamide (1.6×10^{-5} *M*), to the increase in rate above control to histamine alone. o – o 40°C, x – x 26°C. (B) Same as above with diphenhydramine (6.9×10^{-6} *M*) as the antagonist (see Table IV for data). Vertical axis=ratio of $\triangle R_I/\triangle R_C$. Horizontal axis=$\mu$g/ml histamine base. Vertical lines=S.E.M.

competitive with histamine when rabbit atria is the test object. Therefore, we decided to test guinea pig atria under exactly the same conditions, and we have found that the metiamide blockade in guinea pig atria was competitive (Fig. 2 and Table I) as reported by others. We then tested several histamine analogs for their respective effects on the atrial pairs from both species. There was a very large difference in the response of rabbit and guinea pig atria to these three agonists: histamine, 3-(2-aminoethyl) triazole, and 3-(2-amino-ethyl) pyrazole, with respect to the dose needed to cause a half maximum increase in rate and the theoretical maximum increase in rate (see R/G ratio; Table II and Fig. 3). It should be pointed out at this time that in no case did metiamide or diphenhydramine appear to be a competitive inhibitor when used with rabbit atria, but in the case of the guinea pig atria metiamide did appear to competitively inhibit both the histamine and pyrazole response. The results suggest that the activity with the guinea pig atria is primarily, if not completely, due to an activation of H_2 receptor sites. The responses which occur with rabbit atria suggest that only part of the receptor sites responsible for the chronotropic response are of the H_2 type.

McNeill and Verma (1974) using the guinea pig Langendorff preparation reported that very large doses of histamine, 3-(2-aminoethyl)-1,2,4 triazole and 3-(2-aminoethyl) pyrazole all stimulated both inotropic activity and the tissue levels of cAMP. They reported this activity was not blocked by tripelennamine or diphenhydramine. A later paper (McNeill and Verma 1974b) concerning much the same kind of experimentation but using burimamide as the antagonist reported that this H_2 blocker was effective in preventing these responses.

Our results suggested that part of the population of rabbit chronotropic receptors were probably of the H_1 type since there is a very large difference between the dose of histamine required to cause a half maximum response and that needed for 3-(2-aminoethyl) pyrazole (1:286). We then retested various H_1 blocking agents. Diphenhydramine, in a dose that did not depress spontaneous activity, caused some noncompetitive inhibition of the rabbit response (Table IV and Fig. 4) and to a lesser extent the guinea pig atria (Table I and Fig. 5). We feel our evidence strongly suggests that at least rabbit atrial muscle has both H_1 and H_2 receptors which are responsible for the chronotropic response.

Kenakin et al., (1974) and Cook et al., (1975) reported an interconversion of H_1 and H_2 receptors for guinea pig ileum.

It is possible, if rabbit atria have both types of receptors present, an interconversion of the H_1 and H_2 receptors could occur. It is also possible that histamine receptors in this tissue can interact with both H_1 and H_2 blocking agents in varying degrees while some receptors might be more specific for a particular type of antihistamine and others might respond to a spectrum of blocking compounds. A third possibility is that the rabbit cardiac pacemaker

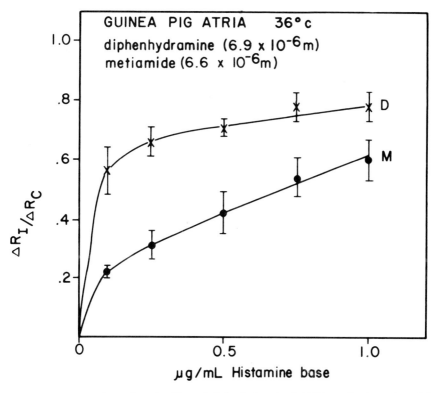

FIG. 5. A comparison of metiamide and diphenhydramine inhibition of guinea pig atrial chronotropic response to histamine at 36° C. Calculation same as Fig. 4 (see Table I for data). x – x D (diphenhydramine 6.9 × 10^{-6} M); o – o M (metiamide 6.6 × 10^{-6} M). Vertical axis=ratio of $\Delta R_I/\Delta R_C$. Horizontal axis=μg/ml of histamine base. Vertical lines=S.E.M.

has specific receptors of both types but contains a relatively larger number of one type than the other.

The first possibility was tested by a series of experiments at various temperatures and using both H_1 and H_2 antagonists. The parameters measured in the presence of metiamide do not appear to change significantly although there was a slight decrease in blockade at 40° C. However, there does seem to be a much greater inhibition of the histamine response in the presence of diphenhydramine at 40° C. This data is certainly not conclusive but could be interpreted as suggesting an increased sensitivity of the H_1 receptors at higher temperatures.

Although much more work is needed to define the receptor complement of rabbit heart, it has some advantages as an experimental tool since it does not contain easily releasable concentrations of histamine, a problem which can cause difficulties when guinea pig atria are used.

ACKNOWLEDGMENTS

This study was supported by U.S. Health Service grant HL16240.

The excellent technical assistance of Rosemary Minervini and Liz Smitten is gratefully acknowledged.

REFERENCES

Black, J.W., Duncan, W.A.M., Emmett, J.C., Ganellin, C.R., Hesselbo, T., Parsons, M.E., and Wyllie, J.H. (1973). Metiamide-an orally active histamine H_2-receptor antagonist. *Agents & Actions* **3**, 133-137.

Black, J.W., Duncan, W.A.M., Durant, C.J., Ganellin, C.R., and Parsons, E.M. (1972). Definition and antagonism of histamine H_2-receptors. *Nature (London)* **236**, 385-390.

Broadley, K.J. (1975). The role of H_1 and H_2-receptors in the coronary vascular response to histamine of isolated perfused hearts of guinea pigs and rabbits. *Brit. J. Pharmacol.* **54**, 511-521.

Cook, D.A., Kenakin, T.P., and Krueger, C.A. (1975). Thermal effects on the histamine receptor system of guinea pig ileum. *Proc. West. Pharmacol. Soc.* **18**, 119-122.

Ercan, Z.S., Bokesoy, T.A., and Turker, R.K. (1974). A study of the histamine H_2-receptors in heart muscle and coronary vessels. *Eur. J. Pharmacol.* **27**, 259-262.

Hughes, M.J., and Coret, I.A. (1972). On specificity of histamine receptors in the heart. *Amer. J. Physiol.* **223**, 1256-1262.

Hughes, M.J., and Coret, I.A. (1974). Effects of tricyclic compounds on the histamine response of isolated atria. *J. Pharmacol. Exper. Ther.* **191**, 252-261.

Hughes, M.J., and Coret, I.A. (1975). A quantitative study of histamine H_2-receptor blockade by burimamide in isolated atria. *Soc. Exper. Biol. Med.* **148**, 127-133.

Kenakin, T.P., Krueger, C.A., and Cook, D.A. (1974). Temperature-dependent interconversion of histamine H_1- and H_2-receptors in guinea pig ileum. *Nature (London)* **252**, 54-55.

Ledda, F., Fantozzi, R., Mugelli, A., Moroni, F., and Mannaioni, P.F. (1974). The antagonism of the positive inotropic effect of histamine and noradrenaline by H_1- and H_2-receptor blocking agents. *Agents & Actions* **4**, 193-194.

Levi, R., and Kuye, J.O. (1974). Pharmacological characterization of cardiac histamine receptors: sensitivity to H_1-receptor antagonists. *Eur. J. Pharmacol.* **27**, 330-338.

Levi, R., Capurro, N., and Chi-Ho, L. (1975a). Pharmacological characterization of cardiac histamine receptors: sensitivity to H_1- and H_2-receptor agonists and antagonists. *Eur. J. Pharmacol.* **30**, 328-335.

Levi, R., Ganellin, C.R., Allan, G., and Willens, H.J. (1975b). Selective impairment of atrioventricular conduction by 2-(2-pyridyl)-ethylamine and 2-(2-thiazolyl)-ethylamine, two histamine H_1-receptor agonists. *Eur. J. Pharmacol.* **34**, 237-240.

Levi, R., Allan, G., and Zavecz, J.H. (1976). Cardiac histamine receptors. *Fed. Proc.* **8**, 1942-1947.

McNeill, J.H., and Muschek, L.D. (1972). Histamine effects on cardiac contractility, phosphorylase and adenyl cyclase. *J.Molec. Cell. Cardiol.* **4**, 611-624.

McNeill, J.H., and Verma, S.C. (1974a). Blockade of cardiac histamine receptors by promethazine. *Can. J. Physiol. Pharmacol.* **52**, 23-27.

McNeill, J.H., and Verma, S. (1974b). Blockade by burimamide of the effects of histamine and histamine analogs on cardiac contractility, phosphorylase activation and cyclic adenosine monophosphate. *J. Pharmacol. Exper. Ther.* **188**, 180-188.

Moroni, F., Ledda, F., Fantozzi, R., Mugelli, A., and Mannaioni, P.F. (1974). Effects of histamine and noradrenaline on contractile force of guinea pig ventricular strips: antagonism by burimamide and metiamide. *Agents & Actions* **4**, 314-319.

Powell, J.R., and Brody, M.J. (1976). Identification and specific blockade of two receptors for histamine in the cardiovascular system. *J. Pharmacol. Exper. Ther.* **196**, 1-14.

Reinhardt, D., Wagner, J., Schümann, H.J. (1974). Differentiation of H_1-and H_2-receptors mediating positive chrono- and inotropic responses to histamine on atrial preparations of the guinea pig. *Agents & Actions* **4**, 217-221.

Reinhardt, D., Wiemann, H.M., and Schümann, H.J. (1976). Effects of the H_1-antagonist promethazine and the H_2-antagonist burimamide on chronotropic, inotropic and coronary vascular responses to histamine in isolated perfused guinea pig hearts. *Agents & Actions* **6**, 683-689.

Steinberg, M.I., and Holland, D.R. (1975). Separate receptors mediating the positive inotropic and chronotropic effect of histamine in guinea pig atria. *Eur. J. Pharmacol.* **34**, 95-104.

PART III
NEURAL
HISTAMINE RECEPTORS

11

Histamine Receptors in Mammalian Brain: Characteristics and Modifications Studied Electrophysiologically and Biochemically

J. C. Schwartz, J. M. Palacios, G. Barbin,
Th. T. Quach, M. Garbarg
Unité de Neurobiologie (U. 109)
Centre Paul Broca de l'I.N.S.E.R.M.
75014 Paris, France

H. L. Haas and P. Wolf
Neurophysiologisches Laboratorium
Neurochirurgische Universitatsklinik
CH 8091 Zurich, Switzerland

INTRODUCTION

There is now reasonable evidence to suggest that histamine (HA) is to be considered as one of the dozen of substances playing a messenger role between neurones in the mammalian brain (for recent reviews see Schwartz, 1975, 1977; Calcutt, 1976; Green et al., 1978,. If this is the case, one should be able to characterize membrane components recognizing specifically the imidazolamine and transducing the message, i.e., eliciting appropriate intracellular changes in the target cells. Such a general definition of HA receptors indicates that both electrophysiologists and biochemists can participate in this task with their own methodology.

In the present work our purpose was first to review the available evidence for the presence in mamalian brain of HA receptors responsible for changes in either neuronal activity or synthesis of the "second messenger," 3′, 5′-cyclic adenosine monophosphate. Meanwhile we have tried to answer the question: Are specific electrophysiological and biochemical effects of HA on target cells in brain linked with one of the two categories of HA receptors defined on peripheral systems? In different ways we have also tried to relate presynaptic events in the histaminergic system with receptor mechanisms. We show the potential usefulness of antagonists of HA receptors in the electrophysiological identification of histaminergic neuronal pathways which, otherwise, has only relied on a purely neurochemical approach. Finally, we have investigated the development of long-term changes in responsiveness of target cells to HA as a consequence of presynaptic modifications.

I. HISTAMINE RECEPTORS IN BRAIN:
ELECTROPHYSIOLOGICAL EVIDENCE

The technique of microiontophoresis allows unit recording and simultaneous application of minute amounts of substances into the immediate environment of single nerve cells, thus, providing an elegant method for investigation of receptors on neuronal membranes *in vivo*. Many neurones in the Central Nervous System were found to be responsive to locally applied histamine and some of its metabolites. It is, however, often difficult to correlate such effects with a natural histaminergic input.

On spinal motoneurones Phillis *et al.,.* (1968a)found depression of cell firing associated with a hyperpolarization. It was recently shown that this hyperpolarization is accompanied by a decrease in membrane conductance, presumably a reduction in resting sodium permeability (Engberg *et al.,* 1976). Intracellular recordings in Aplysia neurones indicate a different mechanism in these invertebrates where HA may also play a transmitter role (Carpenter and Gaubatz, 1975; Weinreich *et al.,* 1975). On cerebral cortical neurones of the cat (Phillis *et al.,* 1968b; Haas and Wolf, 1977), the rat (Haas and Wolf, 1977, Sastry and Phillis, 1976a), and the guinea pig (Haas *et al.,* 1977), the usual response to microiontophoretically applied HA is also depression of firing, but occasionally excitatory or dual effects can be observed. An example of a depressant action is illustrated in Fig. 1. Similar depressant actions were observed on the cuneate nucleus (Galindo *et al.,* 1967), the brain stem reticular formation (Bradley, 1968; Haas *et al.,* 1973), the cerebellum (Siggins *et al.,* 1971), the vestibular nucleus (Kirsten and Sharma, 1976; Satayavivad and Kirsten, 1977), and thalamus and hippocampal cortex (Haas and Wolf, 1977). In contrast to the actions on these structures, many

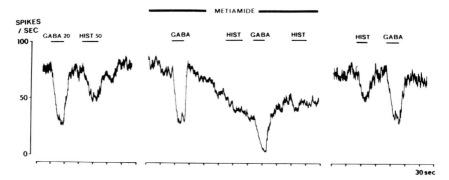

FIG. 1.   Influence of metiamide on depressant actions of histamine and GABA on a neurone from the rat sensorimotor cortex. Firing frequency vs. time diagram during microiontophoretic application of metiamide (50nA) (middle trace), the action of histamine (50nA) but not that of GABA (20nA) is blocked. Recovery is shown 6 minutes after withdrawal of metiamide on the right.

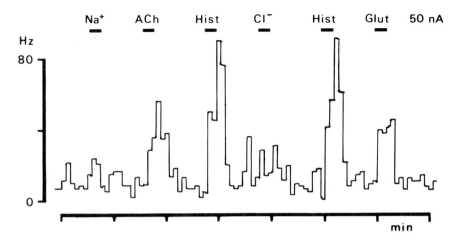

FIG. 2.   Excitation by histamine (50nA), acetylcholine (50nA), and glutamate (50nA) of a neurone of rat anterolateral hypothalamus. Firing frequency/time histogram. Sodium and chloride ions (50nA) are ineffective.

neurones in the hypothalamus, the region with, by far, the highest levels of HA and histidine decarboxylase (HD) activity, are excited by HA (Haas, 1974; Haas *et al.,* 1975; Haas and Wolf, 1977; Renaud, 1976; Geller, 1976). The excited cells include supraoptic neurosecretory neurones, neurones excited by Medial Forebrain Bundle stimulation, neurones projecting to the median eminence and tuberal neurones *in vivo.* Excitatory actions are also found in the lateral vestibular nucleus (Kirsten and Sharma, 1976; Satayavivad and Kirsten, 1977) and in the midbrain central grey (Haas and Wolf, 1977). Two types of excitation were described: a slow time course and a brisk excitation (Haas, 1974; Renaud, 1976). An example of a brisk and powerful excitation of a hypothalamic neurone is illustrated in Fig. 2. On such cells even slow potentials indicating synchronous discharges of a neurone population were observed during and after histamine iontophoresis. On cells which are continuously excited by glutamate, depression of firing is more common (Haas and Wolf, 1977, in press; Renaud, 1976).

    The actions of some related imidazole compounds at the cellular level are of particular interest; imidazole acetic acid, a histidine metabolite is a strong depressant on many central neurones. This action seems to be mediated by GABA receptors (Haas *et al.,* 1973; Godfraind *et al.,* 1973; Haas and Wolf, 1977; Phillis *et al.,* 1968b). The immediate catabolites of histamine 1,4-methylhistamine, and 1,4-methylimidazoleacetic acid are usually ineffective (Fig. 3) or have similar but weaker actions than HA, a finding which supports the view that methylation is the mechanism for transmitter inactivation of HA (Haas *et al.,* 1973; Haas and Wolf, 1977). Definitive clues on the question

SPIKES

/ SEC   **Na** _____   **HIST** _____   **MH** _____

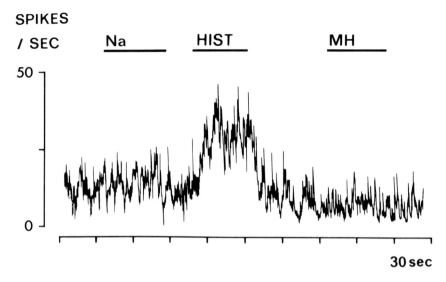

30 sec

FIG. 3. Action of histamine (50nA) and methylhistamine (50nA) on a neurone from the anterolateral hypothalamus of the cat. Firing frequency/time diagram. 1,4-methylhistamine and sodium ions (Na, 50nA) are ineffective.

if HA actions are mediated by cyclic nucleotides cannot yet be derived from microiontophoretic experiments (Anderson et al., 1973; Siggins et al., 1971; Godfraind et al., 1973).

Specific antagonists against the HA actions could be very useful for correlation of the effects with electrical or natural stimulation of possible histaminergic afferences. Pharmacological experiments using gross injections in the ventricles or regions of the brain considered to be relevant for functions like thirst (Leibowitz, 1973), hunger (Gerald and Maickel, 1972), water balance(Bennett and Pert, 1974; Bhargava et al., 1973; Dogterom et al., 1976; Tuomisto and Eriksson, 1974,) thermoregulation (Green et al., 1976; Clark and Cumby, 1976), regulation of the adenohypophysis (Libertun and Mc Cann, 1976), or central emesis (Bhargava et al., 1976) have revealed more or less specific actions of HA on neurone populations.In some of the experiments a clear distinction between effects mediated by H_1 and H_2 receptors was possible but H_1-receptor antagonists have local anesthetic properties which are probably responsible for their nonspecific effects in microiontophoretic experiments (Phillis et al., 1968b; Haas, 1974). In hypothalamic cultures, however, where the antagonist can be applied by perfusion, a specific antagonism between HA actions and diphenhydramine has been observed (Geller, 1976; Geller, personal communication) indicating that excitant actions of HA may be mediated by receptors of the H_1 type. H_2-receptor antagonists do not block and H_2 agonists do not mimick excitatory responses to histamine on hypothalamic (Haas and Wolf, 1977; Renaud, 1976) and vestibular neurones (Satayavivad and Kirsten, 1977). Depressant effects of HA, however, are mimicked by the H_2 agonists betazole and 4-methylhistamine (Haas and Wolf, 1977; Sastry and Phillis, 1976) and also the H_1 agonists 2-pyridylethylamine and 2-methylhistamine (Sastry and Phillis, 1976a). These effects are antagonized in a relatively specific manner by the H_2 antagonist metiamide (Haas and Bucher, 1975; Haas and Wolf, 1977; Sastry and Phillis, 1976a), as the actions of glutamate, GABA, noradrenaline, and serotonin are not equally affected. An example of a cell from the rat sensorimotor cortex is illustrated in Fig. 1. Excitation of cortical neurones by acetylcholine, however, is slightly reduced (Haas and Wolf, 1977; Phillis *et al.*, 1975). On the rabbit superior cervical ganglion an H_1-mediated facilitatory and an H_2-mediated depressant action have been observed (Brimble and Wallis, 1973).

Hence it appears that excitatory actions of HA are more often mediated by receptors resembling the H_1 type from peripheral tissues whereas inhibitory actions might be more often linked with the H_2 receptors. However more systematic work is needed to check whether such a conclusion always holds true.

II. HISTAMINE RECEPTORS IN BRAIN: BIOCHEMICAL EVIDENCE

In recent years, biochemists have participated in the identification of receptors for a variety of putative neurotransmitters in brain. Such identification has relied either on the ability of membrane constituents to specifically bind agonists or antagonists or in the properties of the neurotransmitters to stimulate the production of "second messengers."

The first approach, consisting in measuring the binding of appropriate radioactive ligands, has not yet been illustrated in the case of HA receptors in brain. On the other hand, many studies have already been devoted to the interaction of HA with the cAMP synthesizing system.

The original finding by Kakiuchi and Rall (1968) that HA was one of the most powerful agents in increasing the cyclic adenosine 3′, 5′-monophosphate (cAMP) level in slices from rabbit cerebellum has been repeatedly confirmed in a variety of brain regions and species like the chick (Nahorski *et al.*, 1974), rabbit (Kakiuchi and Rall, 1968; Palmer *et al.*, 1972; Shimizu *et al.*, 1970), guinea pig (Huang and Daly, 1972; Chasin *et al.*, 1971; Chasin *et al.*, 1973; Baudry *et al.*, 1975), pig (Sato *et al.*, 1974), rat (Schultz and Daly, 1973), mouse (Schultz and Daly, 1973; Skolnick and Daly, 1974), and man (Kodama *et al.*, 1973). In addition, HA stimulates cAMP accumulation in cultured glioma cells (Clark and Perkins, 1971). As in the case of other systems, there is no apparent correlation between the HA content of brain regions and their responsiveness, for instance, the hippocampus, which contains a low density of HA nerve-endings, is the most responsive structure in the guinea pig (Chasin *et al.*, 1973). The action of HA appears mediated by receptors distinct from those mediating the response to catecholamines, as indicated by large differences in responsiveness of the two classes of biogenic amines during brain maturation (Palmer *et al.*, 1972) or in various brain regions and, also, by the lack of effect of adrenergic receptor blockers (Chasin *et al.*, 1973).

The discovery by Black *et al.*, (1972) of specific agonists and antagonists of receptors present in peripheral tissues has initiated a new series of works aimed at identifying the nature of HA receptors linked with the cAMP production in brain tissues. Baudry *et al.* (1975) demonstrated in slices of guinea pig cortex that HA stimulation is partially antagonized by either a H_1 antagonist or a H_2 antagonist and totally blocked in the presence of both

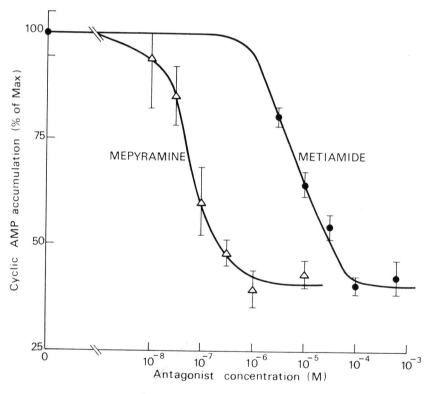

FIG. 4.   Effect of mepyramine and metiamide on the accumulation of cAMP induced by histamine. Slices of guinea pig cerebral cortex incubated in the presence of 50 μM histamine and increasing concentrations of H_1 and H_2 antagonists (reproduced from Baudry *et al.*, *Nature (London)* (1975), **253,** 362.

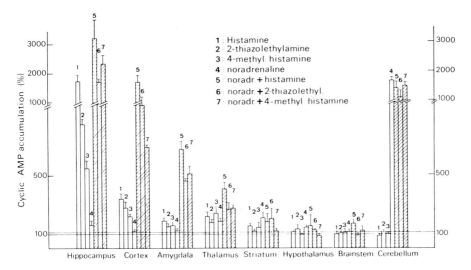

FIG. 5. Cyclic AMP accumulation elicited by histamine, 4-methylhistamine 2-thiazolethyla-mine and noradrenaline, and combinations of the histaminergic agonists with noradrenaline in slices from several areas of the guinea pig brain. Male Hartley guinea pigs (300g) were sacrificed by decapitation, different brain areas dissected and slices (250 μm thick) rapidly prepared with a McIlwain tissue slicer in the cold. Slices from 3–5 animals were pooled, suspended in oxygenated Krebs–Ringer medium, and preincubated for 30 minutes under $O_2:CO_2$ (95/5%). After washing with fresh medium aliquots of 200 μl were preincubated for 10 minutes and, then, incubated for 15 minutes in the presence of the different agents (100 μM). Incubation was stopped by sonication and heating at 95° for 10 minutes. Cyclic AMP was measured in the supernatant of the deproteinazed samples by the method of Brown *et al.* (1971). Results are expressed as percentages of the basal level (slices incubated in the absence of stimulating agent) and represent the means ± S.E.M. of 4–8 separate samples.

agents (see Fig. 4). These data were essentially confirmed by Rogers *et al.* (1975) on slices from guinea pig hippocampus. On the other hand, Hegstrand *et al.* (1976) demonstrated the presence of an HA-stimulated adenylcyclase in homogenates from guinea pig hippocampus which was competitively inhibited by metiamide but on which mepyramine had no effect. In view of the limited specificity of HA antagonists it was important to assess the effects of specific H_1 and H_2 agonists. The H_2 agonist 4-methylhistamine was found to stimulate cAMP synthesis in slices of guinea pig cortex (Baudry *et al.*, 1975; Dismukes *et al.*, 1976) or hippocampus (Dismukes *et al.*, 1976) as well as hippocampal homogenates (Hegstrand *et al.*, 1976). In addition, the H_1 agonists, 2-methylhistamine and 2-thiazolethylamine, were found to have stimulatory actions in guinea pig hippocampal and cortical tissues (Dismukes *et al.*, 1976; Hegstrand *et al.*, 1976).

Taken together all these results suggested that both classes of HA receptors evidenced in peripheral tissues were also present in mamalian brain.

In peripheral tissues H_1 and H_2 receptors appear to be separate molecular entities mediating different physiological responses. The electrophysiological data reported in the preceding section do not reveal in a clearcut manner whether such is the case in cerebral cells.

We reasoned that if H_1 and H_2 receptors were present on different kinds of brain cells, one could expect that one class or another might predominate according to the brain region examined in view of the largely heterogenous cellular composition of the various areas in the brain.

Furthermore, the striking potentiation of HA response by NA (Kakiuchi and Rall, 1968; Huang *et al.*, 1973) offered an additional opportunity to test this hypothesis that H_1 and H_2 receptor are separate entities.

The effects of HA, H_1 and H_2 agonists either alone or in combination with NA (all agents tested at a concentration of 100 μM in several areas of the guinea pig brain) is shown in Fig. 5. The largest cAMP accumulation elicited by HA was found in hippocampus (where histamine produced a 15–30 fold stimulation). Stimulation in cortex and amygdala was less (1.5–3.5 fold) while in thalamus and striatum, HA elicited only a small stimulation. The other regions did not show any significant HA-elicited cAMP accumulation.

These results are in agreement with previously reported distributions of responses to HA (Forn and Krishna, 1971; Chasin *et al.*, 1973; Rogers *et al.*, 1975; Hegstrand *et al.*, 1976). Indeed, the responses to the H_1 and H_2 agonists could only be found in regions responding to HA. Moreover the responses to H_1 and H_2 agonists were roughly parallel in the different areas of the guinea pig brain.

Noradrenaline induced none or marginal accumulation of cAMP in the slices of all brain areas studied with the exception of cerebellum where a 15–30 fold accumulation was found. However in the regions responding to HA, its effects were highly potentiated by noradrenaline. In agreement with the finding of Virion *et al.*, (personal communication) potentiation by NA was observed with either H_1 or H_2 agonists in each region responding to HA. The magnitude of the potentiation by NA was related to the actual HA response and presented a regional variation parallel to that of HA. A supra-additive effect seems to require a clear response to HA but not to NA because in cerebellum where a response to NA (but not to HA) is present, there was no potentiation, while in cortex where the situation is reversed, a clear potentiation was present. The magnitude of the effect was similar with H_1 and H_2 agonists, indicating that the NA potentiation effects are not preferentially associated with a particular class of HA receptors.

Hence, our data show that H_1 and H_2 receptors linked to the cAMP system could not be separated either on a regional basis or on the basis of potentiation by NA; this indicates that the two classes of HA receptors might not represent molecular entities as is apparently the case in peripheral tissues or, alternatively, that the two classes are closely associated in brain tissues.

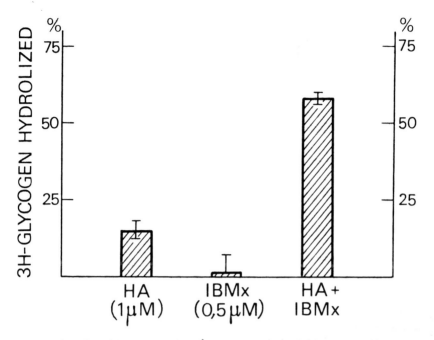

FIG. 6.   Histamine-elicited hydrolysis of ^{3}H-glycogen in mouse cortical slices. Slices from mouse cortex were preincubated at $37°C$ under a stream of $O_2:CO_2$ (95:5) for 15 minutes in a Krebs–Ringer medium containing 3 mM nonradioactive glucose and, thereafter, for 30 minutes in the presence of ^{3}H-glucose. Test substances were added and the slices incubated for a 20-minute period at the end of which they were decanted by a short centrifugation. The tissues were sonicated in cold Krebs–Ringer solution and heated at $95°C$ 10 minutes. ^{3}H-glycogen levels were measured after centrifugation by ethanol precipitation according to the method of Solling and Esmann (1975). Means ± S.E.M. of 3–4 experiments.

The observation that HA does not stimulate markedly cAMP formation in regions where neurochemical studies have provided evidence for histaminergic nerve-endings argues against the idea that receptors linked with cAMP formation represent postsynaptic receptors. However, the failure to observe a stimulatory action in regions containing nerve-endings might be due to technical factors in the process of preparation or incubation of the tissues. This is illustrated by our finding that, in a tissue on which HA has low, hardly apparent stimulatory action on cAMP accumulation, i.e., the mouse cerebral cortex, the amine nevertheless exerts a potent glycogenolytic action (Fig. 6 and 9). The hydrolysis of ^{3}H-glycogen synthesized by mouse cortical slices is accomplished by a rather low HA concentration (EC_{50} = 0.5 ± 0.3 μM) and appears to involve the intracellular production of cAMP inasmuch as this effect is potentiated in the presence of isobutylmethylxanthine, a potent phosphodiesterase inhibitor.

III. NEUROCHEMICAL AND ELECTROPHYSIOLOGICAL EVIDENCE FOR HISTAMINERGIC PATHWAYS IN BRAIN

Various experimental approaches have led, lately, to the idea that HA is present in a specific group of cerebral neurons (see Schwartz 1975, 1977 for reviews). In the absence of a suitable histochemical technique to visualize the putative histaminergic neurons, their anatomical disposition can be investigated by following the neurochemical changes elicited by specific lesions (Garbarg *et al.*, 1976; Barbin *et al.*, 1976; Ben-Ari *et al.*, 1977). Starting from the observation that HA and HD activity had a similar regional distribution as the monoamines and their synthesizing enzymes, lesions were performed in the lateral hypothalamic area in order to interrupt the Medial Forebrain Bundle. They resulted in significant reduction in HD activity in all ipsilateral telencephalic areas investigated, including the hippocampus and cerebral cortex (Table I). The decline in enzyme activity occured with a time-course consistent with anterograde degeneration of nerve-tracts. That the HA synthesizing enzyme in telencephalic areas is contained in terminals from extrinsic neurons is confirmed by its almost complete disappearance after total deafferentation of an area of cat cerebral cortex (Barbin *et al.*, 1975) or of rat hippocampal region (Table I). Selective interruption of dorsal afferents to the hippocampus (comprising fornix superior) resulted in a partial decrease in HD activity in this region (Table I). Although these neuro-chemical data already suggest that ascending histaminergic neurons innervate

Table I
Neurochemical Evidence for Histaminergic Nerve-Terminals in Rat Hippocampus and Cerebral Cortex

Type of lesion	Area analyzed	Change in HD activity (%)
Total deafferentation of the hippocampus	hippocampus	-95 ± 3
Transection of dorsal afferents to the hippocampus (comprising fornix)	hippocampus	-60 ± 6
Lesion of the Medial Forebrain Bundle	hippocampus	-46 ± 8
	cortex	-40 ± 7

[a]The mechanical interruption of hippocampal afferents were performed on male Wistar rats as described by Barbin *et al.* (1976). Medial Forebrain Bundle lesions were placed with a high frequency generator as described by Garbarg *et al.* (1976). *L*-histidine decarboxylase activity (HD) was measured by the radiochromatographic assay.

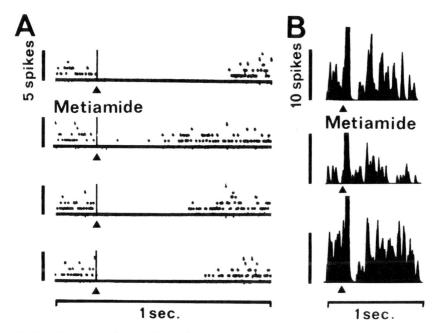

FIG. 7.   Electrophysiological evidence for histaminergic transmission in rat hippocampus and cerebral cortex. Two series of 256 bin peristimulus time histograms computed from 64 sweeps. (A) Hippocampal pyramidal cell. Stimulation of the fornix (3V, 0.2 msec) evoked a long lasting inhibition which was markedly reduced by metiamide (100nA). The third and fourth histograms were taken 1 and 5 minutes after withdrawal of metiamide. (B) Smoothed histograms showing inhibition of rat cerebral cortical neurone after Medial Forebrain Bundle stimulation (3.5V,/0.5 msec). During iontophoretic application of metiamide (25nA), the inhibition is blocked. Lowest histogram shows recovery of the inhibition after 4 minutes.

the cerebral and hippocampal cortices, a confirmation for this hypothesis was searched by a purely electrophysiological approach.

Electrical stimulation of the Medial Forebrain Bundle (Haas and Wolf, 1976, 1977; Sastry and Phillis, 1976b) and the fornix (Haas and Wolf, 1976, 1977) evokes inhibition in neurones of the cerebral and hippocampal cortex respectively. Microiontophoretically applied metiamide reduced these synaptic inhibitions, suggesting that the neurones investigated receive inhibitory histaminergic inputs from fibers ascending in the Medial Forebrain Bundle and the fornix. This is illustrated by two series of peristimulus time histograms in Fig. 7. The observed latencies indicate that the histaminergic fibers have a low conduction velocity (about 0.1 m/second) (Sastry and Phillis, 1976a). Direct cortical inhibition after stimulation of the ipsilateral cortical surface was not equally affected (Haas and Wolf, 1977; Sastry and Phillis, 1976b).

These results illustrate the potential usefulness of selective HA receptor antagonists in the identification of histaminergic pathways in brain.

IV. CHRONIC CHANGES IN RESPONSIVENESS
OF TARGET CELLS TO HISTAMINE
FOLLOWING THEIR DENERVATION.

It is well known that disruption of the normal nerve supply to striated (Axelsson and Thesleff, 1959) or smooth muscles (Trendelenburg, 1966) results in hypersensitivity of the denervated organ to the corresponding neurotransmitter. Various mechanisms appear to be responsible for the observed "hypersensitivity" including synthesis of new receptors and loss of presynaptic inactivation processes. The concept of denervation super sensitivity has been recently extended to the central nervous system in the field of catecholamine receptors (see Ungerstedt 1974; Yarbrough and Phillis, 1975). The discovery of HA synthesizing afferents to cortical regions that could be interrupted in a reproducible manner made it feasible to check whether such process could take place in cerebral cells receiving histaminergic inputs.

Recently, contradictory results were reported in this respect: in the rat the interruption of the Medial Forebrain Bundle resulted in an increased stimulation by HA of cAMP accumulation in neocortical slices (Dismukes *et al.*, 1975) while the same operation did not result in increased responsiveness to a supramaximal concentraion of HA in slices from guinea pig cortex (Dismukes *et al.*, 1976). These results are difficult to interpret because (a) in the rat the response to HA is of low amplitude and the effects of the lesion on histaminergic neurons were not assessed, (b) in the guinea pig brain, where a clear response to HA can be measured, the lesions were reported not to alter HD activity (Dismukes *et al.*, 1976).

We have now investigated the effects of unilateral interruption of the Medial Forebrain Bundle at the level of the lateral hypothalamic area on the responsiveness to HA, evaluated in the guinea pig brain either *in vivo* by microiontophoretic application of the amine or *in vitro* by the accumulation of cAMP.

In agreement with the data obtained in the rat (Table I) such lesions resulted after 8–30 days in significant reductions in HD activity in guinea pig cortex or hippocampus (Tables II, III, and IV).

A clear hypersensitivity to microiontophoretically applied HA (and NA but not GABA) developed in cortical neurones ipsilateral but not contralateral to the lesion (Table II). By constructing dose-response curves for iontophoretic actions it was possible to determine the response threshold and a just maximal response. A threshold response to HA (NA) was usually obtained with about 50nA (30nA) ejecting current on the intact side of lesioned animals and in unlesioned animals. On the lesioned sides the thresholds were about 10nA (10nA). Maximal responses on unlesioned sides were obtained with about 100nA (60nA) but with about 40nA (30nA) on

Table II
Lesions of the Medial Forebrain Bundle: Sensitivity of Guinea Pig Cortical Neurons to Microiontophoretically Applied Histamine and Noradrenaline[a]

Guinea pig	Changes in			
	H.D. activity (%)	D.D. activity (%)	Threshold to HA (%)	Threshold to NA (%)
N° 1	-34		-91	
N° 2	-11		-58	-62
N° 3	-23	-25	-56	-77
N° 4	-29	-51	-85	-58
N° 5	-13	-26	-76	-49
Mean (± S.E.M.)	-22 ± 4	-34 ± 8	-73 ± 7	-62 ± 6

[a]Decrease in H.D. and Dopa-decarboxylase (D.D.) activity and decrease in the response threshold of microiontophoretically applied HA and NA after lesions of the MFB. Thresholds (in nanoamperes ejecting current) for HA (49 cells) and NA (22 cells) were determined from dose-response curves. The changes in enzyme activities and thresholds are expressed as percentage decreases in comparison to the unlesioned side.

lesioned sides. Table II shows percentage decreases of enzyme activities and threshold responses on the lesioned sides as compared to the unlesioned sides.

This clear hypersensitivity of cortical cells to HA after interruption of histaminergic afferents recalls the hypersensitivity of striatal cells to dopamine after degeneration of dopaminergic fibers (Feltz and de Champlain, 1972). In the case of HA, as histaminegic endings do not appear to possess a high affinity uptake system for the amine, this hypersensitivity probably represents a true postsynaptic receptor hypersensitivity developing after denervation.

In contrast with the actions of iontophoretically applied HA (but in agreement with the data of Dismukes *et al.*, 1976) the responsiveness of the cAMP accumulating system to the amine in slices of cerebral cortex did not show any alteration, neither the maximal response to HA nor the EC_{50} of HA

Table III
Lesions of the Medial Forebrain Bundle: Responsiveness to Histamine and Noradrenaline of the cAMP Accumulating System in Guinea Pig Cortical Slices[a]

	N	Intact side	Lesioned side	Change (%)
L-histidine decarboxylase (dpm/mg/h)	18	780 ± 55	221 ± 19	-67 ± 2
cAMP accumulation				
Basal level (pmol/mg prot.)	18	3.93 ± 0.51	4.50 ± 0.67	+15 ± 8
Maximal response to HA[b] (% of basal level)	18	225 ± 18	214 ± 15	-8 ± 12
EC_{50} of HA (μM)	11	17.5 ± 5.0	14.5 ± 3.7	
Response to 100 μM NA (% of basal level)	3	135 ± 34	145 ± 20	+11 ± 15
Response to 100 μM HA + 100μM NA (% of basal level)	3	1086 ± 516	1210 ± 591	+9 ± 28

[a]Unilateral interruptions of the Medial Forebrain Bundle were performed under chloral anesthesia (350mg/kg, i.p.) by delivering a high frequency current (20V during 1 minute) through an electrode lowered at A : +8.3; L : +1.8 and H : +1.2 according to the stereotaxic atlas of Poulain (1971). Male Hartley guinea pigs (300 g) were employed in all the studies.

Animals were sacrificed 8–30 days after lesions placement. L-histidine decarboxylase activity was determined in the cerebral cortex of every animal.Cyclic AMP accumulation was determined in slices as described in Fig. 5.

N represents the number of animals. "Change" indicates the mean percentage (± S.E.M.) of the lesion side as compared to intact side.

[b]Maximal response to histamine represents either the value obtained by plotting the data from a dose-response curve or the response to 100 μM HA.

Table IV

Lesions of the Medial Forebrain Bundle: Responsiveness to Histamine, H_1 and H_2 Agonists and Noradrenaline of the Cyclic AMP Accumulating System in Guinea Pig Hippocampal Slices[a]

	N	Intact side	Lesioned side	Change (%)
L-histidine decarboxylase (dpm/mg/h)	4	636 ± 56	234 ± 24	-62 ± 6
cAMP accumulation Basal level (pmol/mg prot.)	19	4.14 ± 0.41	3.58 ± 0.38	-8 ± 8
Maximal response to HA[b] (% of basal level)	19	2108 ± 288	1974 ± 246	-1 ± 10
EC_{50} of HA (μM)	7	13.3 ± 3.2	16.5 ± 5.2	
Response to 100 μM 2—thiazolethylamine (% of basal level)	3	1343 ± 410	1511 ± 259	+19 ± 24
Response to 100 μM 4-methylhistamine (% of basal level)	5	596 ± 93	628 ± 93	+9 ± 13
Response to 100 μM NA (% of basal level)	4	135 ± 24	194 ± 67	+34 ± 17
Response to 100 μM HA + 100 μM NA (% of basal level)	4	3787 ±453	3231 ± 491	-11 ± 16

[a]Unilateral interruptions of the Medial Forebrain Bundle were performed as described in Table III. L-histidine decarboxylase activity and cAMP accumulation were measured as previously described.

N represents the number of animals. "Change" indicates the mean percentage (± S.E.M.) of the lesion side as compared to the intact side.

[b]Maximal response to HA represents either the value obtained by plotting the data from a dose-response curve or the response to 100 μM HA.

was significantly different in the lesioned side as compared to the intact side in the same animal (Table III). Neither was the response to a combination of HA and NA significantly modified.

Essentially similar conclusions were reached with experiments on hippocampal slices (Table IV). On this preparation the responsiveness to H_1 and H_2 agonists could also be investigated, and the data ruled out that hypersensitivity of a selective class of HA receptors was present. The comparison of the data derived from electrophysiological and biochemical assessment of responsiveness of target cells to HA raises the interesting possibility that different kinds of HA receptors are involved. This could be the case if HA receptors linked with the cAMP generating system were present in nonneuronal cells whereas the response to iontophoretically applied HA indeed involves cortical neurones. In this respect, it must be recalled that HA elicits cAMP accumulation in cultured glioma cells (Clark and Perkins, 1971).

Interestingly, a similar discrepancy between electrophysiological and biochemical data appears to be present in dopaminergic system; selective degeneration of the nigrostriatal bundle is followed by hypersensitivity to iontophoretically applied dopamine (Feltz and de Champlain, 1972) whereas the modification in responsiveness of the dopamine-dependent adenylcyclase is still controversial.

Such discrepancies might be taken as evidence that typical postsynaptic effects do not involve the production of cAMP as a second messenger but the possibility remains that subtle changes in receptor sensitivity are lost during preparation of the tissues for biochemical studies or not detected under our experimental conditions.

V. HYPOSENSITIVITY TO HISTAMINE FOLLOWING RESERPINE TREATMENT

Changes in sensivity to monoamines of target cells in the central nervous system can be observed not only after denervation but also after drug-induced modifications in presynaptic activity. Generally impairment in synaptic transmission results in a few hours in the development of hypersensitivity (see for instance Baudry et al., 1976).

Although treatment with reserpine does not result in extensive depletion of HA stores in brain, the drug releases HA from hypothalamic slices (Taylor and Snyder, 1973; Verdière et al., 1974) and, in vivo, accelerates the disappearance of endogenously synthesized ^{3}H–HA from rat brain (Pollard et al., 1973).

In rats, reserpine treatment elicits the development of hypersensitivity of the cAMP generating system to NA (Dismukes and Daly, 1974; Baudry et al., 1976). It was therefore of interest to investigate whether parallel changes in sensitivity to HA were also occuring.

In fact, the responsiveness to HA was reduced in reserpine-treated guinea pigs; in slices from hippocampus the maximal accumulation of cAMP was significantly lower than in controls, without change in the EC_{50} of the amine (Fig. 8).

A similar result was found concerning the glycogenolytic effect of HA in mouse cortical slices but in this case, the EC_{50} was modified and not the maximal response (Fig. 9). On the other hand, the responsiveness of the glycogenolytic system to dibutyryl-cAMP was not modified in reserpine-treated mice, indicating that the change involved only the cAMP generating step (Fig. 10).

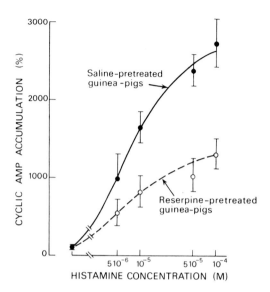

FIG. 8. Histamine-elicited accumulation of cAMP in hippocampal slices from reserpine-pretreated guinea pigs. Male guinea pigs (300 g) were treated with 2.5 mg/kg (i.p.) of reserpine on the first day and 1 mg/kg on the three following days. Controls received the vehicle. Cyclic AMP accumulation was measured 24 hour after the last injection. Results represent means±S.E.M. of data from 6 controls and 5 reserpine-treated animals.

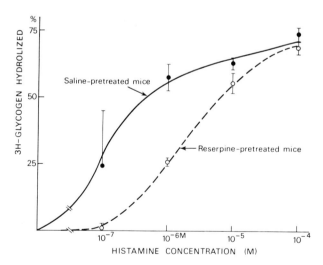

FIG. 9. Histamine-elicited hydrolysis of ^{3}H-glycogen in cortical slices from reserpine-pretreated mice. Groups of 8-12 mice were pretreated by 5 mg/kg on day 1, 2.5 mg/kg on day 2 and sacrificed on the third day. ^{3}H-glycogen hydrolysis was evaluated as described in Fig. 6. Means±S.E.M. of triplicate determinations. The experiment was repeated twice with similar results.

177

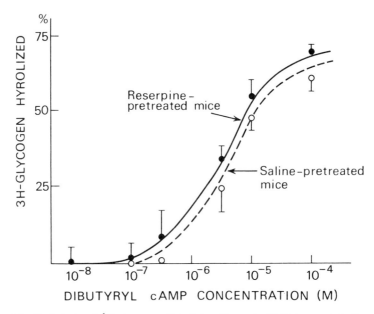

FIG. 1.0 Hydrolysis of ³H-glycogen elicited by dibutyryl-cAMP in cortical slices from reserpine-pretreated mice. Treatment and incubation conditions as described in Fig. 9. Means±S.E.M. from 4 different experiments in which each incubation was triplicated.

These data indicate that the treatment by reserpine results in a state of hyposensitivity to HA which contrasts with the hypersensitivity to catecholamines (including the glycogenolytic action of noradrenaline after the same treatment) (Quach *et al.*, in preparation).

Since hyposensitivity of brain cells to amines generally develops following a drug-induced overstimulation of their receptors (Costentin *et al.*, 1975; Baudry *et al.*, 1976) our data suggest that reserpine treatment elicits a release of unmetabolized HA in the vicinity of histaminergic receptors. This could well be the case because, in contrast to catecholamines, HA is not a substrate for the enzyme monoamine oxidase which is responsible for the deamination of noradrenaline or dopamine occuring intraneuronally after their release by reserpine. This would also account for the lack of extensive HA depletion observed after reserpine.

It would be of interest to check whether reserpine treatment results in a parallel change in sensitivity of brain cells to microiontophoretically applied HA.

CONCLUSION

The present work emphasizes the complementarity of electrophysiological and biochemical approaches in the study of HA receptor mechanisms in brain.

Most of electrophysiological and biochemical data suggest that the two types of HA receptors found in peripheral tissues are also present in the CNS. However a clearcut dissociation of the two types of receptors could not be obtained on the basis of either their regional or cellular localization or the intracellular effects they mediate.

The two experimental approaches led to converging conclusions regarding the identification of histaminergic pathways innervating telencephalic areas. They have also demonstrated that, as in other neuronal systems, the responsiveness of target cells to HA can be modulated according to HA release from its presynaptic stores; denervation hypersensitivity has been demonstrated in microiontophoretic experiments while reserpine-induced hyposensitivity has been demonstrated on the cAMP-generating and glycogen-hydrolyzing systems.

The fact that denervation hypersensitivity can be observed electrophysiologically but not on the cAMP-generating system raises the question of the involvement of cAMP as a second messenger in histaminergic neurotransmission.

REFERENCES

Anderson, E.G., Haas, H.L., and Hosli, L. (1973). Comparison of effects of noradrenaline and histamine with cyclic AMP on brainstem neurones. *Brain Res.* **49**, 471-475.
Axelsson, J., and Thesleff, S.A. (1959). A study of supersensitivity in denervated mammalian skeletal muscle. *J. Physiol. (London).* **147**, 178-193.
Barbin, G., Hirsch, J.C., Garbarg, M., and Schwartz, J.C. (1975). Decrease in histamine content and decarboxylase activities in an isolated area of the cerebral cortex of the cat. *Brain Res.* **92**, 170-174.
Barbin, G., Garbarg, M., Schwartz, J.C., and Storm-Mathisen, J. (1976). Histamine synthesizing afferents to the hippocampal region. *J. Neurochem.* **26**, 259-263.
Baudry, M., Martres, M.P., and Schwartz, J.C. (1975). H_1- and H_2-receptors in the histamine-induced accumulation of cyclic AMP in guinea-pig brain slices. *Nature (London)* **253**, 362-363.
Baudry, M., Martres, M.P., and Schwartz, J.C. (1976). Modulation in the sensitivity of noradrenergic receptors in the CNS studied by the responsiveness of the cyclic AMP system. *Brain Res.* **116**, 111-124.
Ben-Ari, Y., Le Gal La Salle, G., Barbin, G., Schwartz, J.C., and Garbarg, M. (1977). Histamine synthesizing afferents within the amygdaloid complex and bed nucleus of the stria terminalis in the rat. *Brain Res.* **138**, 285-294.
Bennett, C.T., and Pert, A. (1974). Antidiuresis by injections of histamine into the cat supraoptic nucleus. *Brain Res.* **78**, 151-156.
Bhargava, K.P., Kulshrestha, V.K., Santhakumari, G., and Srivastava, Y.P. (1973). Mechanism of histamine-induced antidiuretic response. *Brit. J. Pharmacol.* **47**, 700-706.
Bhargava, K.P., Dixit, K.S., and Palit, G. (1976). Nature of histamine receptors in the emetic chemoreceptor trigger zone. *Brit. J. Pharmacol.* **57**, 211-214,
Black, J.W., Duncan, W.A.M., Durant, C.J., Ganellin, C.R., and Parsons, E.M. (1972). Definition and antagonism of histamine H_2-receptors. *Nature (London)* **236**, 385-390.
Bradley, P.B. (1968). Synaptic transmission in the CNS and its relevance for drug action. *Int. Rev. Neurobiol.* **11**, 1-56.

Brimble, M.J., and Wallis,D.I. (1973). Histamine H_1- and H_2-receptors at ganglionic synapse. *Nature (London)* **246**, 156-158.

Brown, B.L., Albano, J.D.D., Ekins, R.P., Sqherzi, A.M., and Tampion, W. (1971). A simple and sensitive saturation assay method for measurement of adenosine 3′, 5′-cyclic monophosphate. *Biochem. J.* **121**, 561-563.

Calcutt, C.R. (1976). The role of histamine in the brain. *Gen. Pharmacol.* **7**, 15-25.

Carpenter, D.O., and Gaubatz, G.L. (1975). H_1- and H_2 histamine receptors on Aplysia neurons. *Nature (London)* **254**, 343-344.

Chasin, M., Rikvin, I., Mamrak, F., Samaniego, S.G., and Hess, S.M. (1971). Alpha and beta-adrenergic receptors as mediators of accumulation of cyclic adenosine 3′, 5′-monophosphate in specific areas of guinea-pig brain. *J. Biol. Chem.* **246**, 3037-3041.

Chasin, M., Mamrak, F., Samaniego,S.G., and Hess, S.M. (1973). Characteristics of the catecholamine and histamine receptor sites mediating accumulation of cyclic adenosine 3′, 5′-monophosphate in guinea pig brain. *J. Neurochem.* **21**, 1415-1427.

Clark, W.G., and Cumby, H.R. (1976). Biphasic changes in body temperature produced by intracerebroventricular injections of histamine in the cat. *J. Physiol. (London)* **261**, 235-253.

Clark, R.B., and Perkins, J.P. (1971). Regulation of adenosine 3′ ,5′-monophosphate concentration in cultured human astrocytoma cells by catecholamines and histamine. *Proc. Nat. Acad. Sci.* **68**, 2757-2760.

Costentin, J., Protais, P., and Schwartz, J.C. (1975). Rapid and dissociated changes in sensitivities of different dopamine receptors in mouse brain. *Nature (London)* **257**, 405-407.

Dismukes, R.K. and Daly, J.W. (1974). Norepinephrine-sensitive systems generating adenosine 3′ ,5′-monophosphate: increased responses in cerebral cortical slices from reserpine-treated rats. *Mol. Pharmacol.* **10**, 933-940.

Dismukes, R.K., Ghosh, P., Creveling, C.R., and Daly, J.W. (1975). Altered responsiveness of adenosine 3′ ,5′-monophosphate-generating systems in rat cortical slices after lesions of the Medial Forebrain Bundle. *Exper. Neurol.* **49**, 725-735.

Dismukes, R.K., Rogers, M., and Daly, J.W. (1976). Cyclic adenosine 3′ ,5′-monophosphate formation in guinea-pig brain slices: effect of H_1- and H_2-histaminergic agonists. *J. Neurochem.* **26**, 785-790.

Dogterom, J., Van Wimersma Greidanus, T.J.B., and De Wied, D. (1976). Histamine as an extremely potent releaser of vasopressin in the rat. *Experientia* **32**, 659-660.

Engberg, I., Flatman, J.A., and Kadzielawa, K. (1976). Lack of specificity of motoneurone responses to microiontophoretically applied phenolic amines. *Acta Physiol. Scand.* **96**, 137-139.

Feltz, P., and De Champlain, J. (1972). Enhanced sensitivity of caudate neruones to microiontophoretic injections of dopamine in 6-hydroxydopamine treated cats. *Brain Res.* **43**, 601-605.

Forn, J., and Krishna, G. (1971). Effect of norepinephrine, histamine and other drugs on cyclic 3′ ,5′-AMP formation in brain slices of various animal species. *Pharmacology* **5**, 193-104.

Galindo, A., Krnjevic, K., and Schwartz, S. (1967). Micro-iontophoretic studies on neurones in the cuneate nucleus. *J. Physiol. (London)* **192**, 105-118.

Garbarg, M., Barbin, G., Bischoff, S., Pollard, H., and Schwartz, J.C. (1976). Dual localization of histamine in an ascending pathway and in non-neuronal cells evidenced by lesions in the lateral hypothalamic area. *Brain Res.* **106**, 333-348.

Geller, H.M. (1976). Effects of some putative neurotransmitters on unit activity of tuberal hypothalamic neurons *in vitro*. *Brain Res.* **108**, 423-430.

Gerald, M.C., and Maickel, R.P. (1972). Studies on the possible role of brain histamine in behavior. *Brit. J. Pharmacol.* **44**, 462-471.

Godfraind, J.M., Krnjevic, K., Maretic, H., and Pumain, R. (1973). Inhibition of cortical neurones by imidazole and some derivatives. *Can. J. Physiol. Pharmacol.* **51**, 790-797.

Green, M.D., Cox, B., and Lomax, P. (1976). Sites and mechanisms of action of histamine in the central thermoregulatory pathways of the rat. *Neuropharmacology* **15**, 321-324.

Green, J.P., Johnson, C.L., and Weinstein, H. (1978). Histamine as a neurotransmitter in "Psychopharmacology–A Generation of Progress" (M. Lipton, A. Dimascio, and K. Killman, eds.), Raven Press, New York 319-332.

Haas, H.L. (1974). Histamine: action on single hypothalamic neurones. *Brain Res.* **76**, 363-366.

Haas, H.L., and Bucher, U.M. (1975). Histamine H_2-receptors on single central neurones. *Nature (London)* **255**, 634-635.

Haas, H.L., and Wolf, P. (1976). Possible histaminergic pathways in the cat and rat brain. *Pflügers Arch.* **362**, 38.

Haas, H.L., and Wolf, P. (1977). Central actions of histamine: microelectrophoretic studies. *Brain Res.* **122**, 269-279.

Haas, H.L., Anderson, E.G., and Hosli, L. (1973). Histamine and metabolites: their effects and interactions with convulsants on brain stem neurones. *Brain Res.* **51**, 269-278.

Haas, H.L., Wolf, P., Nussbaumer, J.C. (1975). Histamine: action on supraoptic and other hypothalamic neurones of the cat. *Brain Res.* **88**, 166-169.

Haas, H.L., Wolf, P., Garbarg, M., Palacios, J.M., and Schwartz, J.C. (1977). Denervation hypersensitivity of cortical neurons to histamine. *Experientia* **33**, 780.

Hegstrand, L.R., Kanof, P.D., and Greengard, P. (1976). Histamine-sensitive adenylate cyclase in mammalian brain. *Nature (London)* **260**, 163-165.

Huang, M., and Daly, J.W. (1975). Accumulation of cyclic adenosine monophosphate in incubated slices of brain tissue.[1] Structure activity relationship of agonists and antagonists of biogenic amines and of tricyclic tranquilizers and antidepressants. *J. Med. Chem.* **15**, 458-462.

Huang, M., Ho, A.K.S., and Daly, J.W. (1973). Accumulation of adenosine cyclic 3',5'-monophosphate in rat cerebral cortical slices. Stimulatory effects of alpha- and beta-adrenergic agents after treatment with 6-hydroxydopamine, 2,3,5,-trihydroxyphenethylamine and dihydroxytryptamine. *Mol. Pharmacol.* **9**, 711-717.

Kakiuchi, S., and Rall, T.W. (1968). The influence of chemical agents on the accumulation of adenosine 3'-5'-phosphate in slices of rabbit cerebellum *Mol. Pharmacol.* **4**, 367-378.

Kirsten, E.B., and Sharma, J.N. (1976). Microiontophoresis of acetylcholine, histamine and their antagonists on neurons in the medial and lateral vestibular nuclei of the cat. *Neuropharmacology* **15**, 743-753.

Kodama, T., Matsukado, Y., and Shimizu, H. (1973). The cyclic AMP system of human brain, *Brain Res.* **50**, 135-146.

Leibowitz, S.F. (1973). Histamine: a stimulatory effect on drinking behavior in the rat. *Brain Res.* **63**, 440-444.

Libertun, C., Mc Cann, S.M. (1976). The possible role of histamine in the control of prolactin and gonadotropin release. *Neuroendocrinology* **20**, 110-120.

Nahorski, S.R., Rogers, K.J., and Smith, B.M. (1974). Histamine H_2 receptors and cyclic AMP in brain. *Life Sci.* **15**, 1887-1894.

Palmer, G.C., Schmidt, M.J., and Robinson, G.A. (1972). Development and characteristics of the histamine-induced accumulation of cyclic AMP in the rabbit cerebral cortex. *J. Neurochem.* **19**, 2251-2256.

Phillis, J.W., Tebecis, A.K., and York, D.H. (1968a). Depression of spinal motoneurones by noradrenaline, 5-hydroxytryptamine and histamine. *Eur. J. Pharmacol.* **4**, 471-479.

Phillis, J.W., Tebecis, A.K., and York, D.H. (1968b). Histamine and some antihistamines: their actions on cerebral cortical neurones *Brit. J. Pharmacol. Chemother.* **33**, 426-440.

182 SCHWARTZ ET AL

Phillis, J.W., Kostopoulos, G.K., and Odutola, A. (1975). On the specificity of histamine H_2-receptor antagonists in the rat cerebral cortex. *Can. J. Physiol.* **53**, 1198-1218.

Pollard, H., Bischoff, S., and Schwartz, J.C. (1973). Decreased histamine synthesis in the rat brain by hypnotics and anaesthetics. *J. Pharm. Pharmacol.* **25**, 920-921.

Poulain, P. (1971). Atlas stéréotaxique de l'hypothalamus du cobaye. Thèse doctorat 3ème cycle.

Quach, Th.T., Rose, C., and Schwartz, J.C. (1978). ^{3}H-glycogen hydrolysis in brain slices: responses to neurotransmitters and modulation of noradrenaline receptors. *J. Neurochem.* **30**, 1335-1341.

Renaud, L.P. (1976). Histamine microiontophoresis on identified hypothalamic neurons: 3 patterns of response in the ventromedial nucleus of the rat. *Brain Res.* **115**, 339-344.

Rogers, M., Dismukes, K., and Daly, J.W. (1975). Histamine-elicited accumulations of cyclic adenosine 3',5'-monophosphate in guinea-pig brain slices: effect of H_1- and H_2-antagonists. *J. Neurochem.* **25**, 531-534.

Sastry, B.S.R., and Phillis, J.W. (1976a). Depression of rat cerebral cortical neurons by H_1 and H_2 receptor agonists. *Eur. J. Pharmacol.* **38**, 269-273.

Sastry, B.S.R., and Phillis, J.W. (1976b). Evidence for an ascending inhibitory histaminergic pathway to the cerebral cortex. *Can. J. Physiol. Pharmacol.* **54**, 782-786.

Satayavivad, J., and Kirsten, E.B. (1977). Ionotophoretic studies of histamine and histamine antagonists in the feline vestibular nuclei. *Eur. J. Pharmacol.* **41**, 17-26.

Sato, A., Onaya, T., Kotani, M., Harada, A., and Yamada, T. (1974). Effects of biogenic amines on the formation of adenosine 3',5'-monophosphate in porcine cerebral cortex, hypothalamus and anterior pituitary slices. *Endocrinology* **94**, 1311-1317.

Schultz, J., and Daly, J.W. (1973). Accumulation of cyclic adenosine 3',5'-monophosphate in cerebral cortical slices from rat and mouse: stimulation effect of alpha- and beta-adrenergic agents and adenosine. *J. Neurochem.* **21**, 1319-1326.

Schwartz, J.C. (1975). Histamine as a neurotransmitter in brain. *Life Sci.* **17**, 503-518.

Schwartz, J.C. (1977). Histaminergic mechanisms in brain. *Ann. Rev. Pharmacol. Toxicol.* **17**, 325-339.

Shimizu, H., Creveling, C.R., and Daly, J.W. (1970). The effect of histamine and other compounds on the formation of adenosine 3',5'-monophosphate in slices from cerebral cortex. *J. Neurochem.* **17**, 441-444.

Siggins, G.R., Hoffer, B.J., and Bloom, F.E. (1971). Studies on norepinephrine containing afferents to Purkinje cells of rat cerebellum. III Evidence for mediation of norepinephrine effects by cyclic 3',5'-adenosine monophosphate. *Brain Res.* **25**, 535-553.

Skolnick, P., and Daly, J.W. (1974). The accumulation of adenosine 3',5'-monophosphate in cerebral cortical slices of the quaking mouse, a neurologic mutant. *Brain Res.* **73**, 513-525.

Solling, H., and Esmann, U. (1975). A sensitive method of glycogen determination in the presence of interfering substances utilizing the filter-paper technique. *Analyt. Biochem.* **68**, 664-668.

Taylor, K.M., and Snyder, S.H. (1973). The release of histamine from tissue slices of rat hypothalamus. *J. Neurochem.* **21**, 1215-1223.

Trendelenburg, U. (1966). Mechanisms of supersensitivity and subsensitivity to sympathomimetics amines. *Pharmacol. Rev.* **18**, 629-640.

Tuomisto, L., and Eriksson, L. (1974). Central antidiuretic effect of histamine in the unanesthetized goat: effects of H_1- and H_2-antagonists. *J. Pharmacol. (Paris)* **5** (suppl. 2), 101.

Ungerstedt, U. (1974). Functional dynamics of central monoamine pathways "The Neurosciences Third Study Program" (F.O. Schmitt and F.G Worden, eds.), pp.979-988. MIT Press, Cambridge, Mass.

Verdiere, M., Rose, C., and Schwartz, J.C. (1974). Synthesis and release of ^{3}H-histamine in slices from rat brain. *Agents Actions* **4**, 184-185.

Weinreich, D., Weiner, C., and Mc Caman, R. (1975). Endogenous levels of histamine in single neurones isolated from CNS of Aplysia californica. *Brain Res.* **84**, 341-345.

Yarbrough, G.G., and Phillis, J.W. (1975). Supersensitivity of central neurons-a brief review of an emerging concept. *J. Can. Sci. Neurol.* 147-151.

12

Histamine Activation of Adenylate Cyclase in Brain: An H$_2$-Receptor and Its Blockade by LSD

Jack Peter Green, Carl Lynn Johnson, and Harel Weinstein
Department of Pharmacology
Mount Sinai School of Medicine
of the City University of New York
New York, New York

Several bits of evidence are needed to prove that histamine functions as a neurotransmitter in brain. Its distribution *in situ* should be shown; this lack is attributable to the insentivity of the histofluorescent method and to the inability to label the histamine stores because there is no active uptake system for histamine. The turnover of histamine under steady-state conditions needs to be measured, and this requires methods to measure histamine metabolites. Finally, the effects of exogenous histamine on neural structures must be shown to be like those seen after stimulation of nerves.

Other criteria for a neurotransmitter function of histamine have been met (Green, 1964, 1970; Snyder and Taylor, 1972; Dismukes and Snyder, 1974; Schwartz, 1975; Schwartz *et al.*, 1976; Calcutt, 1976; Green *et al.*, 1978). Histamine has a nonuniform regional distribution. It is stored in subcellular fractions containing nerve endings. Specific enzymes for its synthesis and metabolism (methylation) are present in brain. Histamine appears to turn over rapidly. Lesions result in a fall in the activity of the synthesizing enzyme and in the histamine concentration distal to the lesion. Neurons respond to histamine. Histamine is released by potassium ions in a calcium-dependent process. Histamine stimulates adenylate cyclase activity and this effect is blocked by specific antagonists.

Histamine activation of adenylate cyclase activity in many tissues and cells has been described in more than a hundred papers since the initial observation by Kakiuchi and Rall (1968). In many of these studies, notably those on brain slices, both H$_1$ and H$_2$ antagonists were observed to block the effect of histamine in stimulating adenylate cyclase activity. These observations prompted the conclusion that both H$_1$ and H$_2$ receptors mediate the stimulation. The inference seems all the more reasonable in experiments showing H_1 antagonists to be more potent than, or as potent as, the H_2 antagonists.

However, conclusions on the nature of the receptors requires comparison between the concentration of antagonist needed to inhibit the effect of histamine on the enzyme with the concentration of antagonist needed to inhibit the effect of histamine on a system with well defined histamine receptors, e.g., the guinea pig ileum (H_1 receptor) and guinea pig atrium (H_2 receptor). For example, if the pA_2 value (i.e., the negative log of the concentration of antagonist that requires doubling of the agonist concentration to overcome the antagonism) of an antagonist (e.g., mepyramine) on histamine-stimulated adenylate cyclase is 5 and its pA_2 value on the guinea pig ileum is 9, the adenylate cyclase is likely not to be an H_1 receptor. Black (1976: p. 5) described "logical fallacies involving circular arguments" in the interpretation of the actions of antagonists,

"For example, D is estimated to be a competitive antagonist of A on systems P and Q. The homogeneity, and therefore the set, of A receptors is provisionally defined by D. However, D is now classed as a universal A-receptor antagonist, and this is sometimes treated as a separate statement when, without independent tests, it is logically the same statement. A second fallacy often follows from this; the classification of D in terms of tentative set A leads to repeated use of D as an anti-A and the class of A may soon appear to achieve the status of a piece of evidence rather than an assumption. Finally, the classification of D may also begin to appear objective through use and lead to fallacious arguments of the type that effects X and Y are not due to A because they are annulled by D."

Further, in many of the studies on brain slices only one concentration of antagonist was used. In none of these studies were antagonist affinities estimated, nor was competitive antagonism proved. For these purposes, Schild plots (Arunlakshana and Schild, 1959) are extremely useful and were, in fact, used to classify histamine receptors and to define the first H_2 antagonist (Black et al., 1972). With these methods, the adenylate cyclase activity in guinea pig cardiac ventricle was shown to be linked to H_2 receptors (Johnson and Mizoguchi, 1977).

Only a few studies have been reported of the effect of histamine on adenylate cyclase activity in broken cell preparations of brain (Chasin et al., 1974; Spiker et al., 1976; Hegstrand et al., , 1976). Hegstrand et al. (1976) concluded that adenylate cyclase activity in homogenates of the guinea pig hippocampus was associated with H_2 receptors, not H_1 receptors. The conclusion was based on (1) the excellent agreement between the dissociation constant of metiamide for the enzyme and for known H_2 receptors; (2) the ineffectiveness of mepyramine, at a concentration (10^{-8} M) known to inhibit H_1 receptors, to inhibit the adenylate cyclase; (3) the relative potencies of histamine, 4-methylhistamine, and 2-methylhistamine on hippocampal adenylate cyclase correlated with agonist activity on H_2-receptor systems.

Although measuring the relative potencies of agonists on different systems has helped to classify histamine receptors (Ash and Schild, 1966; Black et al., 1972), it is not a dependable criterion, for the relative agonist potencies on different H_2-receptor systems do not always agree. For example, dimaprit, an H_2 agonist, has 17 to 20% of the activity of histamine on the rat uterus and on rat gastric acid secretion, 71% of the activity of histamine on the guinea pig atrium, and 400 to 500% on cat gastric acid secretion (Parsons et al., 1977). 2-Thiazolylethylamine is 0.3 and 3.1% as active as histamine on gastric secretion (Durant et al., 1975a) and atrium (Parsons, 1976), respectively. The corresponding figures for $N\alpha,N\alpha$-dimethylhistamine are 19 and 51% (Durant et al., 1975a; Black et al., 1972).

Our studies were designed to define the histamine receptor associated with adenylate cyclase activity in brain. During the course of the work, we found that D-lysergic acid diethylamide (D-LSD) is a competitive antagonist of H_2 receptors linked to adenylate cyclase, both in the hippocampus and in the heart ventricle.

MATERIALS AND METHODS

Preparation of Tissue

Membrane bound adenylate cyclase was prepared from guinea pig or rat tissues by homogenization in a medium containing 0.32 M sucrose, 5 mM Tris-chloride, 1 mM EGTA, and 1 mM dithiothreitol, pH 7.4. The brain samples were homogenized by three 5-second bursts of a Polytron (Brinkman) followed by motor driven homogenization with a Potter–Elvejhem homogenizer. Brain homogenates were centrifuged at 1000 × g and the supernates were recentrifuged at 27,000 × g. The resulting pellet was washed twice by resuspension in the same medium and recentrifugation. The final pellet was suspended in the same medium at a protein concentration of 0.5 to 0.7 mg/ml. The homogenates from heart ventricle were centrifuged at 1000 × g and the pellet was washed twice. The final 1000 × g pellet was suspended in the same medium at a protein concentration of 1 to 2 mg/ml. Both the brain and cardiac membranes could be quickly frozen with dry ice–acetone and stored at $-70°$C. The cardiac enzyme lost little basal activity or histamine sensitivity on storage. Brain preparations were somewhat less stable: freezing invariably resulting in an increase in basal activity and a decrease in maximal histamine activation, but the agonist potencies (ED_{50} values) and antagonist affinities were not altered by freezing and storage.

Adenylate Cyclase Assay

To facilitate the comparisons of the brain enzyme with our previously published data on the cardiac enzyme (Johnson and Mizoguchi, 1977), the same assay system was used: 75 mM Tris-chloride (pH 7.4), 1 mM ATP, 2 mM MgCl$_2$, 1 mM cAMP, 5 mM phosphocreatine, 0.5 mg/ml creatinephosphokinase, 4 mM theophylline, 10^{-5} M GTP (unless otherwise noted), 0.1 M sucrose, 0.3 mM EGTA, 0.3 mM dithiothreitol, and enzyme protein (30 to 150 μg) in a final volume of 225 μl. All assays were performed in triplicate. All additions were made to the assay tubes on ice. They were then transferred to a 30°C shaking incubator and preincubated for 5 minutes to allow the enzymatic activity to reach a steady state and to eliminate the influence of any lag periods in hormone activation. After the preincubation period, 25μl [α-^{32}P]-ATP (1–2 μCi) were added and in most cases the reaction was allowed to proceed for 10 minutes at which time the reaction was stopped by addition of 100 μl of 1% sodium dodecylsulfate. After addition of 650 μl ^{3}H-cAMP (5000–10,000 CPM) to monitor recovery, the labeled cAMP was isolated with an alumina–Dowex column by the procedure of Saloman et al. (1974). The reaction was linear with protein concentration in the range employed and for at least 15 minutes after the addition of the [α-^{32}P]-ATP. Protein was measured by the method of Lowry et al. (1951).

Treatment of the Data

Curve fitting techniques (Parker and Waud, 1971) were used to estimate the apparent ED$_{50}$ values, maximum stimulation by agonists, and parallelism of the dose-response curves. Antagonism was analyzed by means of Schild plots (Schild, 1947; Arunlakshana and Schild, 1959) in which antagonism is expressed by the dose-ratios (DR) of agonist needed for equal response before and after different concentrations of antagonists (B). Simple competitive antagonism results in a straight line of slope 1 when log (DR-1) is plotted against log (B); and the intercept with the abscissa is –log K_B, where K_B is the apparent dissociation constant for the antagonist-receptor interaction (–log K_B is sometimes referred to as pA_2).

Drugs

All histamine analogs and H$_2$ antagonists were generously provided by Drs. C.R. Ganellin and M. Parsons of Smith Kline and French Laboratories. D-LSD, L-LSD, psilocin, mescaline, and D-2-brom-LSD (BOL) were provided by the National Institute on Drug Abuse. Methysergide was obtained from Sandoz, mepyramine and cyproheptadine from Merck Sharpe and Dohme.

RESULTS

Effects of Histamine Agonists and Antagonists

Dose-response curves to histamine on the guinea pig hippocampal adenylate cyclase were obtained in 38 experiments on 11 different enzyme preparations. In fresh preparations the average basal activity ranged from 70 to 90 pmoles of cAMP formed/minute/mg protein, and this activity always increased by as much as 50% upon freezing and storage. After subtraction of basal activity, maximal histamine stimulation in fresh preparations generally averaged 60 to 100 pmoles of c-AMP formed/minute/mg protein and was somewhat decreased by freezing and storage. The ED_{50} of histamine was 1.43 (± 0.06) $\times$ 10^{-5} M (mean $\pm$S.E.M.). As shown before (Hegstrand et $al.$, 1976), adenylate cyclase activity in the guinea pig cortex is about as sensitive to histamine as that in the hippocampus (Table I).

Rat hippocampal adenylate cyclase, though less sensitive than the guinea pig preparation, is also stimulated by histamine (Table II), in contrast to previous observations (Hegstrand et $al.$, 1976). The enzyme in two rat ventricles was not responsive to histamine.

Dimaprit, a compound with considerable H_2-agonist activity but with less than 0.0001% of the activity of histamine on H_1 receptors (Parson et $al.$, 1977), was active in the same concentration range as was histamine on the guinea pig hippocampal enzyme. The results obtained with this histamine agonist are consistent with the view that the hippocampus contains only an H_2 receptor linked to adenylate cyclase.

Table I
Effect of Histamine on Adenylate Cyclase Activity in
Different Regions of the Guinea Pig Brain[a]

		Adenylate cyclase activity[b]			
			Histamine concentration, M		
Brain area	Basal	10^{-6}	10^{-5}	10^{-4}	10^{-3}
Hippocampus	72.2	78.0	99.8	127.5	140.1
Cortex	48.4	52.5	77.8	99.6	105.1
Striatum	89.4	92.6	99.1	107.9	114.4
Thalamus	18.3	19.7	24.3	27.3	27.4
Hypothalamus	42.9	44.6	47.0	49.5	49.4
Central gray	56.8	58.0	59.6	62.5	61.6

[a]This represents one series of experiments on membranes. Each region was studied at least twice with similar results. A study on whole homogenates gave very similar results.
[b]pmoles of cAMP formed/minute/mg protein.

Table II
Effect of Histamine on Rat Hippocampal Adenylate Cyclase
Activity

| Histamine M | Animal[a] | | |
| | 1 | 2 | 3 |
	pmoles cAMP/minute/mg protein		
0	21.5 ± 0.2	19.6 ± 0.4	19.4 ± 0.2
10^{-6}	21.8 ± 0.1	19.7 ± 0.5	19.6 ± 0.4
10^{-5}	24.5 ± 0.5	21.5 ± 0.1	22.2 ± 0.3
10^{-4}	27.8 ± 0.3	25.0 ± 0.1	25.9 ± 0.4
10^{-3}	30.0 ± 0.5	27.0 ± 0.2	27.6 ± 0.1

[a]The amount of homogenate protein was 193 μg, 187 μg, and 191 μg, respectively, for the three animals. Activity is expressed as pmoles of cAMP formed/minute/mg protein.

More persuasive evidence is provided by studies of the affinities of H_2 and H_1 antagonists. Typical dose response curves are shown for histamine (Fig. 1) and dimaprit (Fig. 2) in the absence and presence of the H_2 antagonist, cimetidine. Cimetidine had no effect on basal enzyme activity. Figure 3 shows the Schild plot for cimetidine with 10 determinations on 4 preparations using histamine as the agonist and with 2 determinations on 1 preparation using dimaprit as the agonist. The slope of the Schild plot was 0.90 ± 0.07, a value not significantly different from the value of 1.0 predicted by assuming simple

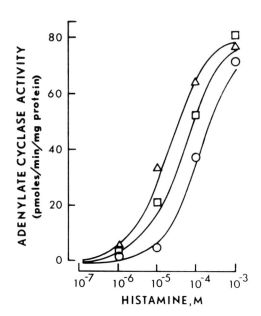

FIG. 1.   Adenylate cyclase activity of the guinea pig hippocampus in response to varying concentrations of histamine in the absence (△) and presence of $10^{-6} M$ (□) or $4 \times 10^{-6} M$ (○) cimetidine. Each point represents the increase in adenylate cyclase activity above basal level (no histamine) and is the mean of triplicate determinations on a single enzyme preparation. Cimetidine alone did not affect basal activity.

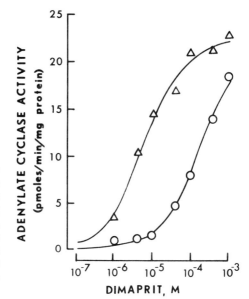

FIG. 2. Adenylate cyclase activity of the guinea pig hippocampus in response to varying concentrations of dimaprit in the absence ($\triangle$) and presence ($\bigcirc$) of 10^{-5} M cimetidine. Each point represents the increase in adenylate cyclase activity above basal level (no histamine) and is the mean of triplicate determinations on a single enzyme preparation.

competitive kinetics. The pA_2 value calculated using all 12 data in the figure was 6.22 ± 0.10 (mean $\pm$ S.E.M.), in essential agreement with the values of 6.10 and 6.09 obtained on the atrium and the uterus, respectively, and very different from the value of 3.4 obtained on H_1 receptors in the ileum (Brimblecombe *et al.,* 1975). The fact that the dose response curves of both histamine and the H_2-selective dimaprit are shifted to the same degree by

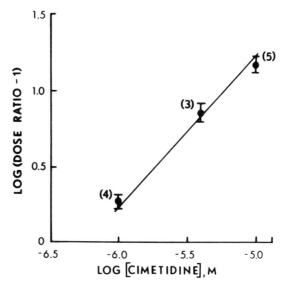

FIG. 3. Schild plot for inhibition by cimetidine of histamine-stimulated adenylate cyclase activity of the guinea pig hippocampus. The dose ratios were calculated as the ratio of the ED_{50} of histamine in the presence of cimetidine to the ED_{50} in the absence of antagonist. The vertical bars represent the S.E.M. for the number of determinations shown in parentheses. The line has unit slope and an X-intercept (pA_2 value) of 6.22.

cimetidine clearly establishes that both agonists are reacting solely with H_2 receptors linked to adenylate cyclase. In two experiments with the H_2 antagonist metiamide we obtained a pA_2 value of 6.06, precisely the value reported by others (Hegstrand *et al.*, 1976), and similar to the values of 6.04, 6.12, and 5.91 obtained on atrial rate, uterine contractility, and gastric secretion, respectively (Black *et al.*, 1974; Bunce and Parsons, 1976).

The H_1-antagonist mepyramine, which has a pA_2 value of 9.4 on H_1 receptors in the ileum (Arunlakshana and Schild, 1959), was reported to be ineffective at 10^{-6} M on hippocampal adenylate cyclase (Hegstrand *et al.*, 1976). At sufficiently high concentration, this compound does act as a competitive antagonist on the guinea pig hippocampal enzyme (Fig. 4) with a pA_2 value of 5.24 (mean of two experiments). This value is in excellent agreement with the estimated value of 5.3 obtained on the H_2 receptors in atria (Trendelenburg, 1960). Mepyramine also blocked the effect of dimaprit, which has virtually no H_1 activity. The pA_2 value of mepyramine was 5.09.

Histamine antagonists were studied for their effects on histamine activated adenylate cyclase in the guinea pig ventricle. The pA_2 values for the ventricle and the hippocampus are very similar (Table III). The pA_2 values of these H_2 antagonists on the cyclase were nearly identical to the pA_2 values on pharmacological preparations (Table III). But the pA_2 values of the H_1 antagonists on these cylcases differed considerably from the pA_2 values on the H_1 receptor (Table III).

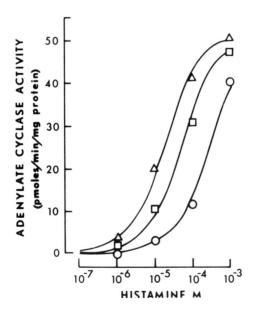

FIG. 4. Adenylate cyclase activity of the guinea pig hippocampus in response to varying concentrations of histamine in the absence ($\triangle$) and presence of 10^{-5} M ($\square$) or 10^{-4} M ($\bigcirc$) mepyramine. Each point represents the increase in adenylate cyclase activity above basal level (no histamine) and is the mean of triplicate determinations on a single enzyme preparation. Cyclase activity was corrected for the slight depression (less than 20%) in basal activity caused by mepyramine alone.

Table III
pA$_2$ Values of Histamine Antagonists

| Antagonists | pA$_2$ on Adenylate Cyclase Activity | | pA$_2$ on Pharmacological Preparations | | | |
| | | | H$_2$ Receptors | | | H$_1$ Receptors |
H$_2$	Ventricle[a]	Hippocampus[a]	atrium[b]	uterus[c]	acid secretion[d]	ileum[e]
Imidazolylpropyl-methylthiourea	3.23 ± 0.09 (3)	3.33 ± 0.02 (2)	3.5[f]			
Nα-guanylhistamine	3.87 ± 0.10 (3)		3.9[g]			3.8[g]
Imidazolylpropyl-guanidine	4.86 ± 0.04 (3)		4.65[h]			
Burimamide	4.96 ± 0.16 (3)		5.11[i]	5.18[i]	5.14[i]	3.5[i]
Thiaburimamide	5.38 ± 0.13 (4)	5.62 ± 0.07 (2)	5.49[j]	5.49[j]		
Metiamide	5.97 ± 0.07 (4)	6.06 ± 0.14 (2)	6.04[k]	6.12[k]	5.91[l]	
Cimetidine	6.14 ± 0.05 (9)	6.22 ± 0.03 (12)	6.10[m]	6.09[m]		3.4[m]
H$_1$						
Mepyramine	5.15 ± 0.04 (3)	5.24 ± 0.03(2)	5.3[n]			9.4[o]
Tripelennamine	5.36 ± 0.30 (3)					8.5[p]

[a]This work, [b]chronotropic effect, [c]histamine inhibition of contractility, rat, [d]rat, [e]contractility, guinea pig, [f]C.R. Ganellin, unpublished. [g]Durant *et al.* (1975b), [h]Parsons *et al.* (1975), [i]Black *et al.* (1972a), [k]Black *et al.* (1974), [l]Bunce and Parsons (1976), [m]Brimblecombe *et al.* (1975), [n]Trendelenburg (1960), [o]Arunlakshana and Schild (1959), [p]Marshall (1955).

193

Effects of LSD and Related Compounds

The hallucinogen D-LSD is a potent antagonist of both histamine-(Fig. 5) and dimaprit-(Fig. 6) activated guinea pig hippocampal adenylate cyclase. D-LSD had no significant effects on basal activity. D-LSD was examined in 17 measurements on 10 preparations, and the Schild plot (Fig. 7) indicated a slope of 1.09 ± 0.03 (mean $\pm$ S.E.M.). Thus, D-LSD has a potency on H_2 receptors similar to that of the potent H_2 antagonists, metiamide and cimetidine. The L-isomer of LSD was without effect on histamine activated adenylate cyclase at a concentration of 10^{-4} M (Table IV); it is thus at least 100 times less potent than D-LSD (higher concentrations were not studied owing to insufficient material). D-2-brom-LSD (BOL), was found to be 10 times more potent than D-LSD (Fig. 8). The histamine-activated ventricular adenylate cyclase showed an identical response to D-LSD and BOL (Table V). The Schild plot for BOL (Fig. 9) had a slope of 1.14 ± 0.10 and the pA_2 value (17 determinations on 7 preparations) was 7.16 ± 0.04 (mean $\pm$ S.E.M.). BOL, unlike D-LSD, consistently depressed basal activity, up to 20% at the highest concentrations tested. This fall in basal activity was subtracted in the analyses shown in Fig. 8 and 9.

Psilocin (10^{-4} M), bufotenine 10^{-5} M), mescaline (10^{-3} M), propranolol (10^{-4} M), methysergide (10^{-5} M) did not antagonize the effects of histamine on guinea pig hippocampal adenylate cyclase. But cyproheptadine acted as a potent competitive antagonist (Fig. 10) with a pA_2 of 7.2 (three determinations on one preparation).

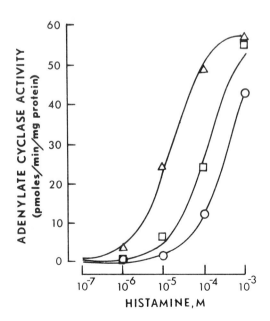

FIG. 5.   Adenylate cyclase activity of the guinea pig hippocampus in response to varying concentrations of histamine in the absence ($\triangle$) and presence of 6×10^{-6} M($\square$) or 2×10^{-5} M ($\bigcirc$) D-LSD. Each point represents the increase in adenylate cyclase activity above basal level (no histamine) and is the mean of triplicate determinations on a single enzyme preparation. D-LSD itself had no effect on basal activity.

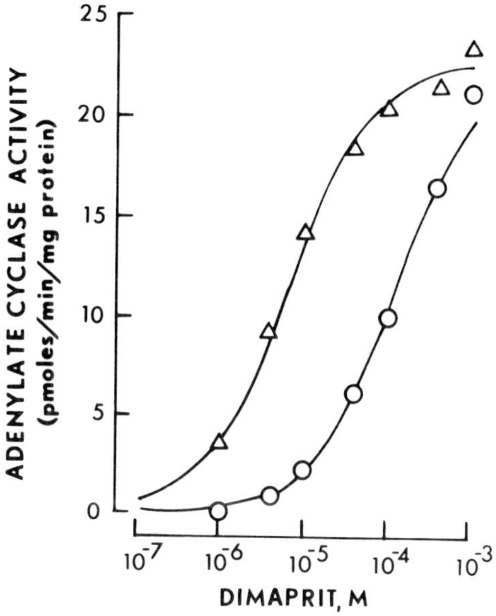

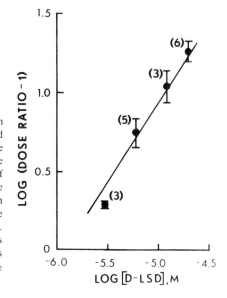

FIG. 6. Adenylate cyclase activity of the guinea pig hippocampus in response to varying concentrations of dimaprit in the absence ($\triangle$) and presence ($\bigcirc$) of 10^{-5} M D-LSD. Each point represents the increase in adenylate cyclase activity above basal level (no histamine) and is the mean of triplicate determinations on a single enzyme preparation.

FIG. 7. Schild plot for inhibition by D-LSD of histamine-stimulated adenylate cyclase activity of the guinea pig hippocampus. The dose ratios were calculated as the ratio of the ED_{50} of histamine in the presence of D-LSD to the ED_{50} in the absence of antagonist. The vertical bars represent the S.E.M. for the number of determinations shown in parentheses. The line has unit slope and an X-intercept (pA_2 value) of 5.95.

Table IV

Effect of L-LSD on Guinea Pig Hippocampal Adenylate Cyclase Activity

| Histamine (M) | Control | Adenylate cyclase activity[a] | | |
| | | L-LSD, (M) | | |
		10^{-6}	10^{-5}	10^{-4}
10^{-6}	6.6	3.0	8.1	4.4
10^{-5}	27.4	25.1	28.5	25.3
10^{-4}	50.8	46.5	52.2	57.4
10^{-3}	63.1	58.8	63.3	62.2

[a]The values, pmoles of cAMP formed/minute/mg protein, are the increase in cyclase activity above basal levels and are the means of triplicate determinations on a single enzyme preparation.

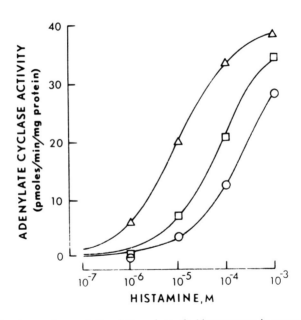

FIG. 8.   Adenylate cyclase activity of the guinea pig hippocampus in response to varying concentrations of histamine in the absence ($\triangle$) and presence of $4 \times 10^{-7}\,M$ ($\square$) or $1.4 \times 10^{-6}\,M$ ($\bigcirc$) D-2-brom-LSD (BOL). Each point represents the increase in adenylate cyclase activity above basal level (no histamine) and is the mean of triplicate determinations on a single enzyme preparation. BOL alone caused slight depressions of basal activity (less than 20%) and this effect was corrected for in the figure.

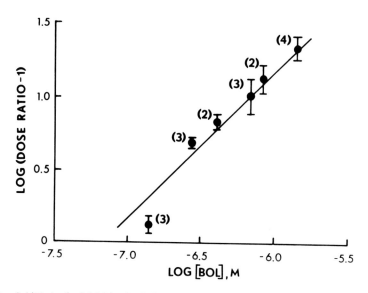

FIG. 9. Schild plot for inhibition by *D*-2-brom-LSD (BOL) of histamine-stimulated adenylate cyclase activity of the guinea pig hippocampus. The dose ratios were calculated as the ratio of the ED_{50} of histamine in the presence of BOL to the ED_{50} in the absence of antagonist. The vertical bars represent the S.E.M. for the number of determinations shown in parentheses. The line has unit slope and an X-intercept (pA_2 value) of 7.16.

FIG. 10. Adenylate cyclase activity of the guinea pig hippocampus in response to varying concentrations of histamine in the absence ($\triangle$) and presence of 10^{-7} M ($\square$) or 10^{-6} M ($\bigcirc$) cyproheptadine. Each data point represents the increase in adenylate cyclase activity above basal level (no histamine) and is the mean of triplicate determinations on a single enzyme preparation. Cyproheptadine alone caused slight depressions of basal activity (less than 20%) and this effect was corrected for in the figure.

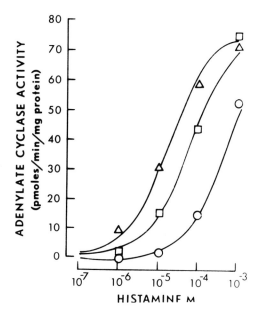

Since LSD and its analogs and cyproheptadine act at some serotonin (5-HT) receptors, we examined the possible interactions between 5-HT and histamine on the guinea pig hippocampal adenylate cyclase. In some experiments. addition of high concentrations of 5-HT (10^{-4} M) or in the presence of histamine resulted in less activation of the hippocampal adenylate cyclase than histamine alone. Although 5-HT may have a low affinity for histamine on the guinea pig hippocampal adenylate cyclase. In some experiments, addition of high concentrations of 5-HT (10^{-4} M) in the presence of histamine resulted in less activation of the hippocampal adenylate cyclase than histamine alone. Although 5-HT may have a low affinity for histamine H_2 receptors, the analysis is complicated by the 5-HT-induced stimulation of activity: in 7 experiments on 5 preparations, 5-HT caused maximal stimulations of 22 to 51% above basal activity (absolute increases of 15.4 to 39.8 pmoles cAMP formed/minute/mg protein). As the actions of 5-HT will be reported in detail elsewhere, only the salient facts are noted: the apparent ED_{50} for 5-HT averaged $3 + 10^{-7}$ M under our standard assay conditions; three substances that blocked histamine in this system—cimetidine (10^{-5} M), cyproheptadine (10^{-6} M) and BOL (10^{-5} M)—had no significant effect on the 5-HT activated cyclase in concentrations 10 times their pA_2 values against histamine; D-LSD, but not L-LSD, acted as a competitive inhibitor of 5-HT with a pA_2 value similar to that for inhibition of histamine.

The histamine-stimulated adenylate cyclase in the hippocampus of the guinea pig is an H_2 receptor, as previously shown (Hegstrand et al., 1976). This is true for the guinea pig ventricle as well (Table V). In both preparations, H_2 antagonists competitively block this effect of histamine, with pA_2 values almost identical to those obtained on known H_2 systems (Table III). The H_1 antagonist, mepyramine, also blocked histamine-activated adenylate cyclase, but the pA_2 values were low, i.e., the concentration of mepyramine needed to block this system was far higher than that needed to block H_1 receptors (Table III). The blockade by mepyramine of dimaprit, an H_2 agonist with almost no H_1 activity (i.e., 0.0001% of that of histamine), clearly shows that high concentrations of H_1 antagonists can block H_2 receptors.

We have not yet examined the effects of histamine antagonists on the histamine-activated adenylate cyclase in other regions of the brain. Electrophysiological studies have revealed only H_2 receptors in various parts of the brain (see Sastry and Phillis, 1976; Haas and Wolf, 1977).

Histamine-sensitive adenylate cyclase was prominent in the hippocampus and cortex (Hegstrand et al., 1976; Table I), which contain far less histamine than other parts of the brain, e.g., hypothalamus, thalamus, caudate nucleus, raphe nucleus, central grey (see tabulation by Green, 1970; more recent studies by Taylor et al., 1972; Abou et al., , 1973). These histamine-rich areas

Table V
Effect of D-LSD and BOL on Guinea Pig Ventricular Adenylate Cyclase Activity

Histamine (M)	Adenylate Cyclase Activity[a]			
	Experiment 1		Experiment 2	
	control	D-LSD $2 \times 10^{-5}\ M$	control	BOL $5 \times 10^{-5}\ M$
10^{-6}	24.7	0.6	25.1	5.7
10^{-5}	93.9	11.0	89.4	27.9
10^{-4}	118.0	48.1	126.4	88.5
10^{-3}	137.2	114.9	148.1	123.5

[a]The values, pmoles of cAMP formed/minute/mg protein, are the increase in cyclase activity above basal levels and are the means of triplicate determinations on a single enzyme preparation.

showed relatively little histamine-stimulated adenylate cyclase activity. The receptors for histamine may be either more abundant or the adenylate cyclase may be more sensitive in the hippocampus and cortex than in other areas of the brain. There have been no published studies of high-affinity binding of histamine in the brain. Based on studies of other systems (Brown et al., 1976; Mukherjee et al., 1976), one can expect that the affinities of H_2 antagonists for the histamine-stimulated adenylate cyclase predict their affinities for the high affinity binding sites for histamine.

The histamine receptors may well have function in the brain. Lesion studies have revealed histaminergic nerve endings in the hippocampus and cortex— the latter from fibers ascending in the medial forebrain bundle, the former from fibers entering by a dorsal route that includes the fimbria and by a ventral route through the amygdala (Barbin et al., 1975, 1976; Garbarg et al., 1976). Hippocampal and cortical neurons, like almost all other neurons in the rat and cat, are depressed by direct application of histamine; only those in the hypothalamus are excited (see Sastry and Phillis, 1976; Haas and Wolf, 1976). Electrical stimulation of the medial forebrain bundle depressed the firing of cortical neurons (Sastry and Phillis, 1976), and electrical stimulation of the fornix depressed the firing of hippocampal cells (Haas and Wolf, 1977). Application of metiamide blocked both these depressions (Sastry and Phillis, 1976; Haas and Wolf, 1977). Metiamide did not block the histamine-induced excitation of the hypothalamic nuclei (Haas and Wolf, 1977). H_1 antagonists blocked neither the effects of histamine nor of electrical stimulation (see Sastry and Phillis, 1976; Haas and Wolf, 1977).

It is intriguing that histamine not only increases cAMP formation but perhaps its destruction as well, for in high concentrations it has been shown to increase the activity of cyclic 3',5'-nucleotide phosphodiesterase (Roberts and Simonsen, 1970). This dual action could serve as a homeostatic control system—release of histamine increases cAMP formation, and a release of large amounts of histamine, by activating the phosphodiesterase, hydrolyzes the cAMP. 3-Methyl-imidazoleacetic acid, the major metabolite of histamine in brain, could contribute to the homeostatic mechanism, for it is potent in increasing phosphodiesterase activity. This metabolite, incidentally, also has effects on neurons, e.g., like histamine, it depresses firing of cat brain stem neurons (Haas *et al.*, 1973) [but not cortical neurons (Godfraind *et al.*, 1973)].

Molecular Considerations in Activation of H₂ Receptors

The molecular structural factors that differentiate between H_1 and H_2 activity of histamine agonists appear to be related to the tautomerism of the imidazole ring (Durant *et al.*, 1975a; Bonnet and Ibers, 1973; Prout *et al.*, 1974). Structural changes, both in the imidazole ring and in the side chain, affect the tautomeric ratio. The effect of these structural modifications can be best understood and predicted if their effect on the electronic structure of histamine is first determined. We showed (Weinstein *et al.*, 1976) that certain characteristic changes appear in the electronic structure of the imidazole ring when the protonated side chain amine in histamine monocation dissociates to yield the free base. These calculations reveal the electronic mechanism responsible for the shift in the tautomeric ratio: the N(3) nitrogen becomes less basic than the N(1) nitrogen when the electronic charge is redistributed in the imidazole ring and the side chain is neutralized. Identical changes in the electronic structure occur when histamine monocation interacts with a negatively charged reagent (such as an OH^- group). The calculations predicted, therefore, that the shift in tautomeric ratio caused by the transition from histamine monocation to histamine free base should also be observed when the monocation is neutralized by interacting with an anionic site.

This finding provides a mechanistic model for the role of imidazole tautomerism in the activation of the H_2 receptor. On this same basis, it was shown that histamine analogs in which the imidazole ring has been modified should differ in their ability to generate a "charge relay" structure in which tautomerism could be responsible for the transport of a proton from one site of the receptor to another. This structure is illustrated for histamine in Fig. 11. It is evident from the theoretical model that the interaction of the protonated side chain amine at site I triggers the transition of a proton from the vicinity of the N(3) nitrogen to site II of the receptor model and from site III of the receptor model to the N(1) nitrogen of hsitamine. Since the interactions are assumed to occur simultaneously at all three sites the proposed mechanism is fully reversible and the imidazole ring would regain its preferred tautomeric

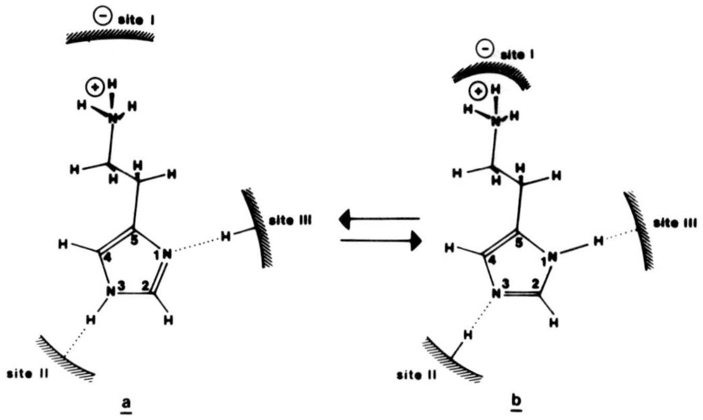

FIG. 11.   Proposed charge-relay mechanism for histamine activation of the H_2 receptor. Histamine reacts with the receptor through its cationic head (i.e., the protonated amino group) at Site I and through the N(3)H and N(1) groups at sites II and III, respectively. Neutralization of the cationic head triggers transition of a proton from N(3)H to site II and transition of a proton from site III of the receptor to N(1).

form when the protonated side chain dissociates from the anionic site I (Weinstein *et al.*, 1976).

The same mechanism can be written for other H_2 agonists, regardless of their atom-to-atom resemblance to histamine, provided that a "proton releasing fragment," a "proton accepting fragment" and a "triggering mechanism" can be identified in their molecular structure. An interesting example is the pure H_2 agonist, dimaprit (Parsons *et al.*, 1977). Due to π-electron conjugation, the isothiourea in dimaprit is strictly planar and sterically fully congruent with the imidazole ring of hsitamine. The charge relay system that can be established by this portion of dimaprit is shown in Fig. 12. The proton at site III is attracted by the highly nucleophilic region generated in the vicinity of the sulfur atom by the two lone pair electrons. Due to the conjugation in the isothiourea moiety, this interaction at the sulfur atom should cause the weakening of the N–H bond at site II and thereby establish the proton transfer (Green *et al.*, 1978). It is well known, however, that the protonated sulfur is an extremely labile species and the entire process is probably rapidly reversed to produce the thermodynamically more stable species; the transient change could be enough to trigger an activation of the receptor.

The proposed system contains all the elements necessary for our dynamic model of receptor activation: the triggering of the change is induced either by an interaction at the anionic site or by the thermodynamical instability of the S–H adduct; the proton accepting and proton releasing moieties are sterically

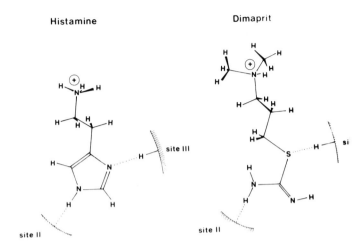

FIG. 12.   Analogy between the charge-relay models for histamine and dimaprit.

equivalent to their counterparts in histamine. The model is supported by experimental data on the activity of several analogues of dimaprit recently tested. Replacement of the sulfur by an NH group abolishes activity (Durant *et al.*, 1977a), presumably because the proton accepting moiety has been removed. Removal of a CH_2 group in the side chain reduces H_2 activity (Durant *et al.*, 1977a); molecular models show that it is difficult to achieve congruency between histamine and this dimaprit analogue, i.e., the histamine N(1) cannot be superimposed on S nor can the histamine N(3) be superimposed on the NH_2 of the analogue.

Another model proposed to account for the activity of dimaprit (Durant *et al.*, 1977a) is untenable. In this model the two nitrogens in dimaprit are not at all congruent with those in the imidazole ring of histamine; the proposed charge relay between the two nitrogens of the isothiourea is independent of any interaction with a receptor site and consequently will have no reason to occur once an interaction at sites II and III has been established. Second, the model lacks a mechanism to trigger proton transfer for the charge relay. These two deficiencies of the model should impair H_2-agonist activity. That congruency is important is clear from the activities of other histamine analogs: 2-thiazolylethylamine, 5-thiazolylethylamine and 3-pyrazolylethylamine (betazole) are all compounds in which slight structural changes in the imidazole ring result in a sharp fall in H_2 activity although tautomerism is still possible, at least in principle (Durant *et al.*, 1975a). That tautomerism controlled charge relay is not enough for agonist activity is clear from the molecular structure of H_2 antagonists: although the imidazole ring is intact, the compounds lack agonist activity. This indicates that a mechanism is necessary to trigger the charge relay when the molecule interacts with the receptor.

The triggering mechanism for histamine and dimaprit has been described above (Weinstein *et al.*, 1976; Green *et al.*, 1978). It can be reduced by eliminating the side chain amino group by or by introducing groups that reduce the effect of interaction at site I on the imidazole ring. Thus, Nα-guanylhistamine is still a partial agonist (Durant *et al.*, 1975b; Table III), but when additional groups are added to the side chain, the resulting burimamide, metiamide, and cimetidine and even their guanidine isostere show only antagonist properties (Durant *et al.*, 1977b). This could result either from the total loss of interaction with site I or from a change in the consequences of that interaction, i.e., the interaction at site I does not cause a charge redistribution in the imidazole ring. Charge redistribution in the imidazole ring can be prevented by the many electronegative and polarizable groups attached to the side chain in the antagonists, e.g., $-C=N-C\equiv N$, $C-S-C$, $-C=S$; the charge is channelled into these groups rather than into the imidazole ring. The triggering mechanism for tautomerism is, thus, lost, even though the imidazole nitrogens could still have acted as proton acceptor and proton donor groups. A model for H_2-receptor activation that invokes tautomerism without a mechanism to trigger it is difficult to accept.

Methylation of the imidazole ring has been shown to affect the tautomeric ratio (Ganellin, 1974). An important qualitative effect of 2- and 4-methylation is the increased differentiation between H_1 and H_2 activity: 4-methyl histamine has an H_1/H_2 activity ratio of 0.005, while 2-methyl histamine is preferentially an H_1 agonist with an H_1/H_2 ratio of 4 (Ganellin *et al.*, 1973). Both compounds, however, have lower H_2 activity than does histamine. This decrease in potency could be related, at least in part, to changes induced by the methyl groups in the proton affinities of the imidazole nitrogens. Our calculations predicted (Green *et al.*, 1978) that the $N(1)$ nitrogen of 4-methylhistamine will have a slightly increased proton affinity compared to $N(1)$ in histamine, while the 2-methyl derivative will have an even more basic $N(1)$ nitrogen. As a result, the calculations indicate that the dication species, in which both ring nitrogens bind hydrogens, will be much more abundant in 2-methylhistamine than in histamine or even in the 4-methyl derivative. The relation between calculations of proton affinity and measured pKa values has been established theoretically (Weinstein *et al.*, 1977). The results are in full accord with measured pKa values (Ganellin, 1974). Further, a recent thermodynamical analysis of the effects of methylation on the measured basicity of the imidazole ring in histamine, histidine, thyrotropin releasing factor and related compounds (Paiva *et al.*, 1976) confirmed our theoretical results: the proton affinity of the imidazole ring in the 2-methyl derivative is about five times that in the 4-methyl derivative. Consequently, the decrease in H_2 activity with $C(2)$ and $C(4)$ methylation can be related to the higher proportion of dication compared to histamine, for the dication cannot interact at site III. The charge relay could be established only by the small fraction of monocation molecules; since this fraction is diminished in the ring methylated derivatives, potency of these compounds should be lower than that of histamine, with 2-methylhistamine being by far the weakest H_2 agonist.

Histamine and the Pharmacology of D-LSD

D-LSD is as potent as cimetidine in blocking the H_2 receptor (compare Fig. 5 and 6 with 1 and 2) and, like cimetidine, it is a competitive antagonist of histamine (cf. Figs. 7 and 3). The pA_2 value of D-LSD was 5.95, very nearly that of cimetidine, 6.22, and of metiamide, 6.06. The L-isomer, which has no measurable hallucinogenic activity (Isbell et al., 1959), did not antagonize the histamine-activated adenylate cyclase (Table IV). The topological congruency of D-LSD and H_2 antagonists is clear, metiamide being shown as the representative H_2 antagonist (Fig. 13). Quantum chemical studies should reveal commonalities between D-LSD and H_2 antagonists as they have between tryptamines and D-LSD (Green et al., 1977). BOL was ten-times more potent than D-LSD in inhibiting histamine-stimulated adenylate cyclase activity (cf. Figs. 8 and 5 and 9 and 7). Interestingly, it did not block the 5-HT-stimulated cyclase, while D-LSD did.

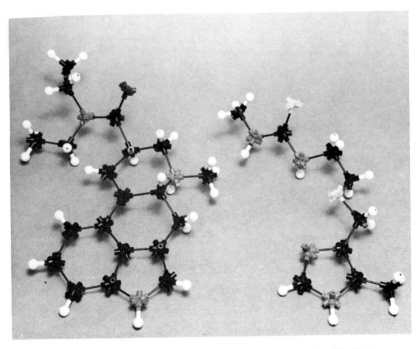

FIG. 13. Topological congruency of D-LSD (left) and metiamide (right).

BOL is not "inactive," as frequently stated. BOL produced D-LSD-like effects in man after intravenous injection of high doses (Schneckloth *et al.*, 1957). After oral administration of high doses, BOL produced mental changes, though not the full effect of D-LSD, notably, visual hallucinations; it was also less active than D-LSD on the knee-jerk, blood pressure, and pupillary diameter (Isbell *et al.*, 1959; Bertino *et al.*, 1959). In rats BOL was one-fifth as potent as D-LSD when tested in a swimming paradigm (Uyeno, 1968) and one-tenth in disrupting bar-pressing (Appel and Freedman, 1965). BOL was much less active than D-LSD in directly inhibiting firing of neurons in the dorsal raphe neurons; high intravenous doses also inhibit (Aghajanian *et al.*, 1970). BOL is slightly less active on postsynaptic sites in the ventral lateral geniculate, and much less active on postsynaptic sites in the amygdala (Aghajanian, 1976) and in blocking 5-HT-inhibition of the hippocampus (Segal, 1976). BOL blocks D-LSD *in vivo* (Corne and Pickering, 1967). BOL has about the same affinities as does D-LSD for the high-affinity binding sites for D-LSD (Bennett and Snyder, 1976; Lovell and Freedman, 1976) and for dopamine, and a greater affinity for the haloperidol binding sites (Creese *et al.*, 1976). It is thus clear that BOL does not produce the total hallucinogenic effect in man of D-LSD, but its agonist and antagonist properties on many neural systems are comparable with those of D-LSD.

Histamine is distinguished in being one of the few putative transmitters that have not been invoked to explain the pharmacology of D-LSD (see review by Freedman and Halaris, 1978). We could find only two studies showing a relationship between D-LSD and histamine. D-LSD appeared to reduce, but not significantly, the lethality of histamine in rats (Weltman and Sackler, 1965). In man, intravenous administration of an H_1 antagonist accentuated the effects of D-LSD (Yamada *et al.*, 1957). The finding that D-LSD is a competitive antagonist of histamine now enlists histamine as an additional substance implicated in the pharmacological effects of D-LSD.

There is no reason to believe that blockade of histamine explains the hallucinogenic or any of the other numerous pharmacological effects of D-LSD. There is also no reason to believe that any other effect of D-LSD on any other single system and site explains the hallucinogenic or any other effect of D-LSD. Any search for a single site and mechanism to explain an effect as complex as hallucinations is likely to be frustrated. More likely, the behavioral and other effects produced by LSD are the final consequences of a concatenation of events at different neural sites occurring by different mechanisms. The search for sites and mechanisms is confounded by the functional interrelations among the different neural systems and their exquisite ability to adapt and to restore and the propensity of drugs to react at more than one site and with more than one receptor. Examples of these complexities were observed in the present study. 5-HT appears to reduce the histamine activation of adenylate cyclase; the inference is not certain since 5-HT itself stimulates the cyclase. Cyproheptadine, which is a 5-HT antagonist in some systems (e.g., Segal, 1975) and is often regarded as a specific 5-HT blocker did not block 5-HT-stimulated cyclase in the hippocampus, but it competitively antagonized histamine-activation (Fig. 10).

The hippocampus as a site of interaction of histamine and D-LSD may have special importance. D-LSD and lesions of the hippocampus produce similar effects. Both interfere with some kinds of habituation, e.g., after these treatments, an animal responds to a stimulus to which it had previously been refractory (Key and Bradlye, 1960; Key, 1964; Isaacson and Pribram, 1975; Kohler, 1976). Both enhance some types of perseveration (Butters, 1966; Isaacson and Pribram, 1975). D-LSD causes seizure discharges from the hippocampus (Killam and Killam, 1960; Adey *et al.*, 1962) and enhances the response of the hippocampus to afferent stimulation (Revzen and Armstrong, 1966). [It is noteworthy that the hippocampal discharges persist for days after a single dose of D-LSD (Adey *et al.*, 1965; Radulovacki and Adey, 1965).] It is known that histamine, perhaps endogenous histamine, depresses the firing of hippocampal cells (Haas and Wolf, 1977). D-LSD may cause discharge of the cells by blocking—among other substances—histamine; perhaps this could account for some of the more subtle effects of D-LSD such as interference with habituation and enhancement of perseveration. The basis for these and other effects of D-LSD will be learnt only after delineation of the many sites and receptors on which it acts—only after a taxonomy of the D-LSD receptors is complete; towards this end, the appropriate model is the work carried out on the taxonomy of the histamine receptors by Schild and Black and their colleagues.

ACKNOWLEDGMENTS

This work was supported by a grant, (MH 17489) from the National Institute of Mental Health and (HL 19495 from the National Heart, Lung and Blood Institute. C. L. J. was a recipient of a Faculty Development Award of the Pharmaceutical Manufacturers Association Foundation.. We are grateful to Dr. W.F. Raub and the Chemical/Biological Information-Handling Program, Division of Research, National Institutes of Health, for providing access to the PROPHET system computer; to Drs. C.R. Ganellin and M. Parsons of Smith Kline and French for providing many of the compounds; to Dr. Robert Willette of the National Institute on Drug Abuse for providing LSD's; to Dr. Stanley D. Glick for dissections and discussions; to Miss Barbara Craddock for excellent assistance; to Miss Linda Crane for drawing figures; to Dr. W. Daniel Edwards for making molecular models.

REFERENCES

Abou, Y.Z., Adam, H.M., and Stephen, W.R.G. (1973). Concentration of histamine in different parts of the brain and hypophysis of rabbit: effect of treatment with histidine, certain other amino acids and histamine. *Br. J. Pharmacol.* **48**, 577–589.

Adey, W.R., Bell, F.R., and Dennis, B.J. (1962). Effects of LSD-25, psilocybin, and psilocin on temporal lobe EEG patterns and learned behavior in the cat. *Neurology* **12**, 591–602.

Adey, W.R., Porter, R., Walter, D.O., and Brown, T.S. (1965). Prolonged effects of LSD on EEG records during discriminative performance in cat; evaluation by computer analysis. *Electroenceph. Clin. Neurophysiol.* **18**, 25–35.

Aghajanian, G.K. (1976). LSD and 2-BROMO-LSD: comparison of effects on serotonergic neurones and on neurones in two serotonergic projection areas, the ventral lateral geniculate and amygdala. *Neuropharmacology,* **15**, 521–528.

Aghajanian, G.K., Foote, W.E., and Sheard, M.H. (1970). Action of psychotogenic drugs on single midbrain raphe neurons. *J. Pharmacol. Exper. Ther.* **171**, 178–187.

Appel, J. B., and Freedman, D.X. (1965). The relative potencies of psychotomimetic drugs. *Life Sci.* **4**, 2181–2186.

Arunlakshana, O., and Schild, H.O. (1959). Some quantitative uses of drug antagonists. *Br. J. Pharmacol.* **14**, 48–58.

Ash, A.S.F., and Schild, H.O. (1966). Receptors mediating some actions of histamine. *Br. J. Pharmacol.* **27**, 427–439.

Barbin, G., Hirsch, J.C., Garbarg, M., and Schwartz, J.-C. (1975). Decrease in histamine content and decarboxylase activities in an isolated area of the cerebral cortex of the cat. *Brain Res.* **92**, 170–174.

Barbin, G., Garbarg, M., Schwartz, J.-C., and Storm-Mathisen, J. (1976). Histamine synthesizing afferents to the hippocampal region. *J. Neurochem.* **26**, 259–263.

Bennett, Jr., J.P., and Snyder, S.H. (1976). Serotonin and lysergic acid diethylamide binding in rat brain membranes: relationship to postsynaptic serotonin receptors. *Mol Pharmacol.* **12**, 373–389.

Bertino, J.R., Klip, G.D., and Weintraub, W. (1959). Cholinesterase, D-lysergic acid diethylamide and 2-bromolysergic acid diethylamide. *J. Clin Exper. Psychopath.* **20**, 218–222.

Black, J.W. (1976). Histamine receptors in, "Proc. Sixth Internat. Congr. Pharmacol. 1975" *Receptors and Cellular Pharmacology* (E. Kling, ed.), Vol. 1, pp. 3–16. Pergamon Press, New York.

Black, J.W., Duncan, W.A.M., Durant, C.J., Ganellin, C.R., and Parsons, M.E. (1972). Definition and antagonism of histamine H_2-receptors. *Nature (London)* **236**, 385–390.

Black, J.W., Durant, G.J., Emmett, J.C., and Ganellin, C.R. (1974). Sulphur-methylene isosterism in the development of metiamide, a new histamine H_2-receptor antagonist. *Nature (London)* **248**, 65–67.

Bonnet, J.J., and Ibers, J.A. (1973). The structure of histamine. *J. Amer. Chem. Soc.* **95**, 4829–4833.

Brimblecombe, R.W., Duncan, W.A.M., Durant, G.J., Emmett, J.C., Ganellin, C.R., and Parsons, M.E. (1975). Cimetidine—A non-thiourea H_2-receptor antagonist. *J. Int. Med. Res.* **3**, 86–92.

Brown, E.M., Fedak, S.A., Woodard, C.J., and Aurbach, G.D. (1976). β-Adrenergic receptor interactions. *J. Biol. Chem.* **251**, 1239–1246.

Bunce, K.T., and Parsons, M.E. (1976). A quantitative study of metiamide, a histamine H_2-antagonist, on the isolated whole rat stomach. *J. Physiol.* **258**, 453–465.

Butters, N. (1966). The effect of LSD-25 on spatial and stimulus perseverative tendencies in rats. *Psychopharmacologia* **8**, 454–460.

Calcutt, C.R. (1976). The role of histamine in the brain. *Gen. Pharmacol.* **7**, 15–25.

Chasin, M., Mamrak, F., and Samaniego, S.G. (1974). Preparation and properties of a cell-free, hormonally responsive adenylate cyclase from guinea pig brain. *J. Neurochem.* **22**, 1031–1038.

Corne, S.J., and Pickering, R.W. (1967). A possible correlation between drug-induced hallucinations in man and a behavioural response in mice. *Psychopharmacologia* **11**, 65–78.

Creese, I., Burt, D.R., and Snyder, S.H. (1976). The dopamine receptor: differential binding of D-LSD and related agents to agonist and antagonist states. *Life Sci.* **17**, 1715–1720.

Dismukes, K., and Snyder, S.H. (1974). Dynamics of brain histamine in "Advances in Neurology," *Second Canadian-Americna Conference on Parkinson's Disease* (F. McDowell and A. Barbeau, eds.) Vol. 5, pp. 101–109, Raven Press, New York.

Durant, G.J., Ganellin, C.R., and Parsons, M.E. (1975a). Chemical differentiation of histamine H_1- and H_2-receptor agonists. *J. Med. Chem.* **18**, 905–909.

Durant, G.J., Parsons, M.E., and Black, J.W. (1975b). Potential histamine H_2-receptor antagonists. 2. Nα-guanylhistamine. *J. Med. Chem.* **18**, 830–833.

Durant, F.J., Ganellin, C.R., and Parsons, M.E. (1977a). Dimaprit, [S-[30(n,N-dimethylamino) propyl]isothiourea]. A highly specific histamine H_2-receptor agonist. Part 2. Structure-Activity Consideration. *Agents Actions,* in press.

Durant, G.J., Emmett, J.C., and Ganellin, C.R. (1977b). The chemical origin and properties of histamine H_2-receptor antagonists, *Proc. Second Internat. Symp. histamine H_2-receptor antagonists.* Excerpta Medica, pp. 1–12.

Freedman, D.X., and Halaris, A.E. (1978). Monamines and the biochemical mode of action of LSD at synapses in "Psychopharmacology—A Generation of Progress" (M. Lipton, A. DiMascio and K. Killam, eds.) Raven Press, New York.

Ganellin, C.R. (1974). Imidazole tautomerism of histamine derivatives, in "Molecular and Quantum Pharmacology" (E.D. Bergmann and B. Pullman, eds.) pp. 43–53. D. Reidel Publ. co., Dordrecht-Holland.

Ganellin, C.R., Port, G.N.J., and Richards, W.G. (1973). Conformation of histamine derivatives. 2. Molecular orbital calculations of preferred conformations in relation to dual receptor activity., *J. Med. Chem.* **16**, 616–620.

Garbarg, M., Barbin, G., Bischoff, S., Pollard, H., and Schwartz, J.-C. (1976). Dual localization of histamine in an ascending neuronal pathway and in non-neuronal cells evidenced by lesions in the lateral hypothalamic area. *Brain Res.* **106**, 333–348.

Godfraind, J.M., Krnjevic, K., Maretic, H., and Pumain, R. (1973). Inhibition of cortical neurones by imidazole and some derivatives. *Can. J. Physiol. Pharmacol.* **51**, 790–797.

Green, J.P. (1964). Histamine and the nervous system. *Fed. proc.* **23**, 1095–1102.

Green, J.P. (1970). Histamine, in "Handbook of Neurochemistry" (A. Lajtha, ed.) Vol. IV, *Control Mechanisms in the Nervous System.* pp. 221–250. Plenum Press, New York.

Green, J.P., Johnson, C.L., and Weinstein, H. (1978). Histamine as a neurotransmitter in "Psychopharmacology—A generation of Progress" (M. Lipton, A. Dimascio, and K. Killman, eds.). Raven Press, New York.

Haas, H.L., and Wolf, P. (1977). Central actions of histamine: microelectrophoretic studies. *Brain Res.* **122**, 269–279.

Haas, H.L., Anderson, E.G., and Hosli, L. (1973). Histamine and metabolites: their effects and interactions with convulsants on brain stem neurones. *Brain Res.* **51**, 269–278.

Hegstrand, L.R., Kanof, P.D., and Greengard, P. (1976). Histamine-sensitive adenylate cyclase in mammalian brain. *Nature (London)* **260**, 163–165.

Isaacson, R.L., and Pribram, K.H., eds. (1975). "The Hippocampus" Vol. 2: Neurophysiology and Behavior. Plenum Press, New York.

Isbell, H., Miner, E.J., and Logan, C.R. (1959). Relationships of psychotomimetic to antiserotonin potencies of congeners of lysergic acid diethylamide (LSD-25). *Psychopharmacologia* **1**, 20–28.

Johnson, C.L., and Mizoguchi, H. (1977). The interaction of histamine and guanylnucleotides with cardiac adenylate cyclase and its relationship to cardiac contractility. *J. Pharmacol. Exper. Ther.* **200**, 174–186.

Kakiuchi, S., and Rall, T.W. (1968). The influence of chemical agents on the accumulation of adenosine 3',5'-phosphate in slices of rabbit cerebellum. *Mol. Pharmacol.* **4**, 367–378.

Key, B.J. (1964). The effect of LSD-25 on the interaction between conditioned and nonconditioned stimuli in a simple avoidance situation. *Psychopharmacologia* **6**, 319–326.

Key, B.J., and Bradley, P.B. (1960). The effects of drugs on conditioning and habituation to arousal stimuli in animals. *Psychopharmacologia* **1**, 450–462.

Killam, K.F., and Killam, E.K. (1960). The action of lysergic acid diethylamide on central afferent and limbic pathways in the cat. *J. Pharmacol. Exper. Ther.* **116**, 35–42.

Kohler, C. (1976). Habituation after dorsal hippocampal lesions: a test dependent phenomenon. *Behav. Biol.* **18**, 89–110.

Lovell, R.A., and Freedman, D.X. (1976). Stereospecific receptor sites for *D*-lysergic acid diethylamide in rat brain: effects of neurotransmitters, amine antagonists, and other psychotropic drugs. *Mol. Pharmacol.* **12**, 620–630.

Lowry, O.H., Rosebrough, N.J., Farr, A.L., and Randall, R.J. (1951). Protein measurement with the Folin phenol reagent. *J. Biol. Chem.* **193**, 265–275.

Marshall, P.B. (1955). Some chemical and physical properties associated with histamine antagonism. *Brit. J. Pharmacol.* **10**, 270–278.

Mukherjee, C., Caron, M.G., Mullikin, D., and Lefkowitz, R.J. (1976). Structure-activity relationships of adenylate cyclase-coupled beta adrenergic receptors: determination by direct binding studies. *Mol. Pharmacol.* **12**, 16–31.

Paiva, A.C.M., Juliano, L., and Boschcov, P. (1976). Ionization of methyl derivatives of imidazole, histidine, thyreotropin release factor and related compounds. *J. Amer. Chem. Soc.* **98**, 7645–7648.

Parker, R.B., and Waud, D.R. (1971). Pharmacological estimation of drug-receptor dissociation constants. Statistical evaluation. I. Agonists. *J. Pharmacol. Exper. Ther.* **177**, 1–12.

Parsons, M. E. (1976). Personal communication.

Parsons, M.E., Blakemore, R.C., Durant, G.J., Ganellin, C.R., and Rasmussen, A.C. (1975). 3-[4(5)-imidazolyl]propylguanidine (SK&F 91486)—a partial agonist at histamine H_2-receptors. *Agents Actions* **5**, 464.

Parsons, M.E., Owen, D.A.A., Ganellin, C.R., and Durant, G.J. (1977). Dimaprit-[S-[3-N,N-dimethylamino)propyl] isothiourea]—A highly specific histamine H_2-receptor agonist. Part I. Pharmacology. *Agents Actions,* **7**, 31–37.

Prout, K., Critchley, S.R., and Ganellin, C.R. (1974). 2-(4-Imidazolyl) ethylammonium bromide (histamine monohydrobromide). *Acta Cryst. Sect B* **30**, 2884–2886.

Radulovacki, M., and Adey, W.R. (1965). The hipposcampus and the orienting reflex. *Exper. Neurol.* **12**, 68–83.

Revzin, A.M., and Armstrong, A. (1966). The effects of LSD-25 on the amplitude of evoked potentials in the hippocampus of the cat. *Life Sci.* **5**, 259–266.

Roberts, E., and Simonsen, D.G. (1970). Some properties of cyclic 3',5'-nucleotide phosphodiesterase of mouse brain: effects of imidazole-4-acetic acid, chlorpormazine, cyclic 3',5'-GMP, and other substances. *Brain Res.* **24**, 91–111.

Salomon, Y., Londos, C., and Rodbell, M. (1974). A highly sensitive adenylate cyclase assay. *Anal. Biochem.* **58**, 541–548.

Sastry, B.S.R., and Phillis, J.W. (1976). Evidence for an ascending inhibitory histaminergic pathway to the cerebral cortex. *Can. J. Physiol. Pharmacol.* **54**, 782–786.

Schild, H. O. (1947). pA, A new scale for the measurement of drug antagonism. *Br. J. Pharmacol.* **2**, 189–206.

Schneckloth, R., Page, I.H., Del Greoo, F., and Corcoran, A.C. (1957). Effects of serotonin antagonists in normal subjects and patients with carcinoid tumors. *Circulation* **16**, 523–532.

Schwartz, J.-C. (1975). Histamine as a transmitter in brain. *Life Sci.* **17**, 503–518.

Schwartz, J.-C., Baudry, M., Bischoff, S., Martres, M.-P., Pollard, H., Rose, C. and Verdiere, M. (1976). Pharmacological studies of histamine as a central neurotransmitter in "Drugs and Central Synaptic Transmission" (P.B. Bradley and B.N. Dhawan, eds.) pp. 371–382. University Park Press, Baltimore.

Segal, M. (1975). Psychological and pharmacological evidence for a serotonergic projection to the hippocampus. *Brain Res.* **94**, 115–131.

Segal, M. (1976). 5-HT antagonists in rat hippocampus. *Brain Res.* **103**, 161–166.

Snyder, S.H., and Taylor, K.M. (1972). Histamine in the. brain: A neurotransmitter? in "Perspectives in Neuropharmacology, A Tribute to Julius Axelrod" (S.H. Snyder, ed.) pp. 43–73. Oxford University Press, New York.

Spiker, M.D., Palmer, G.C., and Manian, A.A. (1976). Action of neuroleptic agents on histamine sensitive adenylate cyclase in rabbit cerebral cortex. *Brain Res.* **104,** 401–406.

Taylor, K.M., Gfeller, E., and Snyder, S.H. (1972). Regional localization of histamine and histidine in the brain of the rhesus monkey. *Brain Res.* **41,** 171–179.

Trendelenburg, U. (1960). The action of histamine and 5-hydroxytrptamine on isolated mammalian atria. *J. Pharmacol. Exper. Ther.* **30,** 450–460.

Uyeno, E.T. (1968). Hallucinogenic compounds and swimming response. *J. Pharmacol. Exper. Ther.* **159,** 216–221.

Weinstein, H., Chou, D., Johnson, C.L., Kang, S., and Green, J.P. (1976). Tautomerism and the receptor action of histamine: a mechanistic model. *Mol. Pharmacol.* **12,** 738–745.

Weinstein, H., Srebrenik, S., Maayani, S., and Sokolovsky, M.A. (1977). A theoretical model study of the comparative effectiveness of atropine and scopolamine action in the central nervous system. *J. Theoret. Biol.* **64,** 295–309.

Weltman, A.S., and Sackler, A.M. (1965). Effect of lysergic acid diethylamide (LSD-25) on growth metabolism and the resistance of male rats to histamine stress. *J. Pharm. Sci.* **54,** 1382–1384.

Yamada, T., Tsunoda, T., and Takashina, K. (1957). Accentuation of LSD$_{25}$ effect through antihistaminica. *Folia Psychiatrica et Neurologica Japonica* **11,** 266–273.

13

Histamine Receptors in the Central Thermoregulatory Pathways

Peter Lomax and Martin D. Green
Department of Pharmacology
School of Medicine and the
Brain Research Institute
University of California
Los Angeles, California

The compelling neurochemical evidences to suggest that histamine may have a role as a central neurotransmitter have encouraged a search for physiological responses to the amine. Effects of central administration of histamine on locomotor function, central autonomic responses and anti-diuretic hormone release have recently been described (Bhargava, 1974; Tuomisto and Erikson; Bennett and Pert, 1974).

That histamine might be involved in neuronal activity in the hypothalamus was suggested by the relatively high concentrations of both histamine and histidine decarboxylase in this part of the diencephalon and also by the observation that lesions of the medial forebrain bundle reduced these levels over a time course compatible with a process of Wallerian degeneration (Garbarg *et al.*, 1974). Of the many functions controlled by the hypothalamus thermoregulatory activity has been most extensively investigated and is perhaps best localized. In all species studied the pre-eminence of the preoptic/anterior hypothalamic nuclei as the major temperature regulating centers has been established. These considerations rendered it likely that histamine might well be involved in the central thermoregulatory neural network.

THE EFFECTS OF HISTAMINE ON BODY TEMPERATURE

Systemic injection of histamine will induce changes in body temperature in several species with the direction being a function of the environmental temperature. For example, in rats and mice histamine (3 mg, s.c.) causes a fall in body temperature at an environmental temperature of 18–20°C whereas a rise occurs at 30°C (Fabinyi and Szebehely, 1949). Since histamine does not readily penetrate the blood/brain barrier these responses are believed to be mediated peripherally and can be attributed to changes in heat exchange consequent to increased cutaneous blood flow (Issekutz et al., 1950).

Direct injection of histamine (1, 2.5, or 5 μg) into the preoptic/anterior hypothalamic nuclei of the rat causes a dose dependent fall in body temperature ranging from 0.5 to 2.0°C (Brezenoff and Lomax, 1970). Pretreatment of the animals with the histamine H_1-antagonist chlotyclizine (5 mg. kg^{-1}, i.p.) blocked the hypothermic response to intracerebral histamine. A fall in body temperature was also reported in mice after injection of histamine (1–10 μg) into a lateral ventricle but this response could not be blocked by chlorcyclizine administered either systemically or intraventricularly (Shaw, 1971).

HISTIDINE LOADING

Since brain histamine is formed locally from l-histidine following decarboxylation by a specific histidine decarboxylase, an alternative to direct injection of histamine into the brain is to increase neuronal levels by systemic histidine loading (Schwartz et al., 1973; Taylor and Snyder, 1972).

In rats pretreated with a peripheral decarboxylase inhibitor (Ro4-4602, 30 mg. kg^{-1}, i.p.) l-histidine (800 mg. kg^{-1}, i.p.) induced a fall in body temperature of 1.9 $\pm$ 0.4°C (mean $\pm$ S.E.M.) at an environmental temperature of 18°C (Green et al., 1975). That the hypothermia was due to centrally formed histamine was confirmed by injecting an inhibitor of brain histidine decarboxylase (McN-A-1293, 40 μg) into the lateral ventricle prior to administration of histidine (800 mg. kg^{-1}, i.p.); this pretreatment prevented the histidine induced fall in temperature (Cox et al., 1976a).

HISTAMINE H₁- AND H₂- ANTAGONISTS

As noted, the hypothermic effect of intracerebral histamine was inhibited by systemic or central injection of H_1-receptor antagonists. However, the fall in temperature after histidine loading was only partially blocked by systemic injection of either pyrilamine or chlorcyclizine (Lomax and Green, 1975). These findings recall the observation of Shaw (1971) that chlorcyclizine was ineffective in antagonizing the hypothermic effect of lateral ventricular injection of histamine. These several observations raised the intriguing possibility that the central thermoregulatory pathways contain both H_1- and H_2-histamine receptors.

The available H_2-antagonists are derivatives of histamine and do not cross the blood/brain barrier. Therefore, Green et al. (1975) investigated the effect of burimamide (120 nmoles), injected into various brain sites, on histidine induced hypothermia. Injection of the H_2-antagonist into the preoptic/anterior hypothalamic nuclei or into the lateral ventricles did not modify the fall in temperature after histidine loading but injections into the third ventricle abolished the response.

From these data it was concluded that there are, at least, two sets of histamine receptors: H_1-receptors in the rostral hypothalamic thermoregulatory centers and H_2-receptors on neurons lying close to the wall of the third ventricle. Consistent with this view was the observation that 4-methylhistamine (a predominantly H_2-agonist) causes a fall in temperature when injected into the third ventricle but not when injected into the lateral ventricles or the rostral hypothalamus (Cox et al., 1976b).

MECHANISMS OF ACTION OF HISTAMINE ON THERMOREGULATION

A change in body temperature may occur as a result of a shift in the thermoregulatory set temperature as occurs, for example, in pyrogen induced fever. Also, any procedure which activates the effector pathways regulating heat loss or heat gain will cause a change in temperature. Observation of core temperature alone will not determine the underlying mechanism. In order to overcome this restriction a behavioral method has been devised (Cox et al., 1975) which allows a distinction to be made between these different types of response. The rationale of the method is that an animal will seek an appropriate environmental temperature so as to maintain the minimum deviation of its body temperature from the thermoregulatory set temperature. Conversely, if the set temperature, or the body temperature are changed (e.g, by administering a drug) the animal will seek or avoid heat so as to reestablish the minimum deviation. By providing a heat source, this environmental selection can be studied.

Following intraventricular injection of histamine (5 μg) a marked fall in core temperature occurs and during the falling phase the rat actively avoids the heat source. It is concluded that in this situation a lowering of the set temperature has occurred.

During the period that the body temperature is declining following histidine loading the animal seeks the heat source so as to counteract the falling temperature. In this case it would appear that the thermostats have been unaffected by the increased central histaminergic activity and that the hypothermia is due to stimulation of effector pathways resulting in heat loss (Green et al., 1975).

The results of these behavioral studies confirm the existence of two sets of histamine receptors: H_1-receptors that lower the set temperature and H_2-receptors on the efferent heat loss pathways. Similar responses to H_1-receptor activation have been reported in the cat (Clark and Cumby, 1975).

CYCLIC ADENOSINE 3′, 5′-MONOPHOSPHATE (cAMP) AND THE THERMOREGULATORY EFFECT OF HISTAMINE

Central neurotransmitters, including norepinephrine, dopamine, and 5-hydroxytryptamine, have been shown to stimulate cAMP formation in brain tissue (see Daly, 1976). Histamine may also increase brain cAMP and both H_1-and H_2-receptors have been implicated in this response (Shimuzu et al., 1970; Palmer et al., 1972; Chasin et al., 1973; Nahorski et al., 1974). Thus, it might be expected that the response to histamine would be enhanced by a phospodiesterase inhibitor such as theophylline.

Rats were prepared for injection directly into the third ventricle by stereotaxic implantation of cannula guides. Intraventricular injection of histamine (20 μg) led to a fall in core temperature and this response was significantly enhanced by pretreatment of the animals with theophylline (10 mg. kg^{-1}, i.p.). These data are seen in Table I.

In these experiments it would be presumed that H_2-receptors had been activated. Whether H_1-receptors in the thermoregulatory centers are also sensitive to changes in cAMP activity remains to be studied.

Table I

The Effect of Theophylline on the Hypothermic Effect of Histamine Injected into the Third Ventricle of the Rat

Drug (dose)	Number of animals	Mean temperature change (°C ± S.E.M.)
0.9 NaCl (1 ml i.p.) + Histamine (20 μg 3rd vent.)	7	−1.2 ± 0.05[a]
Theophylline (10 mg.kg^{-1} i.p.)	5	+0.6 ± 0.26
Theophylline (10 mg.kg^{-1} i.p.) + Histamine (20 μg 3rd vent.)	7	−1.7 ± 0.19[a]

[a]Significantly different (p < 0.05) (Mann Whitney U test).

Table II
The Effect of Blockade of Histamine H_2-Receptors in the Central Heat Loss Pathways on the Hypothermic Effect of Drugs that Lower the Thermoregulatory Set-Point

Drug (dose)	Number of animals	Mean temperature change ($°C \pm$ S.E.M.)
0.9% NaCl (1 μl 3rd vent.) + Histamine (20 μg i.c.)	6	-1.4 ± 0.26
Cimetidine (10 μg 3rd vent.) + Histamine (20 μg i.c.)	6	-1.3 ± 0.14
0.9% NaCl (1 μl 3rd vent.) + Morphine (15 mg.kg^{-1} i.p.)	9	-2.1 ± 0.40
Cimetidine (10 μg 3rd vent.) + Morphine (15 r..g.kg^{-1} i.p.)	9	-2.4 ± 0.57
0.9% NaCl (1 μl 3rd vent.) + Oxotremorine (4 μg i.c.)	14	-2.8 ± 0.19[a]
Cimetidine (10 μg 3rd vent) + Oxotremorine (4 μg i.c.)	7	-1.2 ± 0.27[a]

[a]Significantly different ($p < 0.01$) (Mann Whitney U test).

HISTAMINERGIC PATHWAYS

The histamine H_1-receptors on the neurons of the preoptic/anterior hypothalamic nuclei could represent the terminals of short interneurons acting as neuromodulators involved in the setting of the thermoregulatory centers. Alternatively, they could be the endings of long pathways, as suggested by the studies of Garbarg et al. (1974), conveying information from peripheral thermoreceptors. Analogous long cholinergic pathways have been described by Knox et al. (1973). Whether cutaneous thermal stimulation will increase the firing of histamine sensitive neurons in the rostral hypothalamus remains to be determined. However, Haas (1974) has reported an increase in firing freuqency of hypothalamic neurons in response to histamine H_1-receptor stimulation; these neurons were distinct from adjacent cholinergic neurons. Since the cholinergic pathways appear to modulate the setting of the thermostats (Knox *et al.*, 1973) these several observations are consistent with the view that histaminergic (H_1-) pathways could subserve a similar function.

The H_2-receptors in the efferent heat loss pathways could also be associated with descending long tracts or be located at the termination of short interneurons. No evidence to indicate long descending pathways has yet emerged. Of immediate interest, however, was the question as to whether these histaminergic synapses are part of a common final pathway mediating heat loss following any downward setting of the thermostats. This problem was investigated by studying the effect of a histamine H_2-antagonist, cimetidine, on the hypothermic responses to three agents that lower the thermoregulatory set temperature: histamine (Green *et al.*, 1976), oxo-tremorine (Cox *et al.*, 1975), and morphine (Cox *et al.*, 1976c).

Guides for injection into the preoptic/anterior hypothalamic nuclei and the third ventricle were chronically implanted into rats. Cimetidine was injected into the third ventricle in order to block the H_2-receptors in the efferent pathways coursing through the periventricular grey matter.

Histamine (20 µg) caused a fall in body temperature when injected into preoptic area and the response was unaffected by prior injection of cimetidine (10 µg) into the third ventricle (Table II).

The hypothermic response to morphine sulfate (15 mg. kg^{-1}, i.p.) was also unchanged after H_2-receptor blockade (Table II).

In the case of the cholinomimetic oxotremorine (4 µg, i.c.) the fall in core temperature was significantly attenuated by cimetidine pretreatment (Table II).

These results suggest that the fall in temperature induced by oxotremorine is mediated, at least partly, by the histamine H_2-pathway but that this same efferent route is not activated by injection of histamine or morphine. The

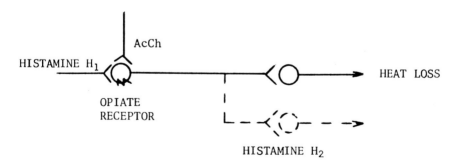

FIG. 1.   Model of histaminergic neurons in the central thermoregulatory pathways. Activation of cholinergic and histamine H_1-receptors, and binding of a narcotic to an opiate receptor, can lower the set temperature of the thermostats. Heat loss effector pathways are activated and these include pathways with a histamine H_2-synapse that can be recruited when maximum responses are required.

three hypothermic agents used all are purported to cause a fall in temperature by a common basic mechanism, viz. by lowering the set temperature of the thermostats. Thus, it is somewhat surprising that a common effector pathways is not involved. The reason for this anomaly may reside in the magnitude of the responses; Oxotremorine, at the dose used, caused the greatest rate, and degree, of fall in temperature. Possibly the histaminergic pathway is only recruited when maximal effects are required—such recruitment is a fundamental feature of central nervous system function. The concept of a parallel histaminergic (H_2-) pathway is illustrated in Fig. 1.

CONCLUSIONS

In the case of histamine the neurochemical and neuropharmacological data for assigning a transmitter role in the central thermoregulatory pathways are impressive. These pathways appear to contain both H_1-and H_2-receptors. An area warranting further investigation is the possible involvement of these pathways during disorders of thermoregulation and in hibernation.

There is no reason to believe that histaminergic neurotransmission is unique within the thermoregulatory system—it merely happens to be a system more readily susceptible to investigation—and evidence for changes in behavior and neuroendocrine function are now emerging. The possible implications in respect to abnormalities of behavior are self-evident but useful clinical applications in central nervous system therapy demand the availability of an H_2-antagonist that can penetrate into the brain after systemic administration.

ACKNOWLEDGMENTS

These studies were supported by Office of naval Research Contract N00014-75-C-0506 P00001. We are grateful to Dr. R. W. Brimblecombe of Smith, Kline and French Laboratories for the supplies of histamine H_2-antagonists.

REFERENCES

Bennett, C.T., and Pert, A. (1974). Antidiuresis produced by injections of histamine into the cat supraoptic nucleus. *Brain Res.* **78**, 151–156.

Bhargava, K.E. (1974). Some neuropharmacological studies with histamine. *J. Pharmacol. (Paris)* **5**, 73.

Brezenoff, H.E., and Lomax, P. (1970). Temperature changes following microinjection of histamine into the thermoregulatory centers of the rat. *Experientia* **26**, 51–52.

Chasin, M., Mamrak, F., Samaniego, S.G., and Hess, S.M. (1973). Characteristics of the catecholamine and histamine receptor sites mediating accumulation of cyclic adenosine 3′,5′-monophosphate in guinea pig brain. *J. Neurochem.* **21**, 1415–1427.

Clark, W.G., and Cumby, H.E. (1975). Biphasic effects of centrally injected histamine on body temperature in the cat. *Pharmacologist* **17**, 256.

Cox, B., Green, M.D., and Lomax, P. (1975)., Behavioral thermoregulatin in the study of drugs affecting body temperature. *Pharmacol. Biochem. Behav.* **3**, 1051–1054.

Cox, B., Green, M.D., and Lomax, P. (1976a). Thermoregulatory effects of histamine. *Experientia* **32**, 498–499.

Cox, B., Green, M.D., Chesarek, W., and Lomax, P. (1976b). The effect of 4-methyl-histamine on temperature regulation in the rat. *J. Thermal Biol.* **1**, 205–207.

Cox, B., Ary, M., Chesarek, W., and Lomax, P. (1976c). Morphine hyperthermia in the rat: an action on the central thermostats. *Europ. J. Pharmacol.* **36**, 33–39.

Daly, J.W. (1976). The nature of receptors regulating the formation of cyclic AMP in brain tissue. *Life Sci.* **18**, 1349–1358.

Fabinyi, M., and Szebehely, J. (1949). The mechanism of desensitization with histamine. *Acta Allerg.* **2**, 233–244.

Garbarg, M., Barbin, G., Feger, J., and Schwartz, J-C. (1974). Histaminergic pathway in rat brain evidenced by lesions of the medial forebrain bundle. *Science* **186**, 833–835.

Green, M.D., Cox, B., and Lomax, P. (1975). Histamine H_1- and H_2-receptors in the central thermoregulatory pathways of the rat. *J. Neurosci. Res.* **1**, 353–359.

Green, M.D., Cox, B., and Lomax, P. (1976). Sites and mechanisms of action of histamine in the central thermoregulatory pathways of the rat. *Neuropharmacol.* **15**, 321–324.

Haas, H.L. (1974). Histamine: action on single hypothalamic neurones. *Brain Res.* **76**, 363–366.

Issekutz, B., Lichtmeckert, I., and Nagy, H. (1950). Effect of capsaicine and histamine on heat regulation. *Arch. Int. Pharmacodyn.* **81**, 35–46.

Knox, G.V., Campbell, C., and Lomax, P. (1973). The effects of acetylcholine and nicotine on unit activity in the hypothalamic thermoregulatory centers of the rat. *Brain Res.* **51**, 215–223.

Lomax, P., and Green, M.D. (1975). Histamine and temperature regulation in "Temperature Regulation and Drug Action" (P. Lomax, E. Schönbaum, and J. Jacob, eds.) pp. 85–94. Karger, Basel.

Nahorski, S.R., Rogers, K.J., and Smith, B.M. (1974). Histamine H_2-receptors and cyclic AMP in brain. *Life Sci.* **15**, 1887–1894.

Palmer, G.C., Schmidt, M.J., and Robinson, G.A. (1972). Development and characteristics of the histamine-induced accumulation of cyclic AMP in the rabbit cerebral cortex. *J. Neurochem.* **19**, 2251–2256.

Schwartz, J-C., Lampart, C., and Rose, C. (1973). Histamine formation in rat brain *in vivo:* effects of histidine loads. *J. Neurochem.* **19**, 801–810.

Shaw, G.G. (1971). Hypothermia produced in mice by histamine acting on the central nervous system. *Brit. J. Pharmacol.* **42**, 205–214.

Shimuzu, H., Creveling, C.R., and Daly, J.W. (1970). The effect of histamine and other compounds on the formation of adenosine 3',5'-monophosphate in slices from cerebral cortex. *J. Neurochem.* **17**, 441–444.

Taylor, K.M., and Snyder, S.H. (1972). Dynamics of the regulation of histamine levels in mouse brain. *J. Neurochem.* **19**, 341–354.

Tuomisto, L., and Eriksson, L. (1974). Central antidiuretic effect of histamine (H) in the unanesthetized goat: effects of H_1- and H_2-antagonists. *J. Pharmacol. (Paris)* **5**, 101.

14

Histamine: Modification of Behavioral and Physiological Components of Body Fluid Homeostasis

Sarah Fryer Leibowitz
The Rockefeller University
New York, New York

Histamine is classically associated with various pathological processes, such as allergy, anaphylaxis, injury, and stress; in these processes, histamine is liberated from mast cells in the body to produce characteristic physiological responses, such as vasodilatation, itching, and edema. Recent evidence, however, has accumulated to suggest a function for histamine in neural control of various physiological processes. Studies will be described here which demonstrate complementary behavioral and physiological effects of histamine in regulation of body fluid homeostasis. These effects, namely, drinking behavior and antidiuresis, are found to occur after injection of histamine directly into particular brain regions, as well as systemically, and are shown to be mediated by H_1- and H_2-histamine receptors.

HISTAMINE-INDUCED DRINKING BEHAVIOR

Introduction

There are very few studies in the literature which have related histamine to the control of behavior. This substance has been shown to produce symptoms of behavioral arousal (Monnier et al., 1970) and to have an inhibitory effect on the rewarding properties of brain stimulation (Cohn et al., 1973). With respect to its effects on ingestive behavior, there is one study in the cat (Clineschmidt and Lotti, 1973) which found intraventricular histamine to produce a small (25%) suppression of food intake. In the rat, we have observed a similar, although more robust, effect with systemic histamine injection (Leibowitz, unpublished data), but, with injection into the lateral hypothalamus, a small increase of food intake was observed (Leibowitz, 1973b). The significance of these effects on feeding behavior is not known, although it is very likely that they are related to, and perhaps secondary to, histamine's potent stimulatory effect on water ingestion.

The first indication that histamine might alter drinking behavior was provided by a study of Gerald and Maickel (1972) in which systemically administered antihistamines were found to markedly suppress the water intake of thirsty rats, and lateral hypothalamic injections of histamine (at relatively large doses of 40–160 μg) were found to potentiate water intake. Shortly thereafter, two independent reports simultaneously appeared in which a potent stimulatory effect of systemically administered histamine on drinking was described (Gutman and Krausz, 1973; Leibowitz, 1973a). In the report from this laboratory, histamine was also injected centrally and found to have a similar effect, although at much lower doses. This increase in water intake phenomenon, observed after central histamine, appeared to be localized to the hypothalamus, most particularly to the rostral portion.

This evidence provides the background for our research on histamine as related to the control of water ingestion in the rat. In this section, we will first describe the effects observed with systemically injected histamine, as a function of dose, in the presence of various receptor blockers, and in nephrectomized animals. We will then describe similar experiments conducted in the brain of rats with chronic cannulas aimed at the hypothalamus. We will follow with a discussion of the significance of these findings, relating histamine's dipsogenic action to its peripheral and central effects on the vasculature and neuronal function.

Studies with Systemic Drug Administration

Abstract

Results described here demonstrate that systemically administered histamine produces a dramatic, dose-dependent increase in drinking behavior in the satiated rat. This effect, which can be observed at doses as low as 0.38 mg/kg, appears to involve both H_1- and H_2-histamine receptors and occurs independently of renal hormone systems.

Description of peripheral histamine-induced drinking

The procedures used in these studies involved, first, a pretreatment period (60 minutes) with fresh water to insure maximal satiation, followed by a second 60-minute period to establish the rats' water intake baseline after vehicle injection, and then a third 60-minute interval to measure the effect of histamine on water intake. All tests were conducted in the absence of food.

In the first series of tests, we examined histamine's effect on water consumption as a function of dose. After subcutaneous injection, this substance produced a vigorous drinking response in the normally satiated rat. The smallest significant effect was 1.7 ml at a dose of 0.38 mg/kg, and this effect increased monotonically to over 14 ml at a dose of 24 mg/kg. (This amount is approximately one-third of what a rat normally consumes over a 24-hour period.) This drinking response proved extremely reliable and robust. Rarely did an animal not respond to histamine; furthermore, the latency to respond, as well as the magnitude of the response, was amazingly consistent from animal to animal. The latency was generally between 5 and 6 minutes at doses up to 3 mg/kg, and between 2 and 4 minutes at the higher doses. The drinking response was quite vigorous, continuing without interruption for 5 to 10 minutes at the lower doses and for 10 to 20 minutes at the higher doses. Control injections of sodium chloride at equimolar concentrations failed to produce any water intake.

These results were obtained with subcutaneous injection of histamine. Tests with other routes of administration revealed a slightly more potent effect with intravenous histamine (tested only at doses below 1 mg/kg) and a somewhat less potent effect with intraperitoneal injection. Our experiments with intracranial administration of histamine will be described below.

Characterization of receptors

After establishing this very clear effect on water intake with peripheral histamine, the next series of experiments was designed to analyze the nature of the receptor(s) mediating this phenomenon. In the periphery, two types of histamine receptors have been pharmacologically characterized in the mammalian species (Ash and Schild, 1966; Black *et al.,* 1972). The first type, referred to as H_1, is found to be selectively stimulated by the compounds 2-methylhistamine and pyridyl ethylamine and selectively blocked by the classical antihistamine agents. The second type, H_2, in contrast, is selectively stimulated by the compounds 4-methylhistamine and dimaprit, and selectively blocked by recently developed H_2-receptor blockers.

To identify the type of receptor(s) mediating the effect of systemic histamine on drinking behavior, we first examined the effects of the histamine agonists, 2-methylhistamine, pyridyl ethylamine, 4-methylhistamine, and dimaprit, on water intake in comparison to the effect of histamine itself. Each of these compounds, after subcutaneous injection, produced a reliable increase in water intake (at least at $p < 0.05$), with a relative potency in the order of histamine > pyridyl ethylamine = 4-methylhistamine = dimaprit > 2-

methylhistamine. At the maximum dose tested (48 mg/kg), the H_2-receptor agonists 4-methylhistamine and dimaprit produced an effect (5–6 ml of water intake) equivalent in magnitude to that observed with 3 mg/kg of histamine; the H_1 agonist pyridyl etmylamine elicited a comparable effect, whereas 2-methylhistamine appeared somewhat less potent, producing a 3.5 ml response, similar to that observed with 1 mg/kg histamine.

These tests, showing a smaller but significant effect with the selective histamine agonists, provide the first indication that both H_1- and H_2- histamine receptors may be involved in the drinking response elicited by systemic histamine. Further evidence in support of this suggestion is provided by our studies with the receptor antagonists subcutaneously injected a few minutes prior to histamine. Our findings with these compounds (Table I) have shown a clear dose-dependent suppression of histamine-induced water intake with several different H_1 antagonists, as well as with the H_2 antagonist cimetidine. This antagonism was partial in each case (approximately 50% inhibition) and competitive in nature. Table I summarizes the results obtained with the various antihistamines, tested not only in combination with histamine itself but also under a variety of conditions, associated with increased drinking, namely, after 22 hours of water deprivation or after subcutaneous injection of the β-adrenergic agonist isoproterenol or intraperitoneal injeciton of hypertonic saline. The purpose of these tests was to examine the specificity of the antihistamine's antagonistic action on histamine-elicited drinking.

In Table I are reported the threshold antagonist doses found to reliably suppress water intake under the different conditions and the magnitude of the effects observed at that dose. From these results, it can be seen that dexbrompheniramine and cimetidine were most specific in their antagonism of histamine's effect, in that they were reliably effective at doses at least ten-fold lower than were found to suppress the other elicited drinking responses. The dose-response curves of these antagonists were parallel, and their ID_{50} (that is, the dose calculated to produce a 50% inhibition of the histamine response) was found to be 4.3 mg/kg for dexbrompheniramine and 6.6 mg/kg for cimetidine. Slightly higher doses produced up to a 60% inhibition; however they also exhibited a reliable suppressive effect on isoproterenol-induced water consumption and occasionally on deprivation-induced drinking. [Gerald and Maickel (1972) similarly reported a general drinking suppressive effect of the antihistamines at high doses.] The ID_{50} values for promethazine hydrochloride and methylchloride were somewhat higher, 8.0 and 10.0 mg/kg, respectively, whereas the ID_{50} for methapyrilene (1.5 mg/kg) and tripelennamine (1.7 mg/kg) were considerably lower. As shown in Table I, however, these latter two antagonists, particularly tripelennamine, appeared to be acting partially in a nonspecific fashion, as evidenced by their significant inhibition of isoproterenol and hyperosmotic drinking at

Table I
Effect of Receptor Antagonists on Drinking Elicited by Histamine, Isoproterenol, Hypertonic Saline, and Water Deprivation

Type of receptor	Antagonist	Threshold dose (TD in mg/kg) and percent inhibition of elicited drinking (%↓)							
		Histamine		Isoproterenol		Hypertonic saline		Water deprivation	
		TD	%↓	TD	%↓	TD	%↓	TD	%↓
H$_1$ Histaminergic	Dexbrompheniramine	0.67	-30[b]	6.0	-46[b]	>6.0	—	>6.0	—
	Promethazine methylchloride	4.30	-40[a]	—	—	—	—	24.0	-32[b]
	Promethazine hydrochloride	4.30	-30[a]	—	—	—	—	24.0	-25[b]
	Methapyrilene	0.37	-32[b]	1.6	-54[c]	3.2	-45[b]	4.5	-40[b]
	Tripelennamine	0.65	-44[b]	0.65	-52[b]	0.65	-35[b]	>5.7	—
H$_2$ Histaminergic	Cimetidine	0.4	-23[a]	>8.0	—	>8.0	—	>8.0	—
β-Adrenergic	dl-Propranolol	0.08	-51[c]	0.08	-51[c]	0.23	-35[b]	0.7	-18[a]
α-Adrenergic	Phentolamine	>3.3	—	>3.3	—	>3.3	—	>3.3	—
Dopaminergic	Haloperidol	0.15	-50[b]	0.15	-73[c]	0.15	-67[c]	0.15	-63[c]
Cholinergic	Atropine	0.5	-33[b]	1.5	-35[c]	0.5	-41[c]	0.5	-27[c]
Serotonergic	Methysergide	>15.0	—	>15.0	—	>15.0	—	>15.0	—

[a] $p < .05$.
[b] $p < .01$.
[c] $p < .001$.

223

relatively low doses. At higher doses, a 70–90% suppression of histamine's effect could be observed with these antagonists. This nearly total inhibition, however, is most likely attributable once again to their strong nonspecific drinking suppression.

To establish further the selectivity of the antihistamines' actions, we tested, in combination with histamine, several other types of receptor antagonists (Table I). We found the α-adrenergic and serotonergic blockers to be ineffective in antagonizing histamine's effect on water intake. The cholinergic blocker atropine and the dopaminergic blocker haloperidol were also ineffective, except at the higher doses tested (0.5–4.5 mg/kg for atropine and 0.15 mg/kg for haloperidol) which caused a general (partial) suppression of drinking induced water deprivation, sodium chloride, and isoproterenol, as well as by histamine. [A similar pattern of results was obtained by Block and Fisher (1975), except that histamine was not tested in that study.]

The final compound tested, dl-propranolol, is an antagonist of β-adrenergic receptors. This drug is of particular interest in light of the potent dipsogenic action exhibited by the β-adrenergic agonist isoproterenol (Lehr et al., 1967) and in light of the possibility that this agonist and histamine, two vasoactive compounds, might be acting through similar mechanisms. The outcome of these tests indicated that dl-propranolol, which at a dose of 6.25 mg/kg abolished isoproterenol-induced drinking (Lehr et al., 1967), can significantly suppress (but not abolish) histamine-induced water intake, at a dose as low as 0.08 mg/kg. The suppression obtained appeared independent of dose, remaining generally constant (at approximately 50%) with doses up to 1.4 mg/kg. [Gutman and Krausz (1973) similarly found 6 mg/kg of propranolol to cause a 50% reduction in histamine drinking.] This dose-response relationship clearly indicates that propranolol's site of action, presumably involving β-adrenergic receptors, is different from that affected by the histamine receptor antagonists. The specificity of this propranolol suppression will need to be carefully evaluated in light of our additional finding that this drug also causes a reliable suppression of hyperosmotic and deprivation-induced thirst as well (see Table I).

These pharmacological studies have clearly demonstrated the involvement of specific H_1- and H_2-histamine receptors in the mediation of drinking behavior elicited by subcutaneous histamine. This response is elicited by different H_1 and H_2 agonists and is selectively (partially) abolished by both H_1 and H_2 antagonists. In a separate series of experiments designed to determine the relationship between the two histamine receptors, we examined the effectiveness of dexbrompheniramine (H_1) and cimetidine (H_2), both separately and together, in suppressing histamine-induced drinking at doses of 0.4 mg/kg to 4.0 mg/kg. When tested separately, these antagonists were each found to reduce the histamine response, in a dose-dependent fashion, by up to 42% ($p < 0.01$) for cimetidine and 48% (p < 0.001) for dexbrompheniramine. When injected in combination, these antagonists did not appear to interact but rather showed an additive inhibition of 45% ($p <$ 0.01) at 0.4 mg/kg and 82% ($p < 0.001$) at 4.0 mg/kg each.

Tests in nephrectomized animals

Water consumption stimulated by a variety of hypotensive agents (including isoproterenol) is believed to involve the renin-angiotensin system of the kidney (Fitzsimons, 1972; see discussion below). To gain insight into the nature of the mechanism mediating histamine-induced drinking, we tested this drug, as well as isoproterenol, in rats deprived of their kidneys. The outcome of these tests clearly differentiated the actions of these two dipsogenic agents. Consistent with previous reports (see Fitzsimons, 1972), isoproterenol-induced drinking was found to be abolished by removal of the kidneys. In contrast, the drinking elicited by histamine remained essentially intact after this operation. At the two doses tested (3 and 6 mg/kg), nephrectomized animals responded significantly to histamine, exhibiting only a small reduction in water intake (16% and 11%, respectively) when compared with their preoperative scores. Gutman and Krausz (1973) obtained similar results in nephrectomized animals, although their post-operative reduction averaged approximately 40%.

We may tentatively conclude from these tests that the renin-angiotensin system mediated through the kidney is not crucial to the histamine-induced drinking effect, in contrast to the responses observed with other hypotensive agents. While the small reduction in water intake observed after nephrectomy (especially in the experiments conducted by Gutman and Krausz [1973]) may imply a partial contribution of this system, the incapacitating effects of the operation, particularly in a hypotensive animal (Stricker, 1977), must be carefully evaluated. Consistent with these findings in a nephrectomized animal are the results obtained with propranolol (see above), which showed only a partial, apparently nonspecific, suppression of histamine-induced drinking, in contrast to a total reduction of drinking elicited by other hypotensive drugs (see Fitzsimons, 1972 and discussion below). From these results, it seems quite clear that, although β-adrenergic and kidney-dependent systems may have an effect on the magnitude of the drinking response elicited by histamine, they are not essential for the response to occur.

Studies with Central Drug Administration

Abstract

Injection of histamine directly into the hypothalamus is found to elicit a drinking response of 5–6 ml in a normally satiated rat. This behavioral effect

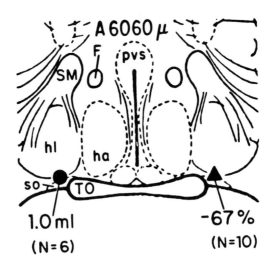

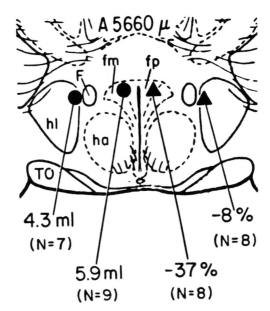

● Water intake ▲ Anti-diuresis

FIG. 1.   Frontal sections of the rat brain illustrating water intake scores (● = ml in 60 minutes)
and antidiuresis scores (▲ = percent suppression of urine output in 60 minutes relative to vehicle
baseline) obtained after histamine injection into the three sites indicated. All values, except the
water intake score for the supraoptic nucleus and the antidiuresis score for the perifornical area,
reached statistical reliability at least at $p < 0.05$. Diagrams (A6060 μ and A5660 μ) are based on
König and Klippel's "Atlas of the Rat Brain"(Williams & Wilkins, 1963). Abbreviations within

is found to be anatomically specific, occurring most readily with injections into the medial–rostral hypothalamic area. At this site, doses of histamine as low as 60 ng (free base) can be seen to produce a reliable response. When tested in combination with receptor antagonists (centrally administered), this drinking response elicited by histamine is selectively, although only partially, inhibited by H_1 and H_2 blockers.

Description of central histamine-induced drinking

The procedures used in these experiments were similar to those described above for peripherally administered histamine, except that animals with stereotaxically implanted brain cannulas were used, and all drugs were injected directly into the brain through these cannulas.

In an earlier study (Leibowitz, 1973a), we discovered that histamine injected into the anterior hypothalamic area, including the lateral hypothalamus and slightly more anterior into the preoptic area, elicited a reliable drinking response of between 5 and 6 ml. Sites in the caudal hypothalamus or in areas outside the hypothalamus were unresponsive. In the present experiment, we examined this phenomenon further, by comparing the effectiveness of histamine in three different brain areas within the rostral hypothalamus, namely, the medial paraventricular nucleus, the lateral perifornical area (1 mm lateral to the paraventricular nucleus), and the supraoptic nucleus (Fig. 1). The results of these tests confirm our original finding of central histamine-induced drinking and provide further information regarding the anatomical localization of this phenomenon. The medial paraventricular nucleus was found to be most sensitive to histamine; at this site, 12.5 to 50 nmoles of histamine (2.3 and 9.2 μg) elicited 4.4 to 5.9 ml of water intake ($p < 0.001$ as compared with 0.0 to 0.5 ml vehicle baseline). The lateral perifornical hypothalamic region yielded a somewhat smaller response (2.3 to 4.3 ml), in contrast to the supraoptic nucleus, which appeared totally unresponsive. The latency of the drinking response observed after paraventricular nucleus injection of histamine generally varied from 2 to 10 minutes. The duration of the response extended up to 30 minutes, during which time more than one bout of drinking was frequently observed.

Tests of threshold doses of histamine

The above results indicate that the stimulatory effect of central histamine on water consumption is anatomically specific. It appears to be associated

---

hypothalamus: fm, nucleus paraventricularis pars magnocellularis; fp, nucleus paraventricularis pars parvocellularis; ha, nucleus anterior; hl, nucleus lateralis; pvs, nucleus periventricularis stellatocellularis; so, nucleus supraopticus; F, columna fornicis; SM, stria medullaris thalami; TO, tractus opticus.

with the rostral hypothalamic region, most particularly the dorsal and medial portion. To evaluate more carefully the sensitivity of this area to lower doses of histamine, we selected a group of rats, with paraventricular nucleus cannulas, which consistently and vigorously responded to histamine at relatively high doses; we then gradually lowered these doses until a reliable drinking response was no longer observed.

In these animals with verified paraventricular cannulas, histamine at 17.3 nmoles produced a drinking response in all animals, averaging 5.4 ml ($p <$ 0.001, as compared with a zero baseline). This response gradually declined to 2.3 ml ($p < 0.001$) at a dose of 2.2 nmoles and to 1.2 ml ($p < 0.05$) observed at a dose of 0.6 nmole. This threshold dose (equivalent to 60 ng free base) for histamine-induced drinking in the paraventricular nucleus is comparable to the threshold doses we have sometimes observed for other brain amine effects on ingestive behavior, although it is somewhat higher than the 1 to 10 ng doses of epinephrine which we find to elicit feeding and suppress drinking after injection into the paraventricular nucleus (Leibowitz, 1973c, 1976, 1978). Since histamine is susceptible to the catabolic action of particular enzymes, it is possible that pretreatment with an inhibitor of these enzymes might lead us to reveal the effectiveness of lower histamine doses. This has been found to be the case with monoamine oxidase inhibitors and catecholamine effects on feeding (Leibowitz, 1978).

Characterization of receptors

Very little research has been done on the problem of identifying the nature of the receptors mediating histamine's effects in the brain. The primary work in this area has derived from biochemical studies investigating a stimulatory effect of histamine on cyclic AMP (cAMP) and glycogenolysis in brain tissue (Chasin et al., 1973; Nahorski et al., 1974; Rogers et al., 1975; Baudry et al., 1975; Nahorski et al., 1975; Hegstrand et al., 1976). These studies have implicated both H_1- and H_2-histamine receptors in the mediation of these phenomena, showing either a partial or complete inhibition with selective H_1 and H_2 antagonists. Iontophoretic studies, generally showing an inhibitory effect of histamine on cortical neurons in contrast to an excitatory effect on hypothalamic neurons, have also found H_1 and H_2 antagonists effective in blocking histamine's actions (Haas, 1974; Haas et al., 1975; Sastry and Phillis, 1976). However, the specificity of this receptor antagonism, especially with respect to the H_1 antagonists, has been questioned (Phillis et al., 1968). Finally, in temperature regulation, the brain also appears to operate through both H_1 and H_2 receptors, although the evidence suggests that these receptors may be located in different parts of the brain (Green et al., 1976).

These studies provide the background for our experiments in the brain on intact, behaving animals. To characterize the receptors mediating histamine's stimulatory effect on water ingestion, we tested in combination with histamine the H_1 antagonists chlorpheniramine, methapyrilene, and tripelennamine, and the H_2 antagonist cimetidine (1 to 15 nmoles). To examine the specificity of these drugs' actions, we also tested a variety of other drugs known to antagonize dopaminergic (haloperidol), β-adrenergic (propranolol), α-adrenergic (phentolamine and tolazoline), and cholinergic (atropine) receptors. All drugs were injected directly into the paraventricular nucleus, with the receptor antagonists administered 5 minutes prior to histamine.

The outcome of these experiments on histamine-induced water ingestion clearly revealed a selective inhibition of this phenomenon with the histamine-receptor antagonists. The blockers of other types of receptors, tested at doses known to produce effective blockade in the brain, had no effect on the drinking elicited by central histamine. In contrast, each of the antihistamines produced a reliable dose-dependent suppression of histamine's action. The blockade was only partial, reaching 50% to 55% ($p < 0.01$) with the H_1 antagonists and only 35% ($p < 0.01$) with the H_2 antagonist. Higher doses of the antagonists failed to produce any further inhibition, and on occasions actually appeared to be less effective than at lower doses. To test the possibility that this partial blockade reflected the additive function of H_1 and H_2 receptors in mediating histamine's action (this was found to be the case for peripherally administered histamine), we tested chlorpheniramine (H_1) and cimetidine (H_2) simultaneously in combination with histamine. These antagonists, when injected together at lower doses, were indeed additive in their effect on histamine-elicited drinking. However, when tested at maximally effective doses, these drugs still produced only a partial blockade of 58% ($p < 0.01$).

These results, consistent with those obtained in the periphery, indicate that the stimulatory effect of central histamine on water intake involves distinct histamine receptors, apparently with H_1 and H_2 properties. Both H_1 and H_2 antagonists significantly suppressed the response, while other types of blockers had no effect. Similar to the findings obtained with peripheral injection, central antihistamines produced only a partial inhibition of histamine-induced drinking. A partial blockade with antihistamines has been reported for a number of effects, including histamine-induced hypothermia (Calcutt, 1976) as well as histamine's stimulatory effect on brain cAMP and glycogenolysis (Chasin et al., 1973; Baudry et al., 1975; Nahorski et al., 1975). The basis for this may lie in a complex interaction between the two distinct histamine receptors, which perhaps may exist on two different cell types (such as glial versus nerve cells), or on cells located in different regions of the brain (see Green et al., 1976). It is quite possible, however, that the complication lies in the actions of the antihistamines themselves; these compounds, in addition to blocking histamine receptors, are known to have potent local anesthetic action, especially at high doses. When tested by themselves in the paraventricular nucleus, these drugs, at the doses used in the above experiments, failed to have any effect on the rats' baseline drinking behavior. However, based on our observation that higher doses of the antihistamines might actually be less effective in blocking histamine's action than somewhat lower doses, it seems possible that the antihistamines are indeed producing additional effects which, at the higher doses, might actually limit the effectiveness of their blockade. The additional possibility, that a total blockade might be obtained with combinations of antihistamines and other types of receptor antagonists, should also be considered.

Discussion of Histamine's Stimulatory Effect on Drinking

These results obtained with systemic and central injection of histamine in the rat reveal a potent stimulatory effect of this substance on water ingestion. The effect is dose-dependent, occurring at doses as low as 100 μg peripherally injected (intravenously) and 60 ng centrally injected (into the hypothalamic paraventricular nucleus). With peripheral administration, this histamine effect is mimicked by selective H_1- and H_2-receptor agonists and, both centrally and peripherally, the effect is selectively and partially suppressed by H_1- and H_2-receptor antagonists. Removal of the kidney is found to have little effect on the drinking response elicited by peripheral histamine.

What is the significance of these findings? What are the physiological mechanisms involved in histamine's actions, and what is the relationship, if any, between histamine's peripheral and central phenomena?

To understand histamine's effect on water intake, it will be necessary to very briefly review our current understanding of the physiological systems controlling thirst (see reviews by Fitzsimons, 1972; Epstein, 1973, 1976; Stricker, 1973; Severs and Summy-Long, 1975). Body water is distributed into two major compartments, intracellular and extracellular fluid. Maintenance of body water constancy requires the function of two types of receptors: (1) one responsive to changes in effective osmolarity of extracellular fluid or to changes in intracellular fluid volume which occur concomitantly; and (2) one responsive to changes in intravascular fluid volume. Such alterations in the distribution and composition of body fluids are compensated for by increased thirst, as well as by decreased urine output. The regulatory mechanisms involved in activating these complementary physiological and behavioral adjustments are believed to be: (1) in the case of intracellular thirst, the osmoreceptors of the brain which are sensitive to their own dehydration; and (2) in the case of extracellular or hypovolemic thirst, the renin–angiotensin hormone system of the kidney and neural afferents located in the capacitance vessels on the low-pressure side of the circulation. These baroreceptors, whose afferents run in the vagus, have been shown to have a role in the control of ADH secretion, as well as the secretion of renal renin and of aldosterone, and it is likely that they provide the signal which leads to extracellular thirst in the absence of renal hormone.

Systemic injection of histamine is known to have dramatic effects on the cardiovascular system (Douglas, 1975). This substance causes a rapid lowering of systemic blood pressure, an effect which involves both H_1- and H_2-histamine receptors (Black et al., 1972; Owen and Parsons, 1974; Brimblecombe et al., 1975; Owen, 1975; Powell and Brody, 1976). This hypotensive effect of histamine, which has been shown to occur in the rat at the histamine doses used in the present investigations (Leenen et al., 1975), may be attributed to its potent vasodilatory action on the minute blood vessels and capillaries. It may also be a consequence of histamine's ability to increase capillary permeability. This effect, which causes an outward passage of plasma protein and fluid into the interstitial space, results in a decreased blood volume and thus hypotension. [It should be noted that this effect on vascular permeability does not appear to occur in the brain or the kidney (Gabbiani et al., 1970; Schwartz and Cotran, 1972; Sinclair et al., 1974).] These effects of histamine on the vasculature, and the consequent changes in composition and distribution of body fluids, would be expected among other things to cause an increase in renin release (Leenen et al., 1975) and a change in baroreceptor activity (Douglas, 1975). As just described above, both of these phenomena have been strongly implicated in the mediation of extracellular thirst and therefore are likely contributors to the drinking response observed with histamine.

The evidence crucial to our evaluation of this suggestion is: (1) the finding that hypotensive drugs consistently cause an increase in water intake associated with an increase in renin release. These effects are abolished by bilateral nephrectomy, as well as by the β-adrenergic blocker propranolol (see Fitzsimons, 1972); and (2) the finding that a decrease in blood volume, caused by injection of either polyethylene glycol or formalin (which produce, respectively, a loss of protein-free and protein-rich plasma fluid from the circulation), stimulates a drinking response which is unaffected by removal of the kidneys (see Fitzsimons, 1972; Stricker, 1973).

Our experiment with histamine in the nephrectomized animal was designed to assess the contribution of the renin–angiotensin system in the mediation of histamine's stimulatory effect on drinking behavior. In contrast to the dependence on this system of other hypotensive agents, the effect of histamine remained essentially intact in the absence of the kidneys. This result would appear to argue against an essential role for renin–angiotensin in histamine-induced water ingestion. Consistent with this finding are the experiments with the β-adrenergic blocker propranolol. This drug, which is known to abolish the release of renin as well as the increase in water consumption elicited by hypotensive drugs (see above), had only a partial suppressive effect on histamine-elicited drinking. This effect of propranolol may be nonspecific, as it appeared to be independent of dose, over a range of 0.08 mg/kg up to 1.4 mg/kg as shown here, and perhaps up to 6 mg/kg as shown by Gutman and Krausz (1973). Furthermore, propranolol, at doses as low as 0.23 mg/kg, has been found in this laboratory to reliably suppress drinking elicited by hypertonic saline (Table I). The nature of this general suppression produced by propranolol, possibly related to its hypertensive action, will need to be examined further. From the available evidence, however, it seems quite clear that, although β-adrenergic and kidney-dependent systems may have an effect on the magnitude of the drinking response elicited by histamine, they are not essential for this response to occur.

Histamine, therefore, appears to be distinguishable from other hypotensive drugs whose actions are critically dependent on kidney and β-adrenergic function. The primary difference would appear to lie in histamine's additional action on vascular permeability. Similar to the effects observed with polyethylene glycol and formalin (Stricker, 1973), histamine, by causing an increase in capillary permeability, would be expected to produce a decrease in blood volume which, through baroreceptor mediation, would lead to the activation of thirst-stimulating mechanisms in the brain. Further work will need to be done to evaluate the contribution of this mechanism to histamine-induced drinking. It appears consistent with the available evidence, however, to postulate at least a partial mediating role for this series of events, perhaps somewhat aggravated by histamine's potent vasodilatory effect.

In considering this possibility, it will be important to bear in mind the results of Gutman and Krausz (1973) obtained with the drug dextran. These authors found that this compound, intravenously administered, produced effects similar to those observed with histamine (increased water consumption, decreased blood volume after loss of protein-rich plasma, and increased renin release). Moreover, they found the increase in water intake to be abolished by the antihistamine diphenhydramine. Dextran's mechanism of action clearly differs from that of histamine, since its drinking response was also abolished by propranolol and nephrectomy. However, in trying to understand histamine's mechanism of action and the role of the histamine receptors in mediating increased water consumption, it is of value to note that diphenhydramine, while blocking the dextran effect on drinking, had no effect on the decrease in blood volume and renin release which acocmpanied the drinking. This dissociation between the physiological and the behavioral effects of dextran would, if nothing else, seem to suggest the existence of histamine receptors which function independently of blood volume to elicit drinking. In the case of histamine-induced water ingestion, we may be dealing with more than one set of receptors; those involved in producing its vascular effects and those with a more direct, perhaps neural, function involved in eliciting drinking. This suggestion is indeed speculative and must be evaluated cautiously, particularly in light of the finding that antihistamines may have a general suppressive effect on a variety of elicited drinking responses (Table I). However, the possibility that histamine receptors have a direct and specific function in mediating drug-elicited, as well as natural, thirst has received little attention, and it would appear to deserve further investigation in light of the results presented above.

In our discussion of the effect of histamine on water ingestion, we have so far neglected consideration of a very important organ, namely, the brain. It is certainly possible that histamine, in producing its effects on behavior, is acting on histamine receptors located somewhere in the central nervous system. Snyder et al. (1964), in analyzing the distribution of C^{14}-histamine after systemic administration, found that relatively little of the amine penetrated into the brain tissue, although a minute amount was detected over and above that expected to lie within the vasculature. While one could argue that this small amount may exist in a particular structure (lying within the blood-brain barrier) which is involved in stimulating drinking, a more reasonable suggestion might be that histamine is acting either on the cerebral vasculature or on brain areas, such as the circumventricular structures, which do not have a barrier.

Our evidence with the antihistamines would appear to favor a site of action for histamine which lies outside the blood-brain barrier. That is, both promethazine methylchloride and cimetidine, which are essentially incapable of penetrating into brain tissue, were found to be very effective in suppressing histamine's elicited drinking response (Table I). Another dipsogenic substance, angiotensin, is believed to produce its effects by acting on a circumventricular organ (Epstein, 1976), and it is possible that histamine might be operating in a similar fashion. In a recent study by Nicolaidis and Fitzsimons (1975), evidence was provided to suggest that angiotensin's thirst-provoking action may be mediated by its effects on mechanoreceptors which respond to alterations in the volume of the cerebral blood vessels. The circumventricular structures are highly vascularized, and the effect of angiotensin in this brain region was found to be antagonized by drugs which decrease vascular motility.

The importance of the vasculature in determining brain function has been seriously ignored and, in light of the numerous vasoactive substances found to alter behavior, this hypothesis deserves careful and thorough consideration. It may have value in understanding histamine's actions, since this drug (as discussed above) has extremely potent effects on the vascular system. With regard to the cerebral vascular bed, in vivo studies have generally found that systemically administered histamine is a potent vasodilator (Sokoloff, 1959; Anderson and Kubicek, 1971; Watters, 1971). These effects of histamine on cerebral blood flow, however, must be interpreted with caution, perhaps as possible artifacts related to histamine's systemic effects, its actions on vascular permeability, or on the extracranial circulation. In vitro studies on the vasomotor response of histamine in various intracranial vessels have usually indicated a contractile effect on the smooth musculature (Politoff and Macri, 1966; Nielsen and Owman, 1971). These actions, however, appear to be highly dependent on the conditions under which histamine is tested (Nielsen and Owman, 1971). Furthermore, it has been argued that this contractile response on cerebral vessels represents a nonspecific effect, in that it requires a relatively high concentration of histamine and is blocked in a noncompetitive manner by an H_1-receptor antagonist (Edvinsson and Owman, 1975). These authors, in fact, observed a vasodilatory effect of histamine at somewhat lower doses, and this response was competitively inhibited by an H_2-receptor blocker.

While this evidence does not permit us to draw any conclusions regarding the direction of histamine's vasomotor action, there appears to be no question that an effect on the cerebral vasculature does indeed occur after systemic histamine injection. A consequence of this action could possibly be the activation (or inhibition) of various brain regions, perhaps those that have direct neural control over drinking behavior.

This discussion brings us to the drinking phenomenon observed with central injection of histamine. What is the relationship between this behavior and the similar response observed with systemic injection? The first point to consider is whether the drinking elicited by centrally injected histamine might actually be due to its leakage from the brain and subsequent activation of peripheral histamine receptors. After comparing the doses required to be effective with central and systemic administration (see results above), it appears quite unlikely that this could be the case. To elicit a drinking response of approximately 5 ml, a dose of 500 μg would be required for systemic (intravenous or subcutaneous) injection, while a dose of less than 5 μg would be effective with central injection. Furthermore, the threshold doses observed for these different routes of administration were found to be 100 μg and 60 ng, respectively.

It is very possible, however, that systemic and central histamine are acting on similar receptors, perhaps located in the cerebral vasculature. As suggested above, these receptors may generate impulses to be transmitted to surrounding neural tissue and then converted into a signal for thirst. Until further experiments are conducted, such as those described by Nicolaidis and Fitzsimons (1975), we cannot evaluate the contribution of such a mechanism. It will be important to bear this idea in mind, however, when considering the additional possibility of histamine's direct action on central neural tissue, perhaps performing the function of a neurotransmitter or neuromodulator.

Several lines of evidence suggest a possible neurotransmitter role for histamine in the brain, as reviewed by Green (1970), Snyder and Taylor (1972), Schwartz (1975), and Calcutt (1976). Briefly, histamine is present in the brain and, together with its specific synthesizing enzyme, histidine decarboxylase, is localized in synaptosomes (pinched-off nerve terminals) prepared from brain homogenates. Endogenous histamine is selectively released from slices of brain tissue by potassium depolarization, accompanied by an increase in histamine synthesis. Its turnover in the brain is very rapid (although not in all cellular compartments), and its formation is found to be accelerated by physiological stress and decreased by barbiturates, hypnotics, and histidine decarboxylase inhibitors. Histamine in mammalian brain is distributed in a nonuniform manner, similar to the catecholamines and serotonin. Its concentration is highest in the hypothalamus, lower in the thalamus and midbrain, and lower still in the telencephalon. The histamine cell bodies are believed to be located in the lower brainstem where they give rise to an ascending bundle which passes through the lateral hypothalamus and projects to the forebrain (particularly the hypothalamus). Specific neuronal receptors to histamine (both H_1 and H_2) are apparently present in the brain, as demonstrated by various electrophysiological and iontophoretic studies, as well as by investigations of histamine's stimulatory effects on cAMP.

This evidence provides a strong foundation for a possible neuromodulatory role of histamine in control of behavior. In the experiments described above, histamine injected into the paraventricular nucleus of the hypothalamus was found to cause an increase in drinking behavior. This effect was anatomically specific, could be observed at doses as low as 60 ng, and was selectively suppressed by H_1- and H_2-receptor antagonists. The paraventricular nucleus and other hypothalamic structures of the rat brain have been found to contain relatively high concentrations of endogenous histamine (Brownstein et al., 1974). Furthermore, when applied iontophoretically to a nearby area, histamine was shown to have an excitatory effect (blocked by an H_2-receptor blocker) on neuronal activity (Haas, 1974; Haas et al., 1975). These findings are consistent with the idea that endogenous histamine has a neurotransmitter role in the control of drinking behavior, and that this control involves specific H_1- and H_2-neuronal receptors. The significance of such a receptor mechanism for maintaining body fluid homeostasis is not known at this time. Further investigations to examine the validity of this working hypothesis will need to employ more extensive pharmacological manipulations, such as drugs that release endogenous histamine, as well as biochemical analyses correlated with behavior. It should be pointed out, however, that in the iontophoretic studies of Haas, the neuronal response elicited by histamine was sometimes slow and variable. Furthermore, in our behavioral studies (see above), the drinking response induced by microinjected histamine had a relatively long latency, varying between 2 and 10 minutes.

There are numerous reasons why histamine might be slow in acting, and three possibilities are the following: (1) Rather than acting at the site of injection (paraventricular nucleus), histamine may produce its effect after diffusion to another brain site, perhaps as a result of spread up the cannula shaft and into the ventricles. While this would provide easy access to the subfornical organ where angiotensin is believed to be acting (Epstein, 1976), it does not explain the anatomical specificity demonstrated for histamine with cannulas which have different target sites but similar penetration of the cerebral ventricles. (2) Another possible explanation for the delay in responding may be that histamine, rather than causing direct activation of thirst-stimulating neurons, is acting indirectly through some other neural mechanism. A possible mediating system may be the thermoregulatory pathway described by Brezenoff and Lomax (1970) and by Green et al. (1976). Histamine injected into the anterior hypothalamus was found to produce hypothermia, which these authors attributed to a lowering of the set-point and activation of efferent heat-loss mechanisms. This effect, mediated through H_1 and H_2 receptors, might be expected to elicit drinking behavior as a component of the heat-loss process (see Fitzsimons, 1972). (3) A delay in drinking might also occur if histamine were acting through another transmitter substance in the brain. Relevant to this point are the studies of Campos and Jurupe (1970a,b) in which electrical stimulation was found to increase release of histamine which then very rapidly accelerated the synthesis of serotonin. A similar relationship was described for acetylcholine and histamine, in which the former was believed to be the stimulus for increased cerebral histamine. These findings are especially intriguing, in light of the evidence suggesting a possible role for both serotonin and acetylcholine in the control of drinking behavior (see Fitzsimons, 1972, for review).

There is accumulating evidence to suggest that, in addition to its neuronal localization, histamine in the brain may also exist in nonneuronal cells, probably mast cells (Martres et al., 1975; Schwartz, 1975; Verdiere et al., 1975; Garbarg et al., 1976). While the function of these cells in the hypothalamus is not known, it is interesting to note that they are especially numerous along blood vessels and meninges, although they are also found in the parenchyma (Ibrahim, 1974). The close proxmity of these histamine-containing cells to the vasculature returns us to the first suggestion that histamine might elicit drinking behavior through its actions on the cerebral blood vessels. This mode of action, which might of course occur in addition to a direct histamine effect on brain neurons, may be a component of the immune or inflammatory processes characteristically associated with mast-cell histamine.

HISTAMINE-INDUCED ANTIDIURESIS

Introduction

Histamine, when systemically administered, has been known for many years to cause a reduction in urine output. This effect was first described by

Dale and Laidlaw (1910) in the cat and was subsequently confirmed by Gilman and Kidd (1938) in the dog and by Bjering (1937) and Reubi and Futcher (1949) in humans. These investigators generally agreed on the specifics of the effect produced by histamine, which, in addition to oliguria, included a decrease in blood pressure accompanied by a reduction in renal blood flow. Until 1950, this change in renal hemodynamics, a consequence of hypotension, was believed to be the critical step in producing antidiuresis after histamine injection. Subsequent to Pickford's review (1952), however, in which this relationship was seriously questioned, Blackmore and his associates (1953) presented evidence for a histamine-induced antidiuresis in the dog which occurred in the absence of any change in the glomerular filtration rate of the kidney and was actually associated with an increase in renal blood flow. This indicated that the effect of histamine on urine output might occur independently of changes in renal hemodynamics and that it might instead (or in addition) result from a change in the rate of water reabsorption by the kidney. To test the possibility of a hormonal mediation of the antidiuresis, Blackmore and Cherry (1955) examined dogs with damaged supraopticohypophysial systems and found these animals to be unresponsive to histamine, suggesting a mediating role for antidiuretic hormone (ADH).

This hypothesis receives direct support from a few recent studies in which histamine was injected centrally as well as peripherally and measurements of plasma ADH were taken. Dogterom et al., (1976), working with rats, found histamine (injected intraperitoneally) to cause a rapid increase in plasma ADH levels at doses of 0.625 to 50 mg/kg. When injected into the cerebral ventricles, histamine produced the same effect, although an extremely high dose of 0.6 mg/kg was used.

Ventricular injection of histamine in the anesthetized dog (at doses of 25 to 200 μg) has similarly been found to release ADH, an effect accompanied by oliguria (Bhargava et al., 1973). There appears to be only one study in which histamine was injected directly into the supraoptic nucleus, and in this study, conducted in the anesthetized cat (Bennett and Pert, 1974), antidiuresis was observed with 15 to 60 μg of histamine. This effect was abolished after destruction of the surpaopticohypophysial tract.

These investigations clearly strengthen the idea that ADH is mediating histamine's effect on urine formation, although the possibility still remains, particularly for peripheral histamine, that renal hemodynamic changes may also be involved. This evidence provides the background for our research on histamine as related to the control of urine excretion in the rat. In this section, we will first describe the effects observed with systemically injected histamine, as a function of dose, in the presence of various receptor blockers, and in hypophysectomized animals. We will then describe similar experiments conducted in the brain, in rats with chronic cannulas aimed at the hypothalamus. We will then attempt to discuss the significance of these findings, relating histamine's antidiuretic action to its peripheral and central effects on the vasculature and neuronal function and its effect on drinking behavior.

Studies with Systemic Drug Administration

Abstract

Results described in this section demonstrate that systemically injected histamine in the hydrated rat produces a dramatic, dose-dependent antidiuresis (increase in urine output and decrease in urine osmolality). This effect, which can be observed at doses as low as 0.125 mg/kg, appears to be selectively mediated by H_1- and, to a lesser extent, H_2-histamine receptors, and can occur in the absence of the pituitary.

Description of peripheral histamine-induced antidiuresis

The procedures used in these experiments were as follows. All tests were carried out on food- and water-satiated rats. At the time of the test, all food and water was removed, and each rat received an intragastric water load, approximately 3.5 ml/100 gm body weight. At 15 minutes after intubation, the rats were subcutaneously injected with histamine or its vehicle, and the volume of urine output 60 minutes after injection was recorded. Urine osmolalities (at 60 minutes) were also determined, cryoscopically with a Fiske osmometer.

As shown in Table II, histamine was found to have a dramatic effect on urine output and osmolality in the hydrated rat. At the lowest dose tested (0.125 mg/kg), a 14% reduction in urine output was observed, accompanied by a 25% increase in urine osmolality. (These differences did not quite reach statistical significance, using a two-tailed *t*-test for dependent means.) At a dose of 0.25 mg/kg, a reliable 23% decrease in urine output was recorded,

Table II
Antidiuresis Produced by Subcutaneous Histamine Injection as a Function of Dose

Histamine (mg/kg)	Urine Output (ml)[a]			Urine Osmolality (mOsm/kg H_2O)[a]		
	Mean ± SEM	% Decrease	p	Mean ± SEM	% Increase	p
0.0	6.4 ± 0.55	—	—	263 ± 27.0	—	—
0.125	5.5 ± 0.88	–14	>0.05	329 ± 43.6	+25	>0.05
0.25	4.9 ± 1.10	–23	<0.01	363 ± 34.7	+38	<0.05
1.25	2.6 ± 0.41	–59	<0.001	494 ± 52.4	+88	<0.01
6.25	0.8 ± 0.47	–88	<0.001	565 ± 79.3	+115	<0.01

[a]Comparisons made relative to vehicle (0.0 mg/kg) baseline.

Table III
Effect of Receptor Antagonists on Antidiuresis Produced by Subcutaneous Histamine Injection

Type of receptor	Antagonist	ID_{50} (mg/kg)[a] Urine output	Urine osmolality
H_1 Histaminergic	Dexbrompheniramine	0.5 ± 0.2	0.3 ± 0.1
	Methapyrilene	1.2 ± 0.6	1.4 ± 0.7
	Tripelennamine	1.4 ± 0.5	2.0 ± 0.8
	Promethazine Hydrochloride	2.4 ± 0.6	3.2 ± 0.6
	Promethazine Methylchloride	2.6 ± 0.8	3.5 ± 0.9
H_2 Histaminergic	Cimetidine	6.3 ± 0.7	6.6 ± 0.2
β-Adrenergic	dl-Propranolol	>5.6	>5.6
α-Adrenergic	Phentolamine	>1.5	>1.5
Dopaminergic	Haloperidol	>0.3	>0.3
Cholinergic	Atropine	>1.5	>1.5
Serotonergic	Cinanserin	>4.0	>4.0

[a] ID_{50}: The antagonist dose calculated, on the basis of a dose-response curve, to produce a 50% inhibition of the antidiuretic response (decrease in urine output and increase in urine osmolality) induced by systemic injection of histamine. For drugs other than the histaminergic antagonists, higher doses than those indicated were not tested with histamine, since they were found to alter dramatically the baseline values in control tests. At the doses indicated or at lower doses, no inhibition and sometimes an enhancement of the histamine effect was observed.

along with a 38% increase in osmolality. These reciprocal effects increased in magnitude with increase in dose up to 6.25 mg/kg. At this highest dose tested, an 88% inhibition of urine excretion and a 115% increase in osmolality were observed. This antidiuretic effect of histamine proved extremely robust at doses of 0.5 mg/kg and higher, appearing in essentially every animal tested. These findings are in agreement with the histamine effects described in the literature and, in addition, show the threshold dose for histamine in the rat to be approximately 0.25 mg/kg subcutaneously administered.

Characterization of receptors

There appear to be no studies in the literature which have attempted to identify the nature of the receptors mediating this antidiuretic response to peripheral histamine. Therefore, to provide a pharmacological analysis of this phenomenon, we tested several different histamine (H_1 and H_2) antagonists, as well as antagonists of other types of receptors, in combination with subcutaneous histamine. The results of these experiments, summarized in Table III, revealed a dose-dependent inhibition of histamine's action with each of the histamine antagonists tested. By comparing the ID_{50} of these compounds, their order of potency in reversing histamine-induced antidiuresis was dexbrompheniramine $>$ methapyrilene $=$ tripelennamine $>$ promethazine hydrochloride $=$ promethazine methylchloride $>$ cimetidine. The dose-response curves were essentially parallel, indicating a similar mechanism of action. The maximum blockade obtained with each antagonist (at least 85% for all drugs except cimetidine which produced only a 50% blockade) was observed at a dose which by itself had no consistent effect on the rats' baseline urine output or osmolality. (Higher doses generally did affect the baseline.)

The partial blockade obtained with cimetidine provides the first evidence that H_2 receptors, in addition to H_1 receptors, might play a role in mediating histamine's effect on urine formation. To further substantiate this possibility, we examined the effects of the selective H_1-receptor agonist 2-methylhistamine and the H_2-receptor agonists 4-methylhistamine and dimaprit at relatively high doses of 7.5 and 15 mg/kg. At these doses, subcutaneous histamine produced a near maximum antidiuretic effect, with 65% to 90% reduction of urine output and 135% to 180% increase in urine osmolality. The selective H_1 and H_2 agonists each mimicked these effects, producing up to a 50% suppression of urine volume and a 150% increase in urine osmolality. The H_1 agonist 2-methylhistamine was clearly most potent, producing approximately twice the effect of the H_2 agonist dimaprit. 4-Methylhistamine was least effective at these doses, yielding a relatively small increase in urine osmolality (30 to 70%) without reliably altering urine flow.

These results obtained with the selective histamine agonists and antagonists strengthen the suggestion that both H_1 and H_2 receptors are involved in mediating histamine-induced antidiuresis, with the H_1 receptor apparently playing a more predominant role. To further establish the selectivity of the antihistamine's actions and determine whether other types of receptors might also be involved, we examined, in combination with histamine, various antagonists of adrenergic (phentolamine and propranolol), cholinergic (atropine), dopaminergic (haloperidol), and serotonergic (cinanserin) receptors. None of these receptor blockers (at doses ranging from 0.1 to 6 mg/kg) had any consistent effect on histamine's action, including the β-adrenergic antagonist propranolol which had been found to suppress (although not abolish) histamine-induced drinking (see above).

Tests in hypophysectomized animals

The pituitary is known to contain dense concentrations of endogenous histamine (Adam and Hye, 1966; Snyder and Taylor, 1972), as well as to take up exogenous histamine from the blood (Adam et al., 1964). In light of this evidence, it is possible that histamine might be acting directly on the pituitary to cause a release of ADH. To determine whether this organ is essential for the

Table IV
Histamine-Induced Antidiuresis in Hypophysectomized and Normal Rats[a]

	Histamine (mg/kg)	Normal		Hypophysectomized	
		Mean ± SEM	p	Mean ± SEM	p
Urine output	4	−61 ± 5.7	<0.001	−47 ± 9.7	<0.01
(% decrease)	8	−84 ± 5.0	<0.001	−59 ± 14.2	<0.001
Urine osmolality	4	+86 ± 15.3	<0.01	+108 ± 12.8	<0.01
(% increase)	8	+121 ± 9.7	<0.01	+149 ± 13.5	<0.001

[a]Completeness of hypophysectomy was determined by histological examination and measurements of food and water intake, body weight, growth, and organ weights.

antidiruetic effect of systemic histamine, we examined the effectiveness of this amine in animals that had been hypophysectomized 1 to 2 weeks prior to testing. The results of this experiment, presented in Table IV, clearly showed the pituitary to be unessential for histamine-induced antidiuresis. After removel of this organ, the animals exhibited a significant suppression of urine output, approximately 30% less than normal rats, and a large increase in urine osmolality, approximately 25% greater than normal. These hypophysectomized animals did not show signs of diabetes insipidus, indicating that ADH was being appropriately released by the brain, either from undegenerated or regenerated supraopticohypophysial fibers which normally project to the neurohypophysis (Rasmussen, 1940; Billenstein and Leveque, 1955; Adams *et al.,* 1968) or to the zona externa of the median eminence (Rothballer and Skoryna, 1960; Defendini and Zimmerman, 1978). The ADH release in the absence of the pituitary was apparently sufficient to reveal the antidiuretic effect of histamine. Moreover, the effectiveness of histamine demonstrtated in these hypophysectomized animals clearly indicates that the pituitary does not contain the critical mediating histamine receptors.

Studies with Central Drug Administration

Abstract

This section describes the effect of centrally administered histamine on urine excretion. When injected into the hypothalamus of the hydrated rat, histamine is found to produce a strong antidiurectic response involving a decrease in urine output and an increase in urine osmolality. This effect is anatomically specific, occurring most readily with injection into the supraoptic nucleus and to a somewhat lesser extent in the paraventricular nucleus. In the supraoptic nucleus, doses of histamine as low as 40 ng (free base) are observed to produce a reliable response. When tested in combination with receptor antagonists (centrally administered), the histamine-induced antidiuresis is found to be suppressed or abolished by H_1- and H_2-histamine antagonists, as well as by an α-adrenergic antagonist.

Description of central histamine-induced antidiuresis

In these experiments, all drugs were administered centrally through stereotaxically implanted brain cannulas, and their effects on urine excretion and osmolality in the hydrated rat were measured. (See previous section for details.) In the first series of tests, the effect of histamine was examined after injection into three different brain areas, namely, the supraoptic nucleus, the paraventricular nucleus, and the perifornical lateral hypothalamus. As shown in Fig. 1, the supraoptic and paraventricular nuclei both responded to histamine by inducing a dose-dependent decrease in urine output, accompanied by an increase in urine osmolality. The supraoptic nucleus appeared to be more sensitive than the paraventricular nucleus, while the perifornical lateral hypothalamus (1 mm lateral to the paraventricular nucleus) was essentially unresponsive. At the highest dose tested (100 nmoles), histamine in these three structures caused, respectively, a 67% ($p < 0.001$), 37% ($p < 0.05$), and 8% reduction in urine output and a 64% ($p < 0.001$), 32% ($p < 0.05$), and 3% increase in osmolality. At the lowest dose of 12.5 nmoles, histamine was still reliably effective in the supraoptic and paraventricular nuclei, producing in them, respectively, a 37% ($p < 0.01$) and 20% ($p < 0.05$) decrease in urine output and a 33% ($p < 0.01$) and 18% ($p < 0.10$) increase in osmolality. This antidiuretic effect of histamine, especially in the supraoptic nucleus, was remarkably robust, consistently associated with reciprocal changes in volume and osmolality.

Tests for threshold doses of histamine

The above results indicate a clear dose-dependent effect of central histamine on urine formation. The response is anatomically specific, associated with the supraoptic nucleus and, to a lesser extent, the paraventricular nucleus. To evaluate more carefully the sensitivity of this area to lower doses of histamine, we selected a group of rats with supraoptic cannulas which consistently and vigorously responded to histamine at relatively high doses, and then gradually lowered these doses until a reliable response was no longer observed.

In these animals with verified supraoptic nucleus cannulas, histamine at 10.8 nmoles produced a strong antidiuretic response in all animals (averaging a 65% suppression of urine volume and 52% enhancement of urine osmolality). This response gradually declined to -52% ($p < 0.01$) and $+ 29\%$ ($p < 0.05$), respectively, at a dose of 1.35 nmoles, and further to -34% ($p < 0.05$) and $+8\%$ ($p < 0.10$) at a dose of 0.34 nmoles. This threshold dose (equivalent to 40 ng free base) for histamine-induced antidiuresis is somewhat higher than the 1 to 10 ng doses found to be effective for norepinephrine or epinephrine in producing a similar antidiuretic effect in the rat supraoptic nucleus (Garay and Leibowitz, 1974). It is at least 200-fold lower than the threshold dose revealed for systemic histamine-induced antidiuresis and approximately equivalent to the threshold dose (60 ng) observed for central histamine-elicited drinking behavior (see previous sections).

Characterization of receptors

To characterize the receptors mediating histamine's effect in the supraoptic nucleus, we examined the effects of the H_1-receptor antagonist, dexbrompheniramine, and the H_2 antagonist, cimetidine. To examine the specificity of these drugs' actions, we also tested a variety of other compounds known to antagonize dopaminergic (haloperidol), β-adrenergic (propranolol), α-adrenergic (phentolamine), and cholinergic (atropine) receptors. All drugs were injected directly into the supraoptic nucleus, with the receptor antagonists administered 5 minutes prior to histamine.

The outcome of these experiments on histamine-induced antidiuresis clearly revealed a dose-dependent suppression of this effect with both the H_1- and H_2-receptor antagonists. [Bhargava *et al.*, (1973) in the dog and Bennett and Pert (1974) in the cat each found an H_1 antagonist to be effective in blocking histamine's actions. An H_2 antagonist was not examined in these tests.] At the highest doses tested (which by themselves had no effect on the baseline urine output of hydrated rats), the H_1 blocker dexbrompheniramine (at 9 nmoles) produced a nearly total blockade (approxiamtely 85%), whereas the H_2 blocker cimetidine (at 14 nmoles) yielded only a partial blockade (approximately 50%). This pattern of results is consistent with the findings obtained with peripheral histamine-induced antidiuresis but contrasts with the results obtained with peripheral or central histamine-induced drinking which was partially antagonized by the H_1-, as well as the H_2-, receptor blockers.

This central injection study indicates for the first time that central H_1 and H_2 receptors, located in the supraoptic nucleus, may be involved in histamine-induced antidiuresis, with the H_1 receptor apparently playing a more predominant role. Additional tests with dopaminergic, β-adrenergic, and cholinergic receptor blockers failed to reveal any effects of these drugs on histamine's antidiuretic response, emphasizing once again the specificity of the histamine receptor action. With the α-adrenergic antagonist, however, a nearly total block of histamine's effect was observed. The doses of phentolamine tested ranged from 15 to 60 nmoles. This result, which clearly distinguishes the antidiuretic response to histamine from its elicited drinking response, which remained unaffected by α-adrenergic blockade, is consistent with the finding of Bhargava *et al.* (1973) that phenoxybenzamine, another α-

adrenergic antagonist, can block the ADH-releasing effect of cerebro-ventricular histamine in the dog. Bennett and Pert (1974), however, did not observe this blockade effect with injection into the supraoptic nucleus of the cat.

Discussion of Histamine's Antidiuretic Effect

These results obtained with systemic and central injection of histamine in the rat demonstrate a potent antidiuretic effect, as revealed by a decrease in urine output and an increase in urine osmolality. The effect is dose-dependent, occurring at doses as low as 125 μg systemically injected and 40 ng centrally injected (into supraoptic nucleus). With peripheral administration, this histamine effect is mimicked by selective H_1- and, to a lesser extent, H_2-receptor agonists and is selectively abolished by H_1-receptor blockers and partially suppressed by an H_2-receptor blocker. Furthermore, this response is found to remain intact in hypophysectomized animals. Centrally, histamine-induced antidiuresis is similarly abolished or partially suppressed, respectively, by H_1 and H_2 blockers but is also antagonized by an α-adrenergic receptor blocker.

In light of these results, what might be said regarding histamine's mode of action; what is the relationship between its effect peripherally and centrally, and between its complementary behavioral (drinking) and physiological (antidiuresis) adjustments in body fluid regulation?

When histamine's action on the kidney is examined independently of changes in systemic blood pressure (such as in the isolated kidney), an increase in renal blood flow is generally observed, accompanied by an increase in urine output and a decrease in osmolality (O'Brien and Williamson, 1971; Sinclair et al., 1974; Campbell and Itskovitz, 1976). This evidence indicates that histamine's antidiuretic effect described above cannot be attributed to a direct action on renal hemodynamics. With regard to the possibility of a reflexive change in renal glomerular filtration as a consequence of histamine-induced decrease in systemic blood pressure, Blackmore et al. (1953) demonstrated a histamine antidiuretic response in the dog under conditions of no change in glomerular filtration rate and actually an increase in renal blood flow. This result, indicating once again the independence of histamine's antidiuretic effect from changes in renal hemodynamics, led these authors to propose an effect on tubular reabsorption of water, presumably via ADH. Subsequent investigations have provided clear support for this view, in demonstrating an actual release of ADH after systemic (Dogterom et al., 1976) as well as central (Bhargava et al., 1973; Dogterom et al., 1976) histamine injection, and also in showing the dependence of histamine's action on an intact supraopticohypophysial system (Blackmore and Cherry, 1955; Bennett and Pert, 1974).

This evidence appears to indicate that both central and peripheral histamine produce their antidiuretic effect through the release of ADH. The important question now is, where are the receptors mediating this phenomenon and, furthermore, are peripheral and central histamine acting via the same receptors? As discussed above in the section on water intake, systemically administered histamine is known to have potent effects on the vasculature. These effects include a decrease in blood pressure, resulting from histamine's vasodilatory action and its ability to increase capillary permeability and thus decrease blood volume. These intravascular changes are known to initiate a variety of reflexive mechanisms which contribute to blood volume regulation; these include cardiovascular adjustments involving the autonomic nervous system and adrenal medullary secretions, intrinsic control by the circulation of blood flow in peripheral tissues, and, as mentioned above, the direct effects of arterial pressure on glomerular filtration (Gauer *et al.,* 1970). In addition, they are believed to activate complementary behavioral (water ingestion) and physiological (antidiuresis) adjustments to help restore normal body fluid volume. The mechanisms involved here include the renin–angiotensin system of the kidney and the baroreceptors located in the capacitance vessels of the low-pressure circulation. These volume regulatory mechanisms are known to release ADH (Gauer and Henry, 1963; Share, 1969; Malvin, 1971), which then acts on the kidney to accelerate the rate of water reabsorption. As discussed earlier, they are also believed to motivate drinking, the behavioral component of the volume-regulatory response to plasma deficits.

Our evidence obtained for histamine-elicited drinking appeared to indicate a greater importance of baroreceptor function, rather than the renin–angiotensin system, in the mediation of this response. The primary evidence favoring this suggestion was the failure of propranolol and nephrectomy, procedures that eliminate renin release, to abolish the histamine drinking response. A similar argument may be applied to the control of ADH secretion, which, as reflected in the antidiuretic response observed with histamine, was found to be unaffected by propranolol even at quite high doses. The importance of histamine's potent effect on capillary permeability and blood volume and the consequent changes in baroreceptor activity will need to be carefully examined in terms of the pharmacological properties of this phenomenon and its predictive ability for histamine-induced antidiuresis. At the moment, this mechanism would appear to provide a reasonable explanation for the effect of peripherally administered histamine on ADH release.

Histamine's actions, however, may not end here, and, as discussed for the elicited drinking response, the phenomenon of antidiuresis may involve an additional set of histamine receptors, perhaps located in a region of the brain. In view of Snyder's *et al.* (1964) results indicating that systemic histamine fails to pass the blood–brain barrier in any significant amounts, histamine's central activity would most likely be confined to structures outside the barrier or perhaps in the cerebral vasculature. Evidence to support this suggestion is provided by our finding that antihistamines (cimetidine and promethazine methylchloride), which are essentially incapable of penetrating the blood–brain barrier, are effective in attenuating or abolishing the antidiuresis produced by systemic histamine.

Based on this argument, it seems that the H_1 and H_2 receptors identified by our central injection studies in the supraoptic and paraventricular nuclei are inaccessible to peripheral histamine, unless of course these receptors exist in or near to the vasculature or in some unique location lying outside the barrier. In view of histamine's potent actions on cerebral vessels (see discussion earlier), the possibility of a nonneuronal site of action, for central as well as peripheral histamine, remains a real possibility. With regard to histamine's actions on neural structures lying outside the blood–brain barrier, the most likely candidates are the circumventricular structures which have been postulated to have a role in the mediation of angiotensin-induced thirst (Epstein, 1976) and the median eminence. The median eminence and the pituitary are found to have the highest concentrations of histamine of any brain regions assayed (Adams and Hye, 1966; Snyder and Taylor, 1972; Browstein et al., 1974). The pituitary, however, does not seem to be essential for the antidiuretic effect (nor presumably the ADH release) elicited by peripheral histamine, since we found this response to occur equally in hypophysectomized and normal animals (see evidence above). The median eminence, in contrast, appears to be a reasonable site for peripheral histamine's receptor action since, in addition to its dense concentration of endogenous histamine and its location outside the blood–brain barrier, the median eminence (zona externa) is believed to play a role in ADH release (Rothballer and Skoryna, 1960; Defendini and Zimmerman, 1978). Blackmore and Cherry (1955) found the destruction of this area to abolish the antidiuresis induced by systemic histamine. This experiment, however, does not allow us to distinguish the possibility that peripheral histamine acts directly on median eminence histaminergic receptors, from the possibility of its acting at some other site which then requires an intact supraopticohypophysial pathway for release of ADH.

The question of whether peripheral histamine acts on H_1 and H_2 receptors located in the supraoptic and paraventricular nuclei cannot be resolved at the present time. This remains a distinct possibility, the above considerations notwithstanding. The pharmacological analyses conducted with peripheral and central drug injections revealed similar results with the H_1- and H_2-receptor blockers. A clear distinction, however, between the antidiuretic effects produced by these two routes of administration was observed with an α-adrenergic blocker which essentially abolished central histamine's actions while leaving intact the effect of subcutaneous histamine. This finding, which is consistent with the results of Bhargava *et al.* (1973) in the dog, suggests that peripheral and central histamine may act at different sites, or at least involve different neurochemical mechanisms. It is possible, of course, that in the supraoptic nucleus, where phentolamine blocked histamine's antidiuretic effect, this α-adrenergic antagonist is exhibiting antihistamine properties. This action, however, was not observed with phentolamine in the paraventricular nucleus in our studies of histamine-elicited drinking. Furthermore, Bhargava *et al.* (1973) also found tetrabenazine, a norepinephrine-depleting agent, to block histamine's actions, suggesting that histamine was operating indirectly through the release of norepinephrine. This is certainly a reasonable possibility, in light of the extensive evidence demonstrating an antidiuretic effect of norepinephrine in the supraoptic and paraventricular nuclei (Bhargava *et al.*, 1972; Garay and Leibowitz, 1974; Kühn, 1974; Milton and Paterson, 1974).

Several lines of evidence, summarized in our discussion of histamine-elicited drinking, suggest that histamine in the brain may act as a neurotransmitter in the control of behavioral and physiological processes. The possibility that histamine's antidiuretic effect in the supraoptic and paraventricular nuclei reflects such a neurotransmitter function in the regulation body fluid homeostasis receives support from the following:

1. These hypothalamic structures are known to have a primary role in the release of ADH. Histamine's antidiuretic action appears to be anatomically specific, localized to these two structures and their vicinity (see above and results described by Bennett and Pert, 1974).
2. The supraoptic and paraventricular nuclei contain high concentrations of endogenous histamine (Brownstein *et al.*, 1974).
3. Relatively low concentrations of exogenous histamine (at least as low as 40 ng) are effective in producing antidiuresis after injection into the supraoptic nucleus (see results described above).
4. Iontophoretic application of histamine increases firing of supraoptic neurosecretory neurons (Haas *et al.*, 1975.)
5. Histamine's actions in the supraoptic nucleus are antagonized by selective H_1- and H_2-receptor blockers (see above).
6. Antidiuresis and ADH release, produced by cerebral injection of hypertonic saline, are found to be selectively blocked by histamine receptor antagonists (Santhakumari, 1974).
7. In addition to producing antidiuresis, central histamine injection elicits a drinking response. This behavioral effect is localized to the paraventricular nucleus where it occurs at relatively low doses (60 ng), and, similar to the antidiuretic response, appears to be mediated by H_1 and H_2 receptors. This phenomenon, together with histamine's antidiuretic action in the supraoptic and paraventricular nuclei, possibly indicates a more general role for histamine in central neural

control of body fluid homeostasis. This mechanism may involve an intimate neuronal communication between the supraoptic and paraventricular nuclei, as well as the interaction with other neurochemical systems (such as norepinephrine) and perhaps with nonneuronal compartments of histamine, such as that contained within cerebral mast cells (Schwartz, 1975).

CONCLUSION

The results presented above provide clear evidence for an effect of histamine on the regulation of body fluid balance. This effect occurs with both central and peripheral histamine injections and involves both H_1 and H_2 receptors. These receptors are possibly located on neuronal tissue where histamine, particularly in the brain, may have a neurotransmitter role in regulating the activity of neurons directly involved in stimulating thirst and releasing ADH. The areas of the brain participating in this function appear to be the supraoptic and paraventricular nuclei. The effects observed with peripheral histamine may also involve these brain regions. However, since histamine generally does not penetrate the blood–brain barrier, it may act on central histamine receptors lying outside the barrier, perhaps within the median eminence and circumventricular organs.

The effects of peripheral as well as central histamine may also involve nonneuronal receptors (perhaps located within or on the vasculature) which may contribute indirectly to changes in central neural activity. Relevant to this possibility is the "intrinsic histamine hypothesis" of Schayer (1965) which proposes a role for endogenous histamine in regulating the microcirculation. Histamine is synthesized within cells of small blood vessels, and its function here may be to make appropriate adjustments in central and peripheral capillaries (dilation and increased permeability) to satisfy particular requirements resulting, for example, from exercise, inflammation, temperature fluctuation, injury, and pregnancy. Each of these phenomena is associated with an increase in histamine, as well as with changes in the distribution and composition of body fluids and appropriate homeostatic adjustments (including drinking and ADH release).

It is possible that a role for histamine in controlling neuronal and vascular functions may have special significance in the developing animal. A uniquely high histamine-forming capacity is present in many tissues (including brain) undergoing rapid growth as well as repair (Kahlson and Rosengren, 1971; Schwartz, 1975). Perhaps, under these circumstances, histamine's function in regulating body fluid homeostasis is one of particular importance.

ACKNOWLEDGMENTS

This research was supported by U.S. Public Health Service Research Grant MH 22879 from the National Institute of Mental Health, by an Alfred P. Sloan Fellowship, and by a grant from the Whitehall Foundation. Dr. Edward M. Stricker's advice during the preparation of this manuscript is gratefully acknowledged.

REFERENCES

Adam, H.M., and Hye, H.K.A. (1966). Concentration of histamine in different parts of brain and hypophysis of cat and its modification by drugs. *Brit. J. Pharmacol.* **28**, 137–152.

Adam, H.M., Hye, H.K.A., and Waton, W.G. (1964). Studies on uptake and formation of histamine by hypophysis and hypothalamus in the cat. *J. Physiol. (London)* **175**, 70P–71P.

Adams, J.H., Daniel, P.M., and Prichard, M.L. (1968). Regrowth of nerve fibers in the neurohypophysis: regeneration of a tract of the central nervous system. *J. Physiol. (London)* **198**, 4P–5P.

Anderson, W.D., and Kubicek, W.G. (1971). Effects of betahistine HCl, nicotinic acid, and histamine on basilar blood flow in anesthetized dogs. *Stroke* **2**, 409–415.

Ash, A.S.F., and Schild, H.O. (1966). Receptors mediating some actions of histamine. *Brit. J. Pharmacol.* **27**, 427–439.

Baudry, M., Martres, M.-P., and Schwartz, J.-C. (1975). H_1 and H_2 receptors in the histamine-induced accumulation of cyclic AMP in guinea pig brain slices. *Nature (London)* **253**, 362–364.

Bennett, C.T., and Pert, A. (1974). Antidiuresis produced by injections of histamine into the cat supraoptic nucleus. *Brain Res.* **78**, 151–156.

Bhargava, K.P., Kulshrestha, V.K., Santhakumari, G., and Srivastave, Y.P. (1973). Mechanism of histamine-induced antidiuretic response. *Brit. J. Pharmacol.* **47**, 700–706.

Bhargava, K.P., Kulshrestha, V.K., and Srivastava, Y.P. (1972). Central cholinergic and adrenergic mechanisms in the release of ADH. *Brit. J. Pharmacol.* **44**, 617–627.

Billenstein, D.C., and Leveque, T.F. (1955). The reorganization of the neurohypophyseal stalk following hypophysectomy in the rat. *Endocrinology* **36**, 704–717.

Bjering, T. (1937). The influence of histamine on renal function. *Acta Med. Scand.* **91**, 267–278.

Black, J.W., Duncan, W.A.M., Durant, D.J., Ganellin, C.R., and Parsons, E.M. (1972). Definition and antagonism of histamine H_2 receptors. *Nature (London)* **236**, 385–390.

Blackmore, W.P., and Cherry, G.R. (1955). Antidiuretic action of histamine in the dog. *Amer. J. Physiol.* **180**, 596–598.

Blackmore, W.P., Wilson, V.E., and Sherrod, T.R. (1953). The effect of histamine on renal dynamics. *J. Pharmacol. Exp. Ther.* **109**, 206–213.

Block, M.L., and Fisher, A.E. (1975). Cholinergic and dopaminergic blocking agents modulate water intake elicited by deprivation, hypovolemia, hypertonicity and isoproterenol. *Pharmacol. Biochem. Behav.* **3**, 251–262.

Brezenoff, H.E., and Lomax, P. (1970). Temperature changes following microinjection of histamine into the thermoregulatory centres of the rat. *Experientia* **26**, 51–52.

Brimblecombe, R.W., Flynn, S.B., and Owen, D.A.A. (1975). Effects of histamine, 2-methylhistamine and 4-methylhistamine on blood pressure and vascular resistance in the cat. *J. Physiol. (London)* **249**, 31P–32P.

Brownstein, M.J., Saavedra, J.M., Palkovits, M., and Axelrod, J. (1974). Histamine content of hypothalamic nuclei of the rat. *Brain Res.* **77**, 151–156.

Calcutt, C.R. (1976). The role of histamine in the brain. *Gen. Pharmacol.* **7**, 15–25.

Campbell, W.B., and Itskovitz, H.D. (1976). Effect of histamine and antihistamines on renal hemodynamics and functions in the isolated perfused canine kidney. *J. Pharmacol. Exp. Ther.* **198**, 661–667.

Campos, H.A., and Jurupe, H. (1970a). A histamine-dependent increase of 5-hydroxytryptamine in the rat brain *in vivo. Experientia* **26**, 613–614.

Campos, H.A., and Jurupe, H. (1970b). Evidence for a cholinergic mechanism inducing histamine increase in the rat brain *in vivo. Experientia* **26**, 746–747.

Chasin, M., Mamrak, F., Samaniego, S.G., and Hess, S.M. (1973). Characteristics of the catecholamine and histamine receptor sites mediating accumulation of cyclic adenosine 3′,5′-monophosphate in guinea pig brain. *J. Neurochem.* **21**, 1415–1428.

Clineschmidt, B.V., and Lotti, V.J. (1973). Histamine: intraventricular injection suppresses ingestive behavior of the cat. *Arch. Int. Pharmacodyn.* **206**, 288–298.

Cohn, C.K., Ball, G.G., and Hirsch, J. (1973). Histamine effect on self-stimulation. *Science* **180**, 757–758.

Dale, H.H., and Laidlaw, P.P. (1910). The physiological action of β-imenazolylethylamine. *J. Physiol. (London)* **41**, 318–344.

Defendini, R., and Zimmerman, E.A. (1978). The magnocellular neurosecretory system of the mammalian hypothalamus. *Res. Publ. Ass. Res. Nerv. Ment. Dis.* (in press).

Dogterom, J., Van Wimersma, Tj. B., and de Wied, D. (1976). Histamine as an extremely potent releaser of vasopressin in the rat. *Experientia* **32**, 659–660.

Douglas, W.W. (1975). Histamine and antihistamines; 5-hydroxytryptamine and antagonists, in "The Pharmacological Basis of Therapeutics," (L.S. Goodman and A. Gilman, eds.), 5th ed., pp. 590–629. Macmillan, New York.

Edvinsson, L., and Owman, Ch. (1975). A pharmacologic comparison of histamine receptors in isolated extracranial and intracranial arteries *in vitro. Neurology* **25**, 271–276.

Epstein, A.N. (1973). Epilogue: retrospect and prognosis, in "The Neuropsychology of Thirst." (A.N. Epstein, H.R. Kissileff, and E. Stellar, eds.), pp. 315–332. V.H. Winston, Washington, D.C.

Epstein, A.N. (1976). The physiology of thirst. *Can. J. Physiol. Pharmacol.* **54**, 639–649.

Fitzsimons, J.T. (1972). Thirst. *Physiol. Rev.* **52**, 468–561.

Gabbiani, G., Badonnel, M.C., and Majno, G. (1950). Intra-arterial injections of histamine, serotonin, or bradykinin: a topographic study of vascular leakage. *Proc. Soc. Exp. Biol. Med.* **135**, 447–452.

Garay, K.F., and Leibowitz, S.F. (1974). Antidiuresis produced by adrenergic receptor stimulation of the rat supraoptic nucleus. *Federation Proc.* **33**, 563 (abstract).

Garbarg, M., Barbin, G., Bischoff, S., Pollard, H., and Schwartz, J.C. (1976). Dual localization of histamine in an ascending neuronal pathway and in non-neuronal cells evidenced by lesions in the lateral hypothalamic area. *Brain Res.* **106**, 333–348.

Gauer, O.H., and Henry, J.P. (1963). Circulatory basis of fluid volume control. *Physiol. Rev.* **43**, 423–481.

Gauer, O.H., Henry, J.P., and Behn, C. (1970). The regulation of extracellular fluid volume. *Annu. Rev. Physiol.* **32**, 547–595.

Gerald, M.C., and Maickel, R.P. (1972). Studies on the possible role of brain histamine in behaviour. *Brit. J. Pharmacol.* **44**, 462–471.

Gilman, A., and Kidd, N.E. (1938). The antidiuretic activity of blood and its possible relation to histamine. *J. Pharmacol. Exp. Ther.* **63**, 10.

Green, J.P. (1970). Histamine, in "Control Mechanisms in the Nervous System." (A. Lajtha, ed.) pp. 221–250. Plenum Press, New York.

Green, M.D., Cox, B., and Lomax, P. (1976). Sites and mechanisms of action of histamine in the central thermoregulatory pathways of the rat. *Neuropharmacology* **15**, 321–324.

Gutman, Y., and Krausz, M. (1973). Drinking induced by dextran and histamine: relation to kidneys and renin. *Eur. J. Pharmacol.* **23**, 256–263.

Haas, H.L. (1974). Histmaine: action on single hypothalamic neurones. *Brain Res.* **76**, 363–366.

Haas, H.L., Wolf, P., and Nussbaumer, J.-C. (1975). Histamine: action on supraoptic and other hypothalamic neurones of the cat. *Brain Res.* **88**, 166–170.

Hegstrand, L.R., Kanof, P.D., and Greengard, P. (1976). Histamine-sensitive adenylate cyclase in mammalian brain. *Nature (London)* **260**, 163–165.

Ibrahim, M.Z.M. (1974). The mast cells of the mammalian central nervous system. 1. Morphology, distribution and histochemistry. *J. Neurol. Sci.* **21**, 431–478.

Kahlson, G., and Rosengren, E. (1971). "Biogenesis and Physiology of Histamine." Edward Arnold, London.

Kühn, E.R. (1974). Cholinergic and adrenergic release mechanism for vasopressin in the male rat: a study with injections of neurotransmitters and blocking agents into the third ventricle. *Neuroendocrinology* **16**, 255–264.

Leenen, F.H.H., Stricker, E.M., McDonald, R.H., Jr., and de Jong, W. (1975). Relationship between increase in plasma renin activity and drinking following different types of dipsogenic stimuli, in "Control Mechanisms of Drinking" (G. Peters, J.T. Fitzsimons, and L. Peters-haefeli, eds.) pp. 84–88. Springer-Verlag, New York.

Lehr, D., Mallow, J., and Krukowski, M. (1967). Copious drinking and simultaneous inhibition of urine flow elicited by beta-adrenergic stimulation and contrary effect of alpha-adrenergic stimulation. *J. Pharmacol. Exp. Ther.* **158**, 150–163.

Leibowitz, S.F. (1973a). Histamine: a stimulatory effect on drinking behavior in the rat. *Brain Res.* **63**, 440–444.

Leibowitz, S.F. (1973b). Central histaminergic control of ingestive behavior in the rat. *Proc. 81st Annu. Convention, Amer. Psychol. Assoc.* pp. 1049–1050.

Leibowitz, S.F. (1973c). Brain norepinephrine and ingestive behaviour, in "Frontiers in Catecholamine Research" (E. Usdin and S. Snyder, eds.) pp. 711–713. Pergamon Press, Oxford, England.

Leibowitz, S.F. (1976). Brain catecholaminergic mechanisms for control of hunger, in "Hunger: Basic Mechanisms and Clinical Implications" (D. Novin, W. Wyrwicka, and G. Bray, eds.), pp. 1–18. Raven Press, New York.

Leibowitz, S.F. (1978). Identification of catecholamine receptor mechanisms in the perifornical lateral hypothalamus and their role in mediating amphetamine and *l*-DOPA anorexia. In "Central Mechanisms of Anorectic Drugs" (S. Garattini and R. Samanin, eds.), Raven Press, New York (in press.)

Malvin, R.L. (1971). Possible role of the renin-angiotensin system in the regulation of antidiuretic hormone secretion. *Federation Proc.* **30**, 1383–1386.

Martres, M.-P., Baudry, M., and Schwartz, J.-C. (1975). Histamine synthesis in the developing rat brain: evidence of a multiple compartmentation. *Brain Res.* **83**, 261–275.

Milton, A.S., and Paterson, A.T. (1974). A microinjection study of the control of antidiuretic hormone release by the suproptic nucleus of the hypothalamus in the cat. *J. Physiol. (London)* **241**, 607–628.

Monnier, M., Sauer, R., and Hatt, A.M. (1970). The activating effect of histamine on the central nervous system. *Int. Rev. Neurobiol.* **12**, 265–305.

Nahorski, S.R., Rogers, K.J., and Smith, B.M. (1974). Histamine H_2 receptors and cyclic AMP in brain. *Life Sci.* **15**, 1887–1894.

Nahorski, S.R., Rogers, K.J., and Edwards, C. (1975). Cerebral glycogenolysis and stimulation of β-adrenoreceptors and histamine H_2 receptors. *Brain Res.* **92**, 529–533.

Nahorski, S.R., Rogers, K.J., and Edwards, C. (1975). Cerebral glycogenolysis and stimulation of β-adrenoreceptors and histamine H_2 receptors. *Brain Res.* **92**, 529-533.

Nicolaidis, S., and Fitzsimons, J.T. (1975). La dépendence de la prise d'eau induite par l'angiotensine II envers la fonction vasomotrice cérébrale locale chez le rat. *C.R. Acad. Sci. (Paris)* **281**, 1417-1420.

Nielsen, K.C., and Owman, Ch. (1971). Contractile response and amine receptor mechanisms in isolated middle cerebral artery of the cat. *Brain Res.* **27**, 33-42.

O'Brien, K.P., and Williamson, H.E. (1971). The natriuretic action of histamine. *Eur. J. Pharmacol.* **16**, 385-390.

Owen, D.A.A. (1975). The effects of histamine and some histamine-like agonists on blood pressure in the cat. *Brit. J. Pharmacol.* **55**, 173-179.

Owen, D.A.A., and Parsons, M.E. (1974). Histamine receptors in the cardiovascular system of the cat. *Brit. J. Pharmacol.* **51**, 123P-124P.

Phillis, J.W., Tebecis, A.K., and York, D.H. (1968). Histamine and some antihistamines: their actions on cerebral cortical neurones. *Brit. J. Pharmacol.* **33**, 426-440.

Pickford, M. (1952). Antidiuretic substances. *Pharmacol. Rev.* **4**, 254-283.

Politoff, A., and Macri, F. (1966). Pharmacologic differences between isolated, perfused arteries of the choroid plexus and of the brain parenchyma. *Int. J. Neuropharmacol.* **5**, 155-162.

Powell, J.R., and Brody, M.J. (1976). Identification and blockade of vascular H_2 receptors. *Federation Proc.* **35**, 1935 (abstract).

Rasmussen, A.T. (1940). Effects of hypophysectomy and hypophysial stalk resection on the hypothalamic nuclei of animals and man. *Res. Publ. Ass. Res. Nerv. Ment. Dis.* **20**, 245-269.

Reubi, F.C., and Futcher, P.H. (1949). The effects of histamine on renal function in hypertensive and normotensive subjects. *J. Clin. Invest.* **28**, 440-446.

Rogers, M., Dismukes, K., and Daly, J.W. (1975). Histamine-elicited accumulations of cyclic adenosine 3',5'-monophosphate in guinea-pig brain slices: effect of H_1- and H_2-antagonists. *J. Neurochem.* **25**, 531-534.

Rothballer, A.B., and Skoryna, S.C. (1960). Morphological effects of pituitary stalk section in the dog, with particular reference to neurosecretory material. *Anat. Rec.* **136**, 5-20.

Santhakumari, G. (1974). Mechanism of hypertonic saline induced antidiuretic response. *Proc. Int. Union Physiol. Sci.* 11, XXVI International Congress, New Delhi p. 371.

Sastry, B.S.R., and Phillis, J.W. (1976). Depression of rat cerebral cortical neurones by H_1 and H_2 histamine receptor agonists. *Eur. J. Pharmacol.* **38**, 269-273.

Schayer, R.W. (1965). Histamine and circulatory homeostasis. *Federation Proc.* **24**, 1295-1297.

Schwartz, J.-C. (1975). Histamine as a transmitter in brain. *Life Sci.* **17**, 503-518.

Schwartz, M.M., and Cotran, R.S. (1972). Vascular leakage in the kidney and lower urinary tract: effects of histamine, serotonin, and bradykinin. *Proc. Soc. Exp. Biol. Med.* **140**, 535-539.

Severs, W.B., and Summy-Long, J. (1975). The role of angiotensin in thirst. *Life Sci.* **17**, 1513-1526.

Share, L. (1969). Extracellular fluid volume and vasopressin secretion, in "Frontiers in Neuroendocrinology" (W.F. Ganong and L. Martini, eds.), pp. 183-210. Oxford University Press, New York.

Sinclair, R.J., Bell, R.D., and Keyl, M.J. (1974). Effect of prostaglandin E_2 and histamine on renal fluid dynamics. *Amer. J. Physiol.* **227**, 1062-1066.

Snyder, S.H., Axelrod, J., and Bauter, H. (1964). The fate of C^{14}-histamine in animal tissues. *J. Pharmacol. Exp. Ther.* **144**, 373-379.

Snyder, S.H., and Taylor, K.M. (1972). Histamine in the brain: a neurotransmitter?, in "Perspectives in Pharmacology (A Tribute to Julius Axelrod)" pp. 43-73. Oxford University Press, New York.

Sokoloff, L. (1959). The action of drugs on the cerebral circulation. *Pharmacol. Rev.* **11**, 1-85.

Stricker, E.M. (1973). Thirst, sodium appetite, and complementary physiological contributions to the regulation of intravascular fluid volume, in "The Neuropsychology of Thirst: New Findings and Advances in Concepts"(A.N. Epstein, H.R. Kissileff, and E. Stellar, eds.), pp. 73–98. V.H. Winston and Sons, Washington, D.C.

Stricker, E.M. (1978). The renin-angiotensin system and thirst: a re-evaluation. II. Drinking elicited in rats by caval ligation or isoproterenol. *J. Comp. Physiol. Psychol.* (in press).

Verdiere, M., Rose, C., and Schwartz, J.-C. (1975). Synthesis and release of histamine studied on slices of rat hypothalamus. *Eur. J. Pharmacol.* **34**, 157–168.

Watters, J.W. (1971). The effects of bradykinin and histamine on cerebral arteries of monkeys. *Radiology* **98**, 299–304.

15

Studies on the Nature of Cerebral Receptors Mediating the Hypotensive Effect of Clonidine in Rats

Heikki Karppanen, Ilari Paakkari, and Pirkko Paakkari
Department of Pharmacology
University of Oulu
SF-90220 Oulu 22, Finland

INTRODUCTION

Since the discovery that the vasoconstrictor drug clonidine (2-(2,6-dichlorophenylamino)-2-imidazoline) induces a paradoxical fall in the blood pressure (Hoefke and Kobinger, 1966) the site and mode of the hypotensive action of this agent have been studied extensively. There is plenty of evidence indicating that clonidine exerts its hypotensive effect by decreasing the sympathetic outflow from the central nervous system (Kobinger, 1967; Sattler and van Zwieten, 1967; Schmitt *et al.*, 1967; Haeusler, 1974). However the exact site and mode of action of clonidine have remained obscure.

α-Receptor Concept

The existence of a cerebral α-adrenergic mechanism which is able to mediate a blood pressure decreasing effect of catecholamines seems to be established (for review, see van Zwieten, 1973, 1975). Clonidine stimulates α-adrenergic receptors in peripheral tissues (Hoefke and Kobinger, 1966; Kobinger and Walland, 1967; Boissier *et al.*, 1968; Kobinger, 1973). The hypotensive effect of clonidine can be antagonized by central administrations of piperoxane, yohimbine, phentolamine, or tolazoline which are known to block α-adrenergic receptors (Schmitt *et al.*, 1971, 1973; Finch, 1975).

Therefore it has been suggested that the hypotensive effect of clonidine is due to a stimulation of α-adrenoceptors in the brain (for review, see van Zwieten, 1975). However, there are some controversial findings which challenge the role of classical α-adrenoceptors in the mediation of clonidine-induced hypotension. The α-adrenoceptor blocking agents are nonspecific drugs which are known to block or stimulate many types of receptors (Nickerson and Collier, 1975). Moreover, an intracerebroventricular administration of the potent and irreversible α-receptor antagonist phenoxybenzamine does not antagonize the hypotensive effect of clonidine in the dog (Bogaievsky et al., 1974). Moreover, Schmitt and Schmitt (1970) reported that intracerebroventricular injections of phentolamine do not antagonize the inhibitory effect of clonidine on vasomotor centers in the dog. It has also been reported that clonidine is an antagonist rather than agonist of cerebral α-receptors (Skolnick and Daly, 1975, 1976). Therefore we have examined whether other mechanisms might be involved in the hypotensive effect of clonidine.

Interaction of Histamine H$_2$-Receptor Antagonists With Some Effects of Clonidine

Walz and van Zwieten (1970) reported that clonidine stimulates the secretion of gastric acid in the anesthetized rat by an unknown mechanism. The imidazoline structure of clonidine suggested to us that the structural similarity with histamine might be the basis for the secretory activity of clonidine. When the histamine H$_2$-receptor antagonist burimamide became available (Black et al., 1972) it was demonstrated that the secretory response to clonidine as well as that to histamine can be abolished by burimamide pretreatment in urethane-anaesthetized rats (Karppanen and Westermann, 1973). Burimamide also antagonized the increase in the gastric mucosal content of cAMP which was induced both by histamine and clonidine (Karppanen and Westermann, 1973). In agreement with this finding it has been shown recently that clonidine activates adenylate cyclase both in the gastric mucosa (Anttila and Westermann, 1976) and in the brain (Audigier et al., 1976) by stimulating histamine H$_2$ receptors. An activation of histamine H$_2$ receptors by clonidine is further suggested by the finding that the clonidine-induced stimulation of the heart is antagonized by burimamide (Csongrady and Kobinger, 1974).

Attenuation of the Hypotensive Effect of Clonidine By Histamine H$_2$-Receptor Antagonists

After an administration of metiamide into the lateral ventricles of the brain the hypotensive effect of intravenously injected clonidine was markedly attenuated (Karppanen et al., 1976; Fig. 1). This finding has been confirmed recently by Finch et al. (1977). In conscious cats metiamide failed to antagonize hypotension after central administration of clonidine (Finch and Hicks, 1976c). In the urethane-anesthetized rats, however, the administra-

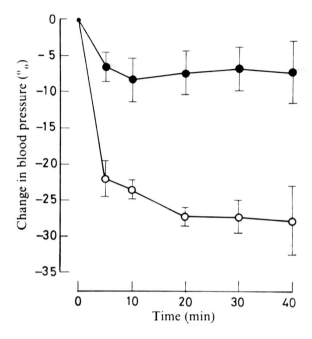

FIG. 1.   Influence of metiamide on the hypotensive effect of clonidine in rats. Metiamide (1.5 μmol per rat) or saline was administered intracerebroventricularly, 10–15 minutes later clonidine (30 μg kg^{-1}) was injected intravenously. Differences between the metiamide (●) and control (○) groups were significant to the $P < 0.001$ level for all measurements except that made at 40 min ($P < 0.02$). The time elapsed after the injection of clonidine is shown on the abscissa. Vertical bars indicate s.e.m. The number of rats was 18 in the control group and 10 in the metiamide group. From Karppanen et al. (1976); reproduced by permission of Nature (London).

tion of metiamide into the lateral ventricle caused a parallel shift of the dose-response curve of clonidine to the right (Paakkari et al., 1976; Karppanen et al., 1977). This finding lends support to the idea that central histamine H$_2$ receptors may be involved in the hypotensive effect of clonidine. However, the relatively selective histamine H$_2$-receptor agonist 4-methylhistamine (Black et al., 1972) did not lower the blood pressure after an administration into the lateral ventricle (Karppanen et al., 1977) or local injections into the posterior hypothalamus (Finch and Hicks,). Moreover, there is no evidence that histamine intracerebroventricularly would under any circumstances lower the blood pressure. On the contrary, histamine intracerebroventricularly exerts a hypertensive effect (Trendelenburg, 1957; White, 1961, 1965; Finch and Hicks, 1976a,b). These findings seem to contradict the existence of sympatho-inhibitory histamine H$_2$ receptors in the brain.

In the present work the interaction of metiamide with the hypotensive effect of clonidine was studied further. In addition, the hypotensive properties of clonidine were compared with those of imidazole acetic acid which is a metabolite of histamine as well as histidine (White *et al.,* 1973). The interaction of metiamide with α-methylnoradrenaline, the centrally acting hypotensive metabolite of the antihypertensive drug α-methyldopa (Henning, 1975), was also studied.

MATERIALS AND METHODS

Male Sprague–Dawley rats, 250–300 gm, were used. For at least one week before the experiments the rats were accommodated to standard ambient conditions. The lights were on from 7 a.m. to 7 p.m. and during the remaining 12 hours the room was completely dark. The temperature was kept at 22° C and relative humidity at 40%. The rats received standard rat pellets (Hankkija Oy, Helsinki) and tap water *ad libitum.*

The rats were anesthetized with urethane (1.5 gm/kg, i.p.). The rectal temperature was kept at 37° C with the help of a heating lamp. The trachea was cannulated with a polyethylene tube and the rats were allowed to breathe spontaneously. The mean blood pressure was measured from the left femoral artery by means of a pressure transducer (Harvard apparatus 377). The heart rate was calculated from the pulse waves. The left femoral vein was cannulated for intravenous injections. The rats were mounted in a stereotaxic instrument and tilted caudally so that the body formed an angle of 10 degrees with the horizontal plane. An injection needle was introduced either into the right lateral ventricle of the brain or into the fourth ventricle. A polyethylene catheter, filled with the drug or control solution to be infused, was attached to the needle. The administration of drugs was not started until the blood pressure remained constant for at least 15 minutes. The desired amount of the solution was allowed to flow slowly by the virtue of hydrostatic pressure. The volume of each infusion was 10 μl into the lateral ventricle and 5 μl into the fourth ventricle during a 2-minute period. At least 8 minutes were allowed to elapse after the completion of the previous infusion before the next infusion was started. The proper position of the needle tip was ascertained at the end of each experiment by an injection of dye (Giemsa solution, Merck) into the cerebral ventricle.

The fall in the blood pressure by hypotensive drugs is proportional to the blood pressure level before the administration of the drug (see Dixon and Johnson, 1976). To minimize the influence on the results of different blood pressure levels before the administration of hypotensive agents, the hypotensive responses were calculated as percentages rather than in absolute values. For obvious reasons the opposite is true as regards the hypertensive responses. Therefore they are expressed in absolute values. Student's t-test was used in the statistical analysis of the results.

The following drugs were used: Clonidine hydrochloride (Boehringer Ingelheim) dissolved in 0.9% (w/v) NaCl; Metiamide (Smith, Kline and French Laboratories Ltd.) dissolved in 1 N HCl and pH adjusted to 6 with 0.1 N NaOH. To obtain a 10^{-1} M solution water was added. Also, dilutions were made with 0.9% (w/v) NaCl. α-Methylnoradrenaline (Sterling-Winthrop) was dissolved in 0.5 N HCl and dilutions were made with saline. Imidazole acetic acid (Sigma Chemicals) was dissolved in 0.9% NaCl (w/v). Control animals received the same volume of the appropriate solvent at the same pH as the drug solution.

RESULTS AND DISCUSSION

Hypotensive Effect of Intravenously Injected Clonidine

In previous studies it has been shown that metiamide or cimetidine intracerebroventricularly antagonize the hypotensive effect of a single intravenous dose (30 μg/kg) of clonidine (Karppanen et al., 1976; Finch et al., 1977). In the present work the antagonism was examined in more detail by using cumulative doses of clonidine intravenously.

In the control rats clonidine induced a dose-related lowering of the blood pressure (Fig. 2). The maximal fall was reached within 20 minutes. Therefore cumulative doses of clonidine were injected at 20-minute intervals to obtain complete dose-response curves. In agreement with previous findings (e.g., Hoefke and Kobinger, 1966; for review, see van Zwieten, 1975) a slight and transient increase in the blood pressure was observed immediately after the injection of the smaller doses (3.75–15 μg/kg) of clonidine. The rise in the blood pressure was much more pronounced when higher doses (30–120 μg/kg) of clonidine were injected during the hypotension induced by the previous doses. In addition to the initial increase, higher doses raised also the long-term level of blood pressure (Fig. 2). The hypertensive effect of clonidine is obviously due to the peripheral vasoconstrictor effect of the drug.

Metiamide pretreatment (1.5 μmol metiamide into the lateral ventricle 20 minutes before the first dose of clonidine) increased the blood pressure on the average by 18 mmHg ($p < 0.05$).

Metiamide shifted the dose-response curve of clonidine to the right but did not affect the maximal effect (Fig. 2). Since metiamide was administered into the lateral ventricle of the brain the interaction probably occurred in the central nervous system. This assumption is further suggested by the finding that after an intravenous injection of metiamide which does not penetrate the blood–brain barrier (Cross, 1973) the hypotensive effect of clonidine is not antagonized (Finch et al., 1977; H. Karppanen, I. Paakkari, and P. Paakkari,

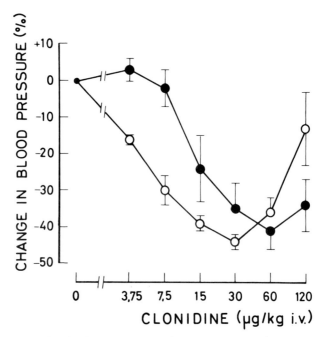

FIG. 2.   Influence of metiamide on the hypotensive effect of clonidine in urethane-anesthetized rats. The infusion of metiamide (1.5 μmol per rat in 60 μl during 15 minutes) or 60 μl of saline into the lateral brain ventricle was completed 20 minutes before the start of the administrations of clonidine. Cumulative doses of clonidine were injected intravenously at 20-minute intervals. The percentage change of blood pressure from the preclonidine level 20 minutes after each clonidine dose is shown. Vertical bars indicate s.e.m. The number of rats was 6 in the control group (o—o) and 5 in the metiamide group (●—●). Differences between the control and metiamide groups were significant to the $P < 0.001$ level at clonidine doses of 3.75 and 7.5 μg/kg.

unpublished results). Moreover, metiamide antagonizes the hypotensive effect of clonidine when both drugs are administered into the lateral ventricles of the brain (Karppanen et al., 1977).

Effects of Metiamide and Clonidine After Administrations Into the Fourth Cerebral Ventricle

Some regions in close vicinity to the floor of the fourth cerebral ventricle are extremely sensitive to the hypotensive action of clonidine (Karppanen et al., 1975; Paakkari et al., 1976) suggesting the role of these regions as a site of action of clonidine. Therefore the interaction of metiamide with the hypotensive effect of clonidine was studied after the administration of the drugs into the fourth ventricle. Metiamide alone induced a dose-related increase in the blood pressure (Fig. 3).

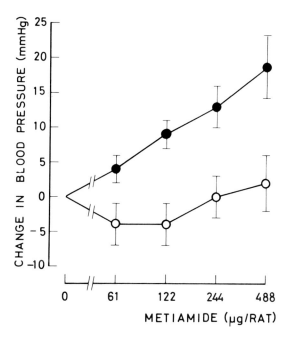

FIG. 3.   Hypertensive effect of metiamide in urethane-anesthetized rats. Cumulative doses of metiamide (●—●) or saline (o—o) were infused into the fourth cerebral ventricle in a volume of 5 μl each. The interval between the infusions was 10 minutes. The changes of blood pressure were calculated with respect to the stabilized level before the start of the infusions of metiamide or saline. The change of blood pressure 10 minutes after each infusion is shown. Vertical bars indicate s.e.m. Differences between the metiamide and saline groups were significant to the $P < 0.05 - < 0.01$ level. The number of rats was 7 in the control group and 8 in the metiamide group.

At doses considerably lower than those injected intravenously clonidine induced a dose-dependent hypotensive response (Fig. 4). No initial rise in the blood pressure was seen by any dose of clonidine. The dose-response curve of clonidine was shifted to the right in metiamide-pretreated rats, but the maximal lowering of the blood pressure following higher doses of clonidine remained unchanged (Fig. 4). This implies further the role of cerebral histamine H_2 receptors in the hypotensive effect of clonidine. However, it has been suggested that clonidine lowers the blood pressure by the same central mechanism as catecholamines do, *viz* by stimulating sympatho-inhibitory α-adrenoceptors (for review, see van Zwieten, 1975). It has been shown that metiamide does not antagonize adrenergic α-receptors either in the peripheral tissues or in the cerebral cortex (Brimblecombe *et al.,* 1976; Phillis, 1975). However, the lack of effect of metiamide on cerebral α-adrenoceptors mediating the hypotensive effect of catecholamines has not been excluded.

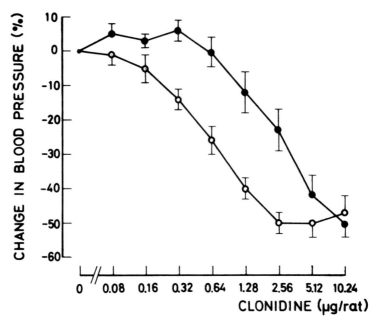

FIG. 4.   Hypotensive effect of clonidine in metiamide-pretreated (●—●) and control (o—o) rats. Both drugs were infused into the fourth cerebral ventricle. The infusions of metidamide (2 μmol in 20 μl) or saline (20 μl) were completed 20 minutes before the start of clonidine administrations. Cumulative doses of clonidine were infused at 20-minute intervals in a volume of 5 μl each. The percentage change of blood pressure from the preclonidine level 20 minutes after each dose of clonidine is shown. Vertical bars indicate s.e.m. The number of rats was 10 in the control group and 8 in the metiamide group. Differences between the control and metiamide groups were significant to the $P < 0.001$ level at clonidine doses of 0.32–2.56 μg/rat.

This possibility was examined by using α-methylnoradrenaline (α-MNA), an established α-adrenergic agonist with central hypotensive action (Henning, 1975).

Effects of α-Methylnoradrenaline After Administrations Into the Fourth Cerebral Ventricle

Metiamide-pretreatment (2 μmol, i.e., 488 μg, into the fourth cerebral ventricle 20 minutes before the start of the administration of α-MNA) enhanced the hypotensive effect of α-MNA (Fig. 5). The dose-response curve was shifted to the left with an increase in the maximal hypotensive effect. This finding indicates that metiamide does not block the central α-adrenoceptors which mediate the hypotensive effect of α-MNA. Drugs which block the neuronal uptake of biogenic amines are known to potentiate the hypotensive

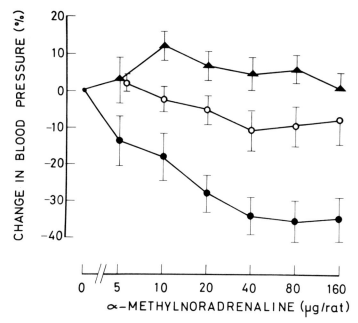

FIG. 5. Hypotensive effect of α-methylnoradrenaline (α-MNA) in metiamide-pretreated (●—●) and control (o—o) rats. The effect of the solvent of α-MNA (▲—▲) was also studied. The metiamide-pretreatment and other experimental design were similar to that described in the legend of Fig. 4. The number of rats was 6 in each group. At the doses of 10–80 μg/rat, α-MNA alone slightly lowered the blood pressure ($P < 0.05$ to < 0.1 vs. solvent). In the metiamide-pretreated rats α-MNA induced a more pronounced fall in the blood pressure so that the differences between the control and metiamide groups were significant to the $P < 0.05$ level at α-MNA doses of 10 and 160 μg/rat and to the $P < 0.01$ level at doses of 20–80 μg/rat.

effect of α-MNA (Heise and Kroneberg, 1973). The mechanism by which metiamide enhanced the hypotensive effect of α-MNA is not known.

However, the opposite effect of metiamide on the central hypotensive responses to clonidine and α-MNA suggests that the mechanism of action of the two drugs is different.

Hypotensive Effect of Intracerebroventricular Imidazole Acetic Acid

Since central administration of histamine does not lower blood pressure the question arises whether some other naturally occurring histamine-related agent could activate the same hypotensive mechanism as clonidine does. Therefore it was interesting that imidazole acetic acid was reported to lower the blood pressure upon intracerebroventricular administration (Walland,

1975). Imidazole acetic acid has been implicated as a possible inhibitory neurotransmitter in the brain (Roberts and Simonsen, 1970). This compound is known to be formed as a metabolite of histamine and also as a transamination product of histidine (White et al., 1973).

The administration of 0.12 mg of imidazole acetic acid per rat into the lateral ventricle lowered the blood pressure (Table I). At the dose of 0.66 mg per rat imidazole acetic acid induced a profound hypotension, and 12 out of 14 control animals died within 20 minutes.

Interestingly, the hypotensive effect of imidazole acetic acid was markedly attenuated by a central pretreatment with metiamide (Table I). Moreover, only one out of 12 metiamide-pretreated rats died during the 20-minute follow-up period after the administration of the higher dose of imidazole acetic acid.

The central hypotensive action of imidazole acetic acid is of particular interest. This compound has been claimed to have little or no pharmacological activity (Douglas, 1975). This may be true of peripheral tissues. However, the present as well as previous findings (Roberts and Simonsen, 1966, 1970; Walland, 1975) indicate that imidazole acetic acid does exert strong effects in the brain. Imidazole acetic acid can be formed from histidine in the brain of

Table I

The effect of imidazole acetic acid on the blood pressure and death rate during the 20-minute follow-up period in control and metiamide-pretreated urethane-anesthetized rats[a]

Drug	Change in blood pressure (%)	Number of deaths per total number of rats studied
Imidazole acetic acid (0.12 mg/rat)	-32 ± 4	0/14
Metiamide (4.5 µmol/rat) + Imidazole acetic acid (0.12 mg/rat)	-6 ± 6^{b}	0/12
Imidazole acetic acid (0.66 mg/rat)	Unreliable because most animals died	12/14
Metiamide (4.5 µmol/rat) + Imidazole acetic acid (0.66 mg/rat)	-40 ± 6	1/12

[a] Metiamide was infused intracerebroventricularly 60–100 minutes before the intracerebroventricular administration of imidazole acetic acid.

[b] $p < 0.001$ vs. imidazole acetic acid (0.12 mg/rat) alone.

the rat (Robinson and Green, 1964). Therefore the possibility exists that imidazole acetic acid might have a physiological role as a central regulatory agent of the blood pressure. It is interesting that upon central administration histamine exerts a hypertensive effect and imidazole acetic acid a hypotensive effect. Therefore it may be warranted to study whether the metabolism of histidine or histamine is altered in hypertension. This possibility is suggested by the finding that in the spontaneously hypertensive rats the content of histamine in the brain stem is two times higher than in the normotensive control rats (Spector et al., 1972).

Since metiamide is considered to be a highly specific antagonist of histamine H_2 receptors, the hypotensive effect of both clonidine and imidazole acetic acid would seem to be due to a stimulation of cerebral histamine H_2 receptors. However, the central hypotensive effect is not shared by the selective agonists of histamine H_2 receptors, 4-methyl-histamine (Karppanen et al., 1977; Finch and Hicks, in press) and dimaprit (H. Karppanen, I. Paakkari and P. Paakkari, unpublished results). Upon intracerebroventricular administrations histamine does not lower the blood pressure even in the presence of central histamine H_1-receptor blockade which antagonizes the hypertensive response (Finch and Hicks, 1976b). These results contradict the existence of cerebral histamine H_2 receptors mediating hypotensive effects.

At the present time it is not possible to explain the controversial results satisfactorily. One possibility would be that histamine and the histamine H_2-receptor agonists do not reach the same site of action as clonidine and imidazole acetic acid do. A more likely explanation would be that the hypotensive receptors involved are similar but not identical to peripheral histamine H_2 receptors. In the latter case metiamide should be able to block a so far unidentified mechanism in the brain, in addition to the histamine H_2 receptors.

Tentative Hypothesis of Cerebral Sympatho-Inhibitory "Imidazole Receptors"

It is certainly premature to implicate a new kind of cerebral receptors in the hypotensive effects of clonidine and imidazole acetic acid. However, the present results could be explained conveniently by imagining the existence of cerebral sympatho-inhibitory "imidazole receptors." An activation of these receptors would bring about a lowering of blood pressure. The hypertensive effect of metiamide could be explained by the blockade of tonically activated "imidazole receptors." The blockade of these receptors by metiamide might, in turn, imply that they are closely related to histamine H_2 receptors. According to the present hypothesis imidazole acetic acid would lower blood pressure by acting as a natural activator of the sympatho-inhibitory "imidazole receptors." The synthetic antihypertensive imidazoline compound clonidine would also be able to stimulate these receptors.

Further studies are needed to elucidate the mechanism by which imidazole acetic acid and clonidine lower blood pressure and by which metiamide antagonizes their effect. The concept of cerebral "imidazole receptors" can only be utilized as a working hypothesis. In future studies the possibility that imidazole acetic acid, clonidine and metiamide might affect some common (intracellular?) biochemical events rather than specific pharmacological receptors should be taken into consideration.

SUMMARY

Intracerebroventricular administrations of metiamide induced a dose-related rise of the blood pressure. Central pretreatment with metiamide antagonized the hypotensive effect of clonidine both upon intravenous and intracerebroventricular administrations of clonidine. The interaction of metiamide with the hypotensive effect of clonidine may be competitive in nature. This is suggested by the parallel shift of the dose-response curves of clonidine to the right without a change in the maximal effect. In contrast to clonidine the hypotensive effect of α-methylnoradrenaline was enhanced by central pretreatment with metiamide. Thus, metiamide does not block the central α-adrenoceptors which mediate the hypotensive effect of catechol-amines. These results suggest that the central hypotensive mechanism of clonidine differs from that of α-methylnoradrenaline.

Imidazole acetic acid which is a metabolite of histamine and can be formed from histidine in the brain, proved to be a potent hypotensive agent upon intracerebroventricular adiminstrations. This may imply a physiological role of imidazole acetic acid in the central control of blood pressure. Central pretreatment with metiamide antagonized the hypotensive effect of imidazole acetic acid, thus, suggesting the involvement of histamine H_2 receptors. However histamine itself or the selective histamine H_2-receptor agonists 4-methylhistamine and dimaprit did not lower the blood pressure upon intracerebroventricular administrations. The results suggest that, in spite of the antagonism by metiamide, the central hypotensive effect of clonidine and imidazole acetic acid is not mediated by receptors identical with peripheral histamine H_2 receptors.

Tentatively the existence of a novel hypotensive "imidazole" mechanism in the brain is suggested as a working hypothesis. Metiamide would block, in addition to the histamine H_2 receptors, also the hypothetical "imidazole" mechanism which is activated by imidazole acetic acid and clonidine but not by histamine. The exact cerebral mechanisms by which clonidine and imidazole acetic acid lower the blood pressure and by which metiamide antagonizes this effect are still far from clear.

ACKNOWLEDGMENTS

This study was done under a contract with Association of Finnish Life Insurance Companies. Our thanks are due to Dr. D.A.A. Owen of Smith Kline and French Laboratories Ltd. for the supply of metiamide, and Mrs. Laimi Mäkelä of Boehringer Ingelheim for the supply of clonidine hydrochloride. α-methylnoradrenaline was kindly donated by Sterling-Winthrop. The skillful technical assistance of Mrs. Sirpa Rutanen and Miss Tiina Heikkinen is gratefully acknowledged. This work was partly supported by grants from the Paavo Nurmi Foundation and Paavo Ilmari Ahvenainen Foundation.

REFERENCES

Anttila, P., and Westermann, E. (1976). Effect of some imidazoline derivatives on the adenylate cyclase activity of guinea pig gastric mucosa in vitro. *Naunyn-Schmiedeberg's Arch. Pharmacol. (Suppl.)* **294,** R 12.

Audigier, Y., Virion, A., and Schwartz, J.-C. (1976). Stimulation of cerebral histamine H_2-receptors by clonidine. *Nature (London)* **262,** 307–308.

Black, J.W., Duncan, W.A.M., Durant, C.J., Ganellin, C.R., and Parsons, E.M. (1972). Definition and antagonism of histamine H_2-receptors. *Nature (London)* **236,** 385–390.

Black, J.W., Duncan, W.A.M., Emmet, J.C., Ganellin, C.R., Hesselbo, T., Parsons, M.E., and Wyllie, J.H. (1973). Metiamide—an orally active histamine H_2-receptor antagonist. *Agents Actions* **3,** 133–137.

Bogaievsky, D., Bogaievsky, Y., Tsoucaris-Kupfer, D., and Schmitt, H. (1974). Blockade of the central hypotensive effect of clonidine by alpha-adrenoreceptor antagonists in rats, rabbits and dogs. *Clin. Expl Pharmacol. Physiol.* **1,** 527–534.

Boissier, J., Giudicelli, J.F., Fichele, J., Schmitt, H., and Schmitt, H. (1968). Cardiovascular effects of 2-(2,6 Dichlorphenylamino)-2-imidazolinhydrochloride (St 155). *Eur. J. Pharmacol.* **2,** 333–339.

Brimblecombe, R.W., Duncan, W.A.M., Owen, D.A.A., and Parsons, M.E. (1976). The pharmacology of burimamide and metiamide, two histamine H_2-receptor antagonists. *Fed. Proc.* **35,** 1931–1934.

Cross, S.A.M. (1973). Distribution of histamine, burimamide and metiamide and their interactions as shown by autoradiography in "International Symposium on Histamine H_2-receptor Antagonists" (C.J. Wood and M.A. Simkins, eds.) p. 73. Smith, Kline & French Laboratories, London.

Csongrady, A., and Kobinger, W. (1974). Investigations into the positive inotropic effect of clonidine in isolated hearts. *Naunyn-Schmiedeberg's Arch. Pharmacol.* **282,** 123–128.

Dixon, G.T., and Johnson, E.S. (1976). Efficacy of antihypertensive drugs. *Lancet* **1,** 515–518.

Douglas, W.W. (1975). Histamine and antihistamines; 5-hydroxytryptamine and antagonists in "The Pharmacological Basis of Therapeutics," (L.S. Goodman and A. Gilman, eds.) pp. 590–629. MacMillan Publishing Co., Inc., New York.

Finch, L. (1975). The central hypotensive action of clonidine and BAY 1470 in cats and rats. *Clin. Sci. Mol. Med.* **48,** 273–276s.

Finch, L., and Hicks, P.E. (1976a). Central hypertensive action of histamine in conscious normotensive cats. *Eur. J. Pharmacol.* **36,** 263–266.

Finch, L., and Hicks, P.E. (1976b). The cardiovascular effects of intraventricularly administered histamine in the anaesthetised rat. *Naunyn-Schmiedeberg's Arch Pharmacol* **293,** 151–157.

Finch, L., and Hicks, P.E. (1976c). No evidence for central histamine-receptor involvement with the hypotensive effect of clonidine in cats. *Eur. J. Pharmacol.* **40,** 365–368.

Finch, L., and Hicks, P.E. (1977). Involvement of hypothalamic histamine receptors in the central cardiovascular actions of histamine. *Neuropharmacol.* **16,** 211–218.

Finch, L., Harvey, C.A., Hicks, P.E., and Owen, D.A.A. (1977). Interaction between histamine H₂-receptor antagonists and the hypotensive effects of clonidine in rats. *Br. J. Pharmacol.,* **59**, 477P.

Haeusler, G. (1974). Clonidine-induced inhibition of sympathetic nerve activity: no indication for a central presynaptic or an indirect sympathomimetic mode of action. *Naunyn-Schmideberg's Arch. Pharmacol.* **286**, 97–111.

Heise, A., and Kroneberg, G. (1973). Central nervous α-adrenergic receptors and the mode of action of α-methyldopa. *Naunyn-Schmiedeberg's Arch. Pharmacol.* **279**, 285–300.

Henning, M. (1975). Central sympathetic transmitters and hypertension. *Clin. Sci. Mol.Med.* **48**, 195s–203s.

Hoefke, W., and Kobinger, W. (1966). Pharmakologische Wirkungen des 2-(2,6 Dichlor-phenylamino)-2-imidazolinhydrochlorids, einer neuen antihypertensiven Substanz. *Arznei-mittel-Forsch. (Drug Res.)* **16**, 1038–1050.

Karppanen, H.O., and Westermann, E. (1973). Increased production of cyclic AMP in gastric tissue by stimulation of histamine H₂-receptors. *Naunyn-Schmiedeberg's Arch. Pharmacol.* **279**, 83–87.

Karppanen, H., Liukkonen, T., and Vainionpää, V. (1975). Hypotensive effects elicited by centrally administered angiotensin and clonidine. *Sixth Int. Congr. Pharmacol., Helsinki.* Volunteer Abstracts, 636.

Karppanen, H., Paakkari, I., Paakkari, P., Huotari, R., and Orma, A.-L. (1976). Possible involvement of central histamine H₂-receptors in the hypotensive action of clonidine. *Nature (London)* **259**, 587–588.

Karppanen, H., Paakkari, I., and Paakkari, P. (1977). Further evidence for central histamine H₂-receptor involvement in the hypotensive effect of clonidine in the rat. *Eur. J. Pharmacol.* **42**, 299–302.

Kobinger, W. (1967). Ueber den Wirkungsmechanismus einer neuen antihypertensiven Substanz mit Imidazolinstruktur. *Naunyn-Schmiedeberg's Arch. Pharmak. Exp. Path.* **258**, 48–58.

Kobinger, W., (1973). Pharmacologic basis of the cardiovascular actions of clonidine in "Hypertension: Mechanisms and Management," (G. Onesti, K.E. Kim, and J.H. Moyer, eds.). pp. 369–380. Grune & Stratton, Inc., New York.

Kobinger, W., and Walland, A. (1967). Kreislaufuntersuchungen mit 2-(2,6 Dichlorphenyl-amino)-2-Imidazolin Hydrochlorid. *Arzneim.-Forsch. (Drug Res.)* **17**, 292–300.

Nickerson, M., and Collier, B. (1975). Drugs inhibiting adrenergic nerves and structures innervated by them in "The Pharmacological Basis of Therapeutics" (L.S. Goodman and A. Gilman, eds.). pp. 533–564. MacMillan Publishing Co., Inc., New York.

Paakkari, I., Karppanen, H., and Paakkari, P. (1976). Site and mode of action of clonidine in the central nervous system. *Acta Medica Scandinavica (suppl.)* **602**, 106–109.

Phillis, J.W., Kostopoulos, G.K., and Odutola, A. (1975). On the specificity of histamine H₂-receptor antagonists in the rat cerebral cortex. *Can. J. Physiol. Pharmacol.* **53**, 1205–1209.

Roberts, E., and Simonsen, D.G. (1966). A hypnotic and possible analgesic effect of imidazoleacetic acid in mice. *Biochem. Pharmacol.* **15**, 1875–1877.

Roberts, E., and Simonsen, D.G. (1970). Some properties of cyclic 3′,5′-nucleotide phosphodiesterase of mouse brain: effects of imidazole-4-acetic acid, chlorpromazine, cyclic 3′,5′-GMP, and other substances. *Brain Res.* **24**, 91–111.

Robinson, J.D., and Green, J.P. (1964). Presence of imidazoleacetic acid riboside and ribotide in rat tissues. *Nature (London)* **203**, 1178–1179.

Sattler, R.W., and van Zwieten, P.A. (1967). Acute hypotensive action of 2-(2,6-dichloro-phenylamino)-2-imidazoline hydrochloride (St 155) after infusion into the cat's vertebral artery. *Eur. J. Pharmacol.* **2**, 9–13.

Schmitt, H., and Schmitt, H. (1970). Interactions between 2-(2,6-dichlorophenylamino)-2-imidazoline hydrochloride (St 155, Catapresan) and alpha-adrenergic blocking drugs. *Eur. J. Pharmacol.* **9**, 7–13.

Schmitt, H., Schmitt, H., Boissier, J.R., and Giudicelli, J.F. (1967). Centrally mediated decrease in sympathetic tone induced by 2-(2,6-dichlorophenylamino)-2-imidazoline (St 155, Catapresan[R]). *Eur. J. Pharmacol.* **2**, 147–148.

Schmitt, H., Schmitt, H., and Fenard, S. (1971). Evidence for an alpha-sympathomimetic component in the effects of catapresan on vasomotor centres: Antagonism by piperoxane. *Eur. J. Pharmacol.* **14**, 98–100.

Schmitt, H., Schmitt, H., and Fenard, S. (1973). Action of alpha-adrenergic blocking drugs on the sympathetic centres and their interactions with the central sympatho-inhibitory effect of clonidine. *Arzneim.-Forsch. (Drug Res.)* **23**, 40–45.

Skolnick, P., and Daly, J.W. (1975). Stimulation of adenosine 3′,5′-monphosphate formation by alpha and beta adrenergic agonists in rat cerebral cortical slices: effects of clonidine. *Molec. Pharmacol.* **11**, 545–551.

Spector, S., Tarver, J., and Berkowitz, B. (1972). Catecholamine biosynthesis and metabolism in the vasculature of normotensive and hypertensive rats in "The spontaneous hypertension. Its pathogenesis and complications" (K. Okamoto, ed.) pp. 41–45. Igaku Shoin Ltd., Tokyo.

Trendelenburg, U. (1957). Stimulation of sympathetic centres by histamine. *Circ. Res.* **5**, 105–110.

van Zwieten, P.A. (1973). The central action of antihypertensive drugs mediated via central receptors. *J. Pharm. Pharmacol.* **25**, 89–95.

van Zwieten, P.A. (1975). Antihypertensive drugs with a central action. *Progr. Pharmacol.* **1**, 1–63.

Walland, A., (1975). cAMP as a second messenger in central blood pressure control. *Naunyn-Schmiedeberg's Arch. Pharmacol.* **290**, 419–423.

Walz, A., and van Zweiten, P.A. (1970). The influence of 2-(2,6-dichlorphenylamino)-2-imidazoline hydrochloride (clonidine) and some related compounds on gastric secretion in the anaesthetized rat. *Eur. J. Pharmacol.* **10**, 369–377.

White, T. (1961). Some effects of histamine and two histamine metabolites in the cat's brain. *J. Physiol. (London)* **159**, 198–202.

White, T. (1965). Peripheral vascular effects of histamine administered into the cerebral ventricles of anesthetised cats. *Experientia* **21**, 132–133.

White, A., Handler, P., and Smith, E.L. (1973). "Principles of Biochemistry." pp. 697–699. McGraw-Hill, New York.

PART IV
HISTAMINE RECEPTORS LINKED TO NEUCLEOTIDE CYCLASES

16

Cardiac Histamine Receptors and Cyclic AMP: Differences between Guinea Pig and Rabbit Heart

John H. McNeill and Subhash C. Verma
Division of Pharmacology and Toxicology
Faculty of Pharmaceutical Sciences
University of British Columbia
Vancouver, Canada

The positive inotropic action of histamine on the heart was first reported in 1910 by Dale and Laidlaw. The cardiac actions of this amine then appear to have been ignored for nearly half a century. Trendelenburg (1960) clearly demonstrated that histamine had a direct positive inotropic and chronotropic effect on cat, guinea pig, and rabbit atria. These data have subsequently been confirmed many times and it is now clear that histamine acts directly on its own receptors in the heart since its effects are not affected by pretreatment with cocaine, reserpine, monamine oxidase inhibitors, or β-adrenergic blocking agents such as dichloroisoproterenol, pronethalol, or propranolol (Pepeu *et al.,* 1958; Burn and Rand, 1958; Trendelenburg, 1960; Mannaioni, 1960; Bartlett, 1963; Flacke *et al.,* 1967; Dean, 1968).

Prior to 1972, it had been reported from many laboratories that the cardiac effects of histamine were not blocked well by classical antihistaminic agents such as diphenhydramine, pyrilamine, tripelennamine, promethazine, or triprolidine (see Verma and McNeill, 1976). Ash and Schild (1966) had previously proposed that there were two histamine receptors since the classical antihistamines available at that time did not block the effects of histamine on the heart, on gastric acid secretion, or on the rat uterus. The discovery by Black and his colleagues (1972) of a new group of antihistamines that are capable of blocking, for example, the cardiac and gastric secretory actions of histamine has greatly clarified the picture. Thus, the division of histamine receptors into H_1 and H_2 receptors has been developed based on whether the effect is blocked by classical antihistamines (H_1) or by the newer agents, burimamide, metiamide, or cimetidine (H_2). The classification has been strengthened by the recent introduction of agonists with selective histamine receptor effects. Compounds such as 2-methylhistamine, 2-(2-pyridyl) ethylamine (PEA), and 2-(2-thiazolyl) ethylamine show a high selectivity for H_1 receptors. Other compounds such as 4-methylhistamine and S-[3-(N, N-dimethylamino) propyl] isothiourea (dimaprit) exhibit greater selectivity for H_2 receptors (Black et al., 1972; Durant et al., 1975; Bergmann, 1974; Beaven, 1976).

The cardiac actions of histamine and its analogs and attempts to elucidate the type of histamine receptor involved have been the subject of considerable interest recently. Pöch and Kukovetz (1967) and Dean (1968) both suggested that histamine might produce its effects on the heart by stimulating adenylate cyclase and elevating cyclic AMP (cAMP) in a manner analagous to that reported by Robison et al., (1965) for the adrenergic amines. The first step in the investigation of this possibility was the work of Klein and Levey (1971). These workers showed that histamine could stimulate adenylate cyclase prepared from guinea pig, cat, and human heart. McNeill and Muschek (1972), while confirming that histamine could stimulate guinea pig heart adenylate cyclase, were able to demonstrate that diphenhydramine and tripelennamine were unable to competitively block the action of histamine. Neither antagonist could block the inotropic action of histamine in the perfused heart. Later work from McNeill's laboratory (McNeill and Verma, 1973; 1974a; McNeill et al., 1973) showed that stimulation of cardiac adenylate cyclase by histamine could be blocked by burimamide. The studies also revealed that:

(1) histamine and two histamine analogs, betazole and 3-(β-aminoethyl)-1, 2, 4-triazole (TD), could stimulate adenylate cyclase in homogenates and increase force of contraction, cAMP, and phosphorylase activity in the isolated perfused guinea pig heart.

(2) The order of potency for all events was histamine $>$ TD $>$ betazole.

(3) All of the effects of the agonists were competitively antagonized by burimamide.

(4) The increase in cAMP occurred prior to the increase in force of contraction.

Based on this evidence it was suggested that the inotropic effect of histamine in guinea pig heart was mediated through stimulation of H_2 receptors. Since cAMP increased prior to the change in force it was further suggested that the increase in cyclic nucleotide might be involved in the inotropic effect. (McNeill and Verma 1973, 1974a, b).

The data of McNeill and Verma were challenged by two groups of workers. Reinhardt et al., (1974) and Steinberg and Holland (1975) were both able to demonstrate, using appropriate blocking agents, that the inotropic effect of histamine in the guinea pig left atrium was due to stimulation of H_1 receptors while the chronotropic effect in the right atrium was due to H_2-receptor stimulation. Using guinea pig right ventricle strips, Moroni et al., (1974) and Ledda et al., (1974) have shown that the histamine inotropic receptor is of the H_2 type. In an attempt to resolve the differences between the observations outlined above, Verma and McNeill (1977a) carried out a series of experiments using isolated guinea pig right and left atria and right ventricle. In addition to employing specific H_1- and H_2-blocking agents, a specific H_1 agonist (PEA) and H_2 agonist (4-methylhistamine) were employed in order to characterize the histamine receptors in the heart.

Data obtained in the study showed that in the right atrium and right ventricle H_2 receptors were present. The receptors were stimulated by histamine and 4-methylhistamine and blocked by burimamide. Furthermore, cAMP rose in both tissues prior to either the inotropic or chronotropic effect. The increase in cyclic nucleotide was also blocked by burimamide. Thus, H_2 receptors were not just associated with changes in rate but also with cAMP. In the left atria, histamine and PEA produced a positive inotropic effect that was blocked by promethazine and not by burimamide. No increase in cAMP was found in this tissue with either agonist. 4-methylhistamine did not have either a mechanical or biochemical effect in left atria. Thus, in agreement with Reinhardt et al., (1974) and Steinberg and Holland (1975), it was shown that left atria contain only H_1 receptors. Stimulation of H_1 receptors in the heart, as elsewhere (Verma and McNeill, 1975), does not produce an increase in cAMP. It was further shown that some H_1 receptors do exist in the right ventricle. These receptors were clearly revealed only in the presence of high concentrations of PEA. The data obtained in the study (Verma and McNeill, 1977a) have been added to in two later reports (Verma and McNeill, 1977b; 1977c). Using two additional agonists tolazoline and clonidine it was found that tolazoline possesses, like histamine, both H_1- and H_2-agonist properties. Clonidine, on the other hand, appears to possess only H_2-agonist effects on histamine receptors. These data also indicate that increases in cAMP are not a sine qua non for histamine-induced inotropism. However, it is also apparent that H_2 receptors and cAMP appear to be linked in some manner.

In an attempt to further investigate cardiac histamine receptors we have carried out a study similar to that of Verma and McNeill (1977a) using the rabbit heart. Previous work involving histamine in the rabbit heart has been limited and has concentrated on the chronotropic effect (Trendelenburg, 1960). From data in the literature the chronotropic receptor has the characteristics of an H_2 receptor although this has not been absolutely determined. We have therefore investigated the chronotropic effect of histamine in right atria. The inotropic receptor in rabbit has not been previously investigated. Therefore histamine inotropism was investigated in left atria, right ventricle, and papillary muscles. Since cGMP as well as cAMP has been implicated in the inotropic actions of drugs it was decided to monitor levels of both nucleotides in the present study. Receptors were characterized using promethazine and metiamide as the antagonists and dimaprit, 4-methylhistamine, PEA, and histamine as the agonists.

MATERIALS AND METHODS

New Zealand White Rabbits (1.75–2.5 kg) of either sex were injected with heparin sodium (8 mg/kg, s.c.) 60 minutes before sacrifice. Animals were sacrificed by a blow to the head and their hearts were quickly excised and placed in Chenoweth–Koelle solution (Chenoweth and Koelle, 1946). The composition of the Chenoweth–Koelle solution in mEq/L was : NaCl 119, KCl 5.6, $CaCl_2 \cdot 2H_2O$ 3.2, $MgCl_2 \cdot 6H_2O$ 2.0, dextrose 10 mM, and $NaHCO_3$ 25 mM. Each heart was placed in a dissecting dish containing Chenoweth–Koelle solution, bubbled with 95% O_2 and 5% CO_2. The atria were carefully dissected away from the ventricles by cutting along the atrioventricular groove. The right atrium was separated from the left atrium. The fat and excess tissue was cut away and the atria were suspended in a 20 ml volume bath containing Chenoweth–Koelle solution, pH 7.4 at 35° C and bubbled with 95% O_2 and 5% CO_2.

A suture was placed in one end of the left atrium for recording and the other end was tied to a platinum electrode. Force of contraction was recorded on a Grass model 7 polygraph using a Grass force displacement transducer. Approximately 1 gm of tension was put on the atria. The muscle was electrically driven at a rate of 1 Hz at a voltage approximately twice threshold. The tissue was allowed to equilibrate at 35° for at least 60 minutes prior to the use of drugs. During this time the bathing solution was changed every 5 minutes. When the preparation was stable the effects of agonists were studied. The spontaneously beating right atrium was suspended, as described for the left atrium, and equilibrated for 60 minutes changing the bathing solution every 5 minutes. At the end of 60 minutes the effects of the drugs were tested.

In order to prepare the right ventricle strips, animals were sacrificed and the heart was quickly removed and transferred to the dissecting dish containing oxygenated bathing fluid. While in the bathing medium, the right ventricle was cut into two strips. The strips were suspended in a 20 ml bath containing Chenoweth–Koelle solution at 35° C as described for the left atrial preparations. The ventricle strips were electrically stimulated at a frequency of 2.5 Hz at double the threshold voltage. A resting tension of 1.0 gm was applied and kept constant by readjustment during the equilibration period. The bathing fluid was frequently changed and after a steady base line was obtained, the effects of the drugs were studied. Papillary muscles were removed from the right ventricle and suspended in buffer solution. The muscles were placed under 1.0 gm resting tension and stimulated at 2.5 Hz and 2 × threshold.

Dose-response curves on the force of contraction were obtained from electrically stimulated left atria, right ventricles, and papillary muscles. Chronotropic effects were recorded from the right atrium. The data are presented as percent increase in force over control vs. dose and as change in heart rate in beats/minute vs. dose. In some experiments, metiamide (1×10^{-6} M) and promethazine (3×10^{-6} M) were added to the bathing solution 15 minutes prior to the addition of the agonists histamine, dimaprit [S-[3-(N, N-dimethylamino propyl] isothiourea], 4-methylhistamine or 2-pyridylethyl-amine (PEA).

The dose of histamine, dimaprit, and 2-pyridyethylamine, which produced the maximum response on force of contraction was selected for the cyclic nucleotide studies. The agonists were added to the bath and at 20 seconds following drug administration the tissues were frozen with Wollenberger clamps (Wollenberger *et al.*, 1960) that had been previously cooled in a mixture of alcohol and dry ice. This time was selected on the basis of our previous experience using preparations from guinea pig heart (Verma and McNeill, 1977a). Changes in contractile force were just beginning in the various preparations at this time interval. The frozen tissues thus obtained were stored at $-80°C$ until analyzed for cyclic nucleotides. The cAMP was measured by a competitive protein binding assay using a cAMP kit TRK 432 obtained from Amersham-Searle. The method employed is essentially that described by Gilman (1970). The only difference is that charcoal rather than millipore filters is used to separate bound from free cAMP. The assay is reproducible and specific for cAMP in the range of 0.2–16 pmoles. Cyclic GMP was analyzed using a radioimmunoassay kit obtained from Schwarz-Mann. The drugs used in the study were as follows: histamine dihydrochloride (Sigma Chemical Co., St. Louis, Mo.), dimaprit, 4-methylhistamine, 2-pyridylethylamine, burimamide [N-methyl-N'-(4,5-imidazolyl) butyl thiourea] (Smith Kline and French Laboratories Ltd., Welwyn Garden City, Herts, England) and promethazine HCl (Poulenc, Montreal, Canada).

RESULTS

Initial studies were carried out using histamine as the agonist. Inotropic dose-response curves were obtained in left atria (Fig. 1), right ventricle (Fig. 2), and papillary muscle (Fig. 3). In agreement with previous work in guinea pig left atria (Reinhardt *et al.*, 1974; Steinberg and Holland, 1975; Verma and McNeill, 1977a) the inotropic effect of histamine in this preparation was found to be due to stimulation of H_1 receptors. The histamine dose-response curve was shifted to the right by promethazine but was unaffected by metiamide. Similar effects were noted in right ventricle and papillary muscle

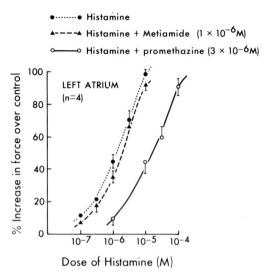

FIG. 1. The effect of metiamide (1×10^{-6} M) and promethazine (3×10^{-6} M) on the inotropic response to histamine in rabbit left atria. Each point represents the mean ± S.E.M. of 4 determinations. Antagonists were added to the bath 15 minutes prior to the addition of histamine.

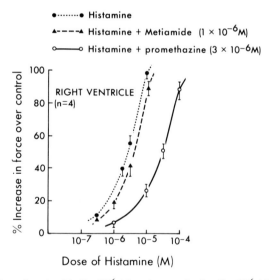

FIG. 2. The effect of metiamide (1×10^{-6} M) and promethazine (3×10^{-6} M) on the inotropic response to histamine in rabbit right ventricle. Each point represents the mean ± S.E.M. of 4 determinations. Antagonists were added to the bath 15 minutes prior to the addition of histamine.

276

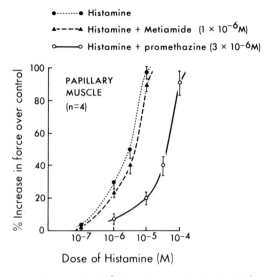

FIG. 3.   The effect of metiamide (1×10^{-6} M) and promethazine (3×10^{-6} M) on the inotropic response to histamine in rabbit papillary muscle. Each point represents the mean $\pm$ S.E.M. of 4 determinations. Antagonists were added to the bath 15 minutes prior to histamine addition.

(Fig. 2 and 3). Confirmation of the presence of H_1 receptors was obtained in experiments in which the specific H_1 agonist PEA was studied (Fig. 4-6). PEA produced a positive inotropic effect on all three preparations. The maximum response was obtained with a concentration of 10^{-4} M, a concentration ten-fold higher than was necessary for the maximum histamine response. In all three preparations the inotropic effect of PEA was competitively antagonized by promethazine and unaffected by metiamide.

In the next set of experiments the inotropic action of the specific H_2 agonists, 4-methylhistamine and dimaprit, was investigated and compared to PEA. As we had noted before, PEA produces an inotropic response in left atria, right ventricle, and papillary muscle (Fig. 7-9). Neither H_2 agonist appeared capable of producing an inotropic response in any of the three preparations.

Experiments in which the chronotropic effect of the agonists was studied in right atria did reveal the presence of H_2 receptors in the rabbit heart (Fig. 10). Histamine, 4-methylhistamine, and dimaprit produced increases in atrial rate. In the case of the latter two drugs the positive chronotropic response was almost completely blocked by metiamide. Metiamide reduced the histamine response but the response was further reduced by the addition of promethazine. Surprisingly PEA (Fig. 10D) also had a chronotropic effect. As with other PEA-induced responses the effect on rate was blocked by promethazine and not by metiamide.

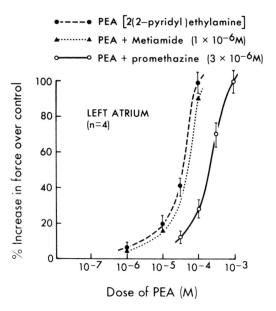

FIG. 4. The effect of metiamide (1×10^{-6} M) and promethazine (3×10^{-6} M) on the inotropic response to PEA in rabbit left atrium. Each point represents the mean $\pm$ S.E.M. of 4 determinations. Antagonists were added to the bath 15 minutes prior to the addition of PEA.

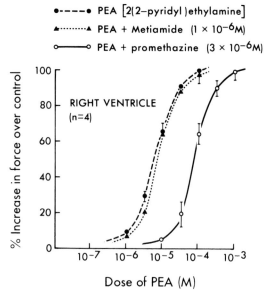

FIG. 5. The effect of metiamide (1×10^{-6} M) and promethazine (3×10^{-6} M) on the inotropic response to PEA in rabbit right ventricle. Each point represents the mean $\pm$ S.E.M. of 4 determinations. Antagonists were added to the bath 15 minutes prior to the addition of PEA.

278

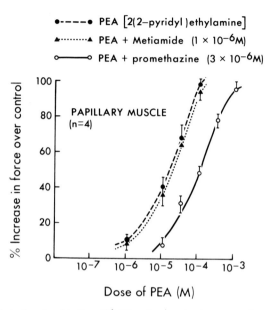

FIG. 6. The effect of metiamide (1×10^{-6} M) and promethazine (3×10^{-6} M) on the inotropic response to PEA in rabbit papillary muscle. Each point represents the mean ± S.E.M. of 4 determinations. Antagonists were added to the bath 15 minutes prior to the addition of PEA.

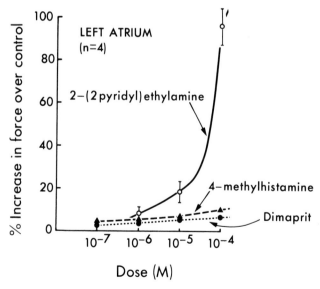

FIG. 7. The effect of PEA, 4-methylhistamine, and dimaprit on force of contraction in rabbit left atria. Each point represents the mean ± S.E.M. of 4 determinations.

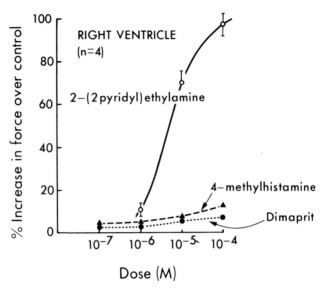

FIG. 8.   The effect of PEA, 4-methylhistamine, and dimaprit on force of contraction in rabbit right ventricle. Each point represents the mean ± S.E.M. of 4 determinations.

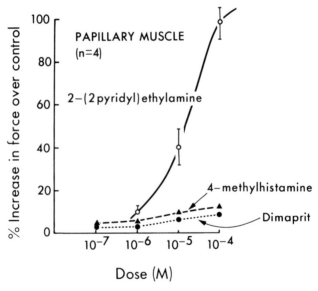

FIG. 9.   The effect of PEA, 4-methylhistamine, and dimaprit on force of contraction in rabbit papillary muscle. Each point represents the mean ± S.E.M. of 4 determinations.

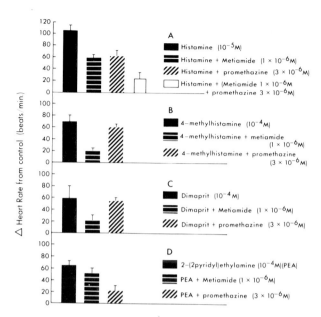

FIG. 10. The effect of metiamide $(1 \times 10^{-6} M)$ and promethazine $(3 \times 10^{-6} M)$ on the chronotropic response produced by $10^{-5} M$ histamine (Panel A), $10^{-4} M$ 4-methylhistamine (Panel B), $10^{-4} M$ dimaprit (Panel C) and $10^{-4} M$ PEA (Panel D) in rabbit right atria. Each bar represents the mean increase in heart rate (beats/minute) ± S.E.M. of 4 determinations. Antagonists were added 15 minutes prior to agonists.

Table I
Cyclic Nucleotide Levels in Various Rabbit Heart Preparations Following
Exposure to Histamine, PEA, and Dimaprit[a]

	Drug treatment (N = 6)	Cyclic GMP (pmol/mg tissue)	Cyclic AMP (pmol/mg tissue)
Left atria	None	0.020 ± 0.002	0.19 ± 0.03
	Histamine $(10^{-5} M)$	0.019 ± 0.003	0.21 ± 0.04
	PEA $(10^{-4} M)$	0.024 ± 0.001	0.22 ± 0.01
	Dimaprit $(10^{-5} M)$	0.019 ± 0.002	0.23 ± 0.01
Right atria	None	0.018 ± 0.001	0.24 ± 0.03
	Histamine $(10^{-5} M)$	0.020 ± 0.002	0.60 ± 0.04[b]
	PEA $(10^{-4} M)$	0.017 ± 0.002	0.26 ± 0.02
	Dimaprit $(10^{-4} M)$	0.019 ± 0.001	0.52 ± 0.02[b]
Right ventricle	None	0.020 ± 0.002	0.22 ± 0.02
	Histamine $(10^{-5} M)$	0.018 ± 0.006	0.26 ± 0.02
	PEA $(10^{-4} M)$	0.019 ± 0.002	0.30 ± 0.04
	Dimaprit $(10^{-4} M)$	0.020 ± 0.001	0.26 ± 0.01

[a]Tissue was exposed to the agonist for 20 seconds and then frozen using precooled tongs.
[b]Significantly greater than no drug treatment (P < 0.05).

The effect of the various agonists and the interaction with antagonists on cAMP and cGMP is illustrated in Table I. None of the agonists affected the levels of cGMP. Cyclic AMP levels were increased by histamine and dimaprit only in the right atria.

DISCUSSION

Previous work from our laboratory using various preparations from guinea pig heart has established that H_2 receptors appear to mediate the inotropic effect of histamine in right ventricle, right atria, and the perfused whole heart as well as the chronotropic effect of histamine in the right atria. The effects of histamine in the above preparations were blocked by burimamide and not by H_1 antagonists. Similarly the effect of histamine could be mimicked in right atria and ventricle by 4-methylhistamine but not by PEA (McNeill and Verma, 1974a, b; Verma and McNeill, 1977a). Data obtained in the above and previous studies (McNeill and Muschek, 1972; McNeill and Verma, 1974a, b) also implicated the adenylate cyclase-cAMP system in the cardiac H_2 actions of histamine. Adenylate cyclase could be stimulated by histamine and other H_2 agonists. The order of potency was the same if either enzyme stimulation or contractile force was monitored. Both events were blocked by H_2 blocking agents. Finally, increases in cAMP occurred prior to the increase in contractile force. Thus the evidence strongly indicated a role for cAMP in the inotropic effect of histamine. In guinea pig left atria, however, it was possible to dissociate inotropism from cAMP. In left atria, histamine receptors are of the H_1 type. Inotropic effects can be produced by H_1 agonists such as PEA and are blocked by H_1 antagonists such as promethazine. Therefore increases in cAMP are not absolutely necessary for the inotropic action of histamine.

In the present study, using the rabbit heart, it was found that histamine receptors regulating the inotropic action of histamine in left atria, ventricle, and papillary muscle were of the H_1 type. The inotropic effect of histamine was mimicked in all preparations by PEA and blocked by promethazine. H_2-receptor agonists were incapable of producing an inotropic response in the rabbit heart preparations. H_2 receptors were found in right atria and again appeared to be associated with cAMP. Increases in atrial rate could be produced by dimaprit and 4-methylhistamine and the effect was blocked by metiamide, as was the increase in cAMP. It is also apparent, however, that H_1-receptor stimulation can lead to a positive chronotropic response in rabbit heart since PEA could also produce the response. Promethazine blocked the PEA chronotropic effect. A combination of promethazine and metiamide was necessary to block the chronotropic response to histamine. In a limited number of experiments, cGMP was measured. No changes in the levels of this nucleotide were found.

It is thus apparent that cardiac histamine receptors vary between species. In the guinea pig heart the receptors are predominantly H_2 while in the rabbit heart they appear to be predominantly H_1. Powell and Brody (1976) have previously reported that histamine receptors in the dog heart are of the H_1 type. There are also differences in histamine receptors within hearts of a particular species. The left atria of the guinea pig has only H_1 receptors while other areas have H_2. Stimulation of either receptor results in an inotropic response and, thus far, it has proved impossible to dissociate increases in cAMP from H_2-receptor stimulation. It should be noted that a parallel situation occurs with the adrenergic amines. Stimulation of either α or β receptors in the heart can lead to an increase in force of contraction. However, only β receptor stimulation has been associated with changes in cAMP. (Martinez and McNeill, 1975; 1977).

REFERENCES

Ash, A.S.F., and Schild, H.O. (1966). Receptors mediating some actions of histamine. *Br. J. Pharmac.* **27**, 427-439.

Bartlett, A.L. (1963). The action of histamine on the isolated heart. *Br. J. Pharmac. Chem.* **21**, 450-461.

Beaven, M.A. (1976). Histamine. *New Eng. J. Med.* **294**, 30-36.

Bergmann, F. (1974). Introductory remarks on pharmacological receptors in "molecular and quantum pharmacology," (E.D. Bergmann and B. Pullman, eds.).pp. 1-7. D. Riedel Publishing Co., Dordrecht-Holland.

Black, J.W., Duncan, W.A.M., Durant, C.J., Ganellin, C.R., and Parsons, E.M. (1972). Definition and antagonism of histamine H_2-receptors. *Nature (London)* **236**, 385-390.

Burn, J.H., and Rand, M.J. (1958). The action of nicotine on the heart. *Br. Med. J.* **1(5063)**, 137-139.

Chenoweth, M.B., and Koelle, F.S. (1946). An isolated heart perfusion system adapted to the determination of non-gaseous metabolites. *J. Lab. Clin. Med.* **31**, 600-608.

Dale, H.H., and Laidlaw, P.P. (1910). The physiological action of β-iminazolethylamine. *J. Physiol. (London)* **41**, 318-344.

Dean, P.M. (1968). Investigation into the mode of action of histamine on the isolated rabbit heart. *Br. J. Pharmac. Chem.* **32**, 65-77.

Durant, G.J., Gavellin, C.R., and Parsons, M.E. (1975). Chemical differentiation of histamine H_1 and H_2-receptor agonists. *J. Med. Chem.* **18**, 905-909.

Flacke, W., Atanackovic, D., Gillis, R.A., and Alper, M.H. (1967). The actions of histamine on the mammalian heart. *J. Pharmacol. Exper. Ther.* **155**, 217-278.

Gilman, A.G. (1970). A protein binding assay for adenosine 3':5'-cyclic monophosphate. *Proc. Natl. Acad. Sci.* **67**, 305-312.

Klein, I., and Levey, G.S. (1971). Activation of myocardial adenyl cyclase by histamine in guinea pig, cat and human heart. *J. Clin. Invest.* **50**, 1012-1015.

Ledda, F., Fantozzi, R., Mugelli, F., Moroni, F., and Mannaioni, P.F. (1974). The antagonism of the positive inotropic effect of histamine and noradrenaline by H_1 and H_2-receptor blocking agents. *Agents Actions* **4**, 193-194.

McNeill, J.H., and Muschek, L.D. (1972). Histamine effects on cardiac contractility, phosphorylase and adenyl cyclase. *J. Mol. Cell. Cardiol.* **4**, 611-624.

McNeill, J.H., and Verma, S.C. (1973). Blockade of the cardiac effects of histamine. *Clin. Res.* **21**, 238.

McNeill, J.H., and Verma, S.C. Blockade by burimamide of the effects of histamine and histamine analogs on cardiac contractility, phosphorylase activation and cyclic adenosine monophosphate. *J. Pharmacol. Exper. Ther.* **188**, 180-188.

McNeill, J.H., and Verma, S.C. (1974b). Blockade of cardiac histamine receptors by promethazine. *Can. J. Phy. and Pharmacol.* **52**, 23-27.

McNeill, J.H., Verma, S.C., and Lyster, D.M. (1973). Blockade of the cardiac biochemical and mechanical effects of histamine and histamine analogues. *Fed. Proc.* **32**, 808.

Mannaioni, P.F. (1960). Interaction between histamine and dichloroisoproterenol. hexamethonium, pempidine and diphenhydramine in normal and reserpine-treated heart preparations. *Br. J. Pharmac. Chem.* **15**, 500-505.

Martinez, T.T., and McNeill, J.H. (1975). Comparison of changes in contractility and cyclic AMP in both paced and spontaneously beating rat atria in response to norepinephrine and phenylephrine. *Pharmacologist* **17**, 112.

Martinez, T.T., and McNeill, J.H. (1977). Cyclic AMP and the positive inotropic effects of norepinephrine and phenylephrine. *Can J. Phy. and Pharmacol.* **55**, 279-287.

Moroni, F., Ledda, F., Fantozzi, R., Mugelli, A., and Mannaioni, P.F. (1974). Effects of histamine and noradrenaline on contractile force of guinea pig ventricle strips: Antagonism by burimamide and metiamide. *Agents Actions.* **4**, 314-319.

Pepeu, G., Mannaioni, P.F., and Giotti, A.L. (1958). L'effutto della reserpina sulla resposta degli atri di caria alla nicotina, istamina 5-idronsi-triptamina ed alle amine simpaticomimetiche. *Boll. Soc. It. Biol. Sper.* **34**, 1326-1328.

Pöch, G., and Kukovetz, W.R. (1967). Drug-induced release and pharmacodynomic effects of histamine in the guinea pig heart. *J. Pharmacol. Exper. Ther.* **156**, 522-527.

Powell, J.R., and Brody, M.J. (1976). Identification and specific blockade of two receptors for histamine in the cardiovascular system. *J. Pharmacol. Exper. Ther.* **196**, 1-14.

Reinhardt, D., Wagner, J., and Schumann, H.J. (1974). Differentiation of H_1 and H_2-receptors mediating positive chrono and inotropic responses to histamine on atrial preparations of the guinea pig. *Agents Actions* **4**, 217-221.

Robinson, G.A., Butcher, R.W, Oye, I., Morgan, H.E., and Sutherland, E.W. (1965). The effect of epinephrine on adenosine 3',5'-phosphate levels in the isolated perfused rat heart. *Mol. Pharmacol.* **1**, 168-177.

Steinberg, M.I., and Holland, D.R. (1975). Separate receptors mediating the positive inotropica and chronotropic effect of histamine in guinea pig atria. *Eur. J. Pharmacol.* **34**, 95-104.

Trendelenburg, U. (1960). The action of histamine and 5-hydroxytryptamine on isolated mammalian atria. *J. Pharmacol. Exper. Ther.* **130**, 450-460.

Verma, S.C., and McNeill, J.H. (1975). Non-involvement of cyclic AMP following H_1-receptor stimulation. *IRCS Medical Science* **3**, 387.

Verma, S.C., and McNeill, J.H. (1976). Cardiac histamine receptors and cyclic AMP. *Life Sciences* **19**, 1797-1801.

Verma, S.C., and McNeill, J.H. (1977a). Cardiac histamine receptors: Differences between left and right atria and right ventricle. *J. Pharmacol. Exper. Ther.* **200**, 352-362.

Verma, S.C., and McNeill, J.H. (1977b). Investigations into the cardiac effects of tolazoline in guinea pig atria and ventricular stips. *Agents Actions* **7**, 191-197.

Verma, S.C., and McNeill, J.H. (1977c). H_2-histaminergic activity of clonidine in the guinea pig heart. *J. Cyclic Nuc. Res.* **3**, 95-106.

Wollenberger, A., Ristan, O., and Schoffa, G. (1960). Eine einfache Technik der extremen schnellen Abkulung grosserer Gewebstucke. *Arch. Ges. Physiol.* **270**, 339-412.

17

Prostaglandin and Histamine Effects on Cyclic AMP Levels in Parietal Cells

Peter Scholes, Joan Lee, John Major, and Michael Walters
Imperial Chemical Industries Limited
Pharmaceuticals Division
Department of Biochemistry
Alderley Park, Macclesfield
Cheshire, England

INTRODUCTION

The status of histamine as a physiological stimulant of gastric acid secretion has been the subject of several controversies (Code, 1965; Johnson, 1971). The demonstration that H_2-receptor blocking agents (Black et al., 1972) are potent inhibitors of gastric acid secretion induced by gastrin, histamine, and cholinergic stimuli (Wyllie et al., 1973; Grossman and Konturek, 1974) has established a role for histamine in the normal processes of gastric acid secretion. However, the mechanism by which histamine stimulates the parietal cell remains a subject of debate.

In amphibia and rats, histamine increases gastric mucosal levels of cyclic AMP (cAMP) and there is good evidence that in these species cAMP is a "second messenger" in the control of gastric acid secretion (Kimberg, 1974). The finding that histamine adenylate cyclase systems from gastric mucosa of several species, including rat (McNeill and Verma, 1974), guinea pig (Dousa and Code, 1974), rabbit (Sung et al., 1973), and dog (Ruoff and Sewing, 1976, Scholes et al., 1976) are inhibited by H_2-receptor blocking agents has been used as supporting evidence that the elevation of cAMP in gastric mucosa is an important component of stimulus secretion coupling in the parietal cell. However, this hypothesis has not gone unquestioned, indeed Mao et al. (1972, 1973) failed to find evidence for an involvement of cAMP in gastric acid secretion in dog, and recent reports in other species support these findings (Thurston et al., 1976; Thompson et al., 1976). Rosenfeld et al. (1976) found that membranes from rat gastric mucosa contained binding sites for metiamide but were unable to detect a histamine stimulated adenylate cyclase. Other data which is used as evidence against the involvement of a histamine H_2-adenylate cyclase system in the stimulation of gastric acid secretion has come from studies designed to understand the mechanism of inhibition of gastric acid secretion by prostaglandins.

Way and Durbin (1969) showed that prostaglandin E_1 (PGE_1) inhibited gastric acid secretion in an *in vitro* bullfrog preparation when gastrin or histamine were stimulants but not when secretion was induced by cAMP. These authors concluded that PGE_1 inhibited the rise in cAMP induced by histamine, thus, explaining why cAMP induced secretion escaped inhibition. However, subsequent observations that prostaglandins stimulate cAMP in preparations from gastric mucosa (Perrier and Laster, 1970; Perrier and Griessen, 1976; Wollin *et al.*, 1976; Dozois *et al.*, 1977, Rosenfeld *et al.*, 1976; Tao *et al.*, 1976) have been used as evidence against this interpretation. It has also been reported that histamine stimulation of adenylate cyclase is additive with prostaglandin stimulation (Wollin et al., 1976) indicating that two separate systems are involved and demonstrating that under the conditions employed prostaglandins did not inhibit the histamine H_2-adenylate cyclase system. The observation that prostaglandins are inhibitors of gastric acid secretion but are frequently associated with increases of cAMP has been used in support of an alternative hypothesis which attempts to correlate an elevation of gastric mucosal cAMP concentration with an inhibition of gastric acid secretion (Amer, 1972; Rosenfeld *et al.*, 1976; Thurston *et al.*, 1976). Other evidence cited in support of this hypothesis includes stimulation of phosphodiesterase activity by secretogogues (Amer, 1971; Amer and McKinney, 1972) and failure to detect histamine stimulated adenylate cyclase in gastric mucosa under some experimental conditions (Rosenfeld *et al.*, 1976; Thompson *et al.*, 1976; Sung *et al.*, 1973). Furthermore, characterization of histamine stimulated adenylate cyclase in some preparations has revealed inhibition by H_1-receptor blockers as well as H_2-receptor blockers, which suggests that this system could not account for the stimulation of gastric acid secretion (Perrier and Griessen, 1976; Sung *et al.*, 1973).

This paper attempts to clarify the complex findings of these conflicting reports by demonstrating:

(1) An H_2-receptor system in cells from dog gastric mucosa.
(2) Localization of the H_2-receptor adenylate cyclase system in parietal cells.
(3) Localization of the prostaglandin adenylate cyclase system in either chief cells or mucous neck cells but not parietal cells.
(4) Inhibition of the parietal cell H_2-receptor adenylate cyclase system by prostaglandins.

METHODS

Preparation of Cells

Suspensions of gastric mucosal cells were prepared as described previously (Scholes et al., 1976). Briefly, gastric muscosa was obtained from control beagle dogs used in toxicological studies and the fundic mucosa was stripped from the underlying tissues and washed in a phosphate buffered saline solution (NaCl 137 mM; KCl 2.7 mM; Na$_2$HPO$_4$ 0.8 mM; KH$_2$PO$_4$ 1.5 mM; CaCl$_2$ 0.9 mM; MgCl$_2$ 0.5 mM; glucose 1 mg/ml and adjusted to pH 7.4 with 1 M NaOH). Surface mucous cells were removed and the tissue was chopped finely using a McIllwain Tissue Chopper (Mickle Laboratory Engineering Company, Gomshall, Surrey, U.K.).

Free cells were prepared from the chopped tissue by incubating with the buffered saline containing protease (Type V from *Streptomyces griseus*, Sigma) and collagenase (Type I from *Clostridium histolyticum*, Sigma). Following incubation, the cell suspension was filtered through nylon gauze (50–60 μm pore size) to remove undispersed tissue fragments and the free cells were harvested by centrifugation at 400 g$_{max}$ for 4 minutes. The cells were washed once by resuspension in buffered saline containing 2% w/v bovine serum albumin (Fraction V, Armour) followed by centrifugation and were then incubated for 30 minutes at 35° C in 100 ml of buffered saline containing 10 mg of DNAase (Sigma) and 2% w/v albumin. A washed cell pellet was obtained by resuspending the cells twice in buffered saline containing 2% w/v albumin and three times in buffer without albumin.

Separation of Cell Types

Free cells prepared from dog gastric mucosa are heterogenous in size and fractionation can be accomplished, therefore, by velocity sedimentation. An effective way of exploiting differences in the velocity of sedimentation is to layer a suspension of cells on top of a density gradient in a suitable chamber and to allow sedimentation to proceed under the influence of unit gravity. The literature contains a variety of designs for suitable apparatus based on this principle.

The sedimentation chamber used in the present study is based on the design described by Tulp and Bont (1975). The apparatus was filled with a nonlinear gradient by mixing 0.3% w/v Ficoll (100 ml), 1% w/v Ficoll (600 ml), and 4% w/v Ficoll (600 ml). Ficoll 400 was purchased from Pharmacia Fine Chemicals, Uppsala, Sweden, and was dissolved in phosphate buffered saline. The gastric muscosal cells ($\simeq 10^7$ per ml) suspended in 100 ml of 0.3% Ficoll solution were then layered on top of the gradient. This was achieved by allowing the cell suspension to flow from a small separating funnel onto a polythene membrane pierced by numerous small holes and held at the surface of the gradient. The membrane may then be removed by allowing a small volume of the gradient to flow from the chamber such that the liquid level falls below the level of the perforated polythene. This procedure, in our hands, proved superior to the nylon sieve used by Tulp and Bont (1975).

After removal of the membrane, the conical top section is attached to the cylinder and the cells allowed to sediment for 2–3 hours. During this period, the cell band resolved into two distinct regions, an upper pale band and a lower yellowish area. In many instances, complete separation of two distinct bands of cells was achieved. When an adequate separation had been obtained, the gradient was fractionated by upward displacement using either 6% Ficoll solution or 6% sucrose. Forty-milliliter fractions were collected and the cells sedimented by low-speed centrifugation (400 g_{max}). The cells were then resuspended in buffer and examined by phase contrase microscopy. Parietal cells were identified by size and intracellular granulation while the smaller cell types were identified as chief cells and mucous neck cells. The very small cells which sediment more slowly than chief cells have not been identified. The correct identification of parietal cells has been confirmed by electron microscopy.

Gradient fractions containing mainly parietal cells were combined as were those containing mainly chief cells. Fractions containing the slowly sedimenting cells were also combined. A chief/parietal cell mixture was prepared by combining the cell fractions lying between the main parietal and chief cell bands. Using the procedure described, parietal cell preparations can be obtained which contain up to 95% parietal cells. For practical purposes where larger numbers of cells are required, it was necessary to compromise and accept preparations of lower purity, e.g. $\simeq 70\%$.

Drugs

Histamine acid phosphate was obtained from British Drug Houses Limited, Poole, Dorset, U.K. Natural prostaglandins E_1, E_2, and $F_2\alpha$ were obtained from Ono Pharmaceutical Company, Osaka, Japan. Metiamide (Black *et al.*, 1973), dimaprit (Parsons *et al.*, 1977), and racemic 16,16-dimethyl prostaglandin E_2 were prepared in our own laboratories. Burimamide (Black *et al.*, 1972) was a gift from Smith, Kline and French Laboratories Limited (Welwyn Garden City, Hertfordshire, U.K.). A potent phosphodiesterase inhibitor, 2-amino-6-methyl-5-oxo-4-n-propyl-4,5-dihydro-S-triazolo(1,5-α)pyrimidine (ICI 63,197) (Somerville, 1973) was added to each test incubation at a concentration of 5×10^{-5} M.

Incubations, Cyclic Nucleotide
Extraction, and Assay

Test incubations (5 minutes at 30° C) were started by the addition of 500 μl of cell suspension to buffered saline containing combinations of phosphodiesterase inhibitor, histamine, and prostaglandins as appropriate. Incubations were terminated by addition of 300 mM HCl (100 μl) followed by heating at 100° C for 10 minutes. Precipitated protein was removed by centrifugation at 5000 g_{ave} for 10 minutes. Aliquots of the supernatant solutions were neutralized with 2 M Tris. The cAMP content of suitable aliquots (usually 50 μl) of the neutralized cell extract was determined by the competitive protein-binding method described by Brown et al. (1971).

RESULTS

We have reported (Scholes et al., 1976) that in the presence of a phosphodiesterase inhibitor, histamine causes a dose-dependent elevation of cAMP concentration when incubated with suspensions of mixed cells from dog gastric mucosa. The histamine analogues, 4-methylhistamine and 2-methyl histamine, and the specific H_2-agonist dimaprit give dose-response curves which are displaced to the right of the histamine dose-response indicating lower potency, but all agents give the same maximum response. The relative activities of these agents calculated from the dose required to give 50% of the maximum response are shown in Table I. The relative activities of 4-methyl histamine and 2-methyl histamine in this system are in both cases rather less than the values reported by Black et al. (1972) for the other H_2-receptor systems, guinea pig atrium, rat uterus, and rat gastric acid secretion. However, the potency of 4-methyl histamine is much greater than 2-methyl

Table I
Relative activity of histamine agonists on the elevation of
cAMP concentration in cells from dog gastric mucosa
calculated on the basis of ED_{50}

Agonist	Relative activity
Histamine	100
4-methyl Histamine (5)[b]	21.6 ± 4.6 (14.1–25.6)
2-methyl Histamine (4)[b]	1.0 ± 0.5 (0.5–1.6)
Dimaprit[a]　　　　(1)[b]	41.0

[a] In this experiment the value for 4 methyl histamine was 24.0.
[b] Numbers in parentheses are number of experiments.

histamine which distinguishes this system from H_1-receptor systems in which 2-methyl histamine is more active than 4-methyl histamine. The relative activity of dimaprit in this system is intermediate between values of 19.5 for gastric acid secretion, 17.5 for rat uterus, and 70.7 for guinea pig atrium, but this agent has very low potency in H_1-receptor systems (Parsons *et al.*, 1977).

This histamine stimulated elevation of cAMP concentration in the mixed cells from dog gastric mucosa is competitively inhibited by burimamide, metiamide (Scholes *et al.*, 1976), and by cimetidine (Scholes and Walters, unpublished observations). By calculating dose ratios (DR) and using the expression log (DR–1) = log (*B*) – log (K_B), where *B* is the antagonist concentration and K_B the apparent dissociation constant of the antagonist-receptor interaction, we have constructed plots of log(DR–1) against log(*B*). These plots give slopes close to unity indicating competitive inhibition (Scholes *et al.*, 1976), and the intercept on the X axis where log (DR–1) = 0 gives apparent K_B values for metiamide and burimamide in this system. These values are shown in Table II for comparison with apparent K_B values reported in the literature for metiamide and burimamide in other H_2- and also H_1-receptor systems. The values obtained with the cells from dog gastric mucosa are generally lower than those reported for other H_2 systems except the K_B metiamide for rat acid secretion, which is very close to that obtained with this mixed cell system. The K_B values for metiamide and burimamide in this system like those in other H_2 systems are several orders of magnitude lower than K_B values reported for H_1-receptor systems (Black *et al.*, 1972).

Table II shows that the H_1-receptor blockers, mepyramine and chlorpheniramine, do not inhibit the cAMP response to histamine, 4-methyl histamine, or 2-methyl histamine. Interestingly, promethazine (3×10^{-5} *M*) does inhibit this system but is less effective than equal concentrations of metiamide. The inhibition by promethazine unlike that of burimamide or metiamide (Scholes *et al.*, 1976) is not overcome by increasing the dose of histamine. Furthermore, we have found that drugs which, like promethazine, prevent

Table II
Apparent K_B values for metiamide and burimamide obtained with the cell system from dog gastric mucosa compared with values obtained in H_1- and H_2-receptor systems

	K_B Metiamide	K_B Burimamide
Gastric mucosal cells (dog)	3.5×10^{-7}	2.3×10^{-6}
Guinea pig atrium	9.2×10^{-7a}	$7.8 \times 10^{-6} M^b$
Rat uterus	7.5×10^{-7a}	$6.6 \times 10^{-6} M^b$
Rat gastric acid secretion	3.6×10^{-7a}	
Guinea pig ileum (H_1)	1.2×10^{-3a}	$2.8 \times 10^{-4} M^b$

[a]Data from Parsons, 1973.
[b]Data from Black *et al.*, 1972.

Table III

The effect of H_1 and H_2 antagonists on the cAMP levels of cells from dog gastric mucosa induced by histamine, 4-methyl histamine, and 2-methyl histamine[a]

	+ 10^{-6} M Histamine	+ 10^{-5} M 4Me Histamine	+ 10^{-4} M 2ME Histamine
No addition	45.6 ± 4.7	65.9 ± 4.7	61.0 ± 7.5
3×10^{-5} M chlorpheniramine	42.5 ± 4.1	63.9 ± 10.2	57.4 ± 4.7
3×10^{-5} M mepyramine	45.1 ± 3.6	58.4 ± 8.2	57.7 ± 6.6
3×10^{-5} M promethazine	26.3 ± 4.5	37.6 ± 5.0	27.9 ± 4.4
3×10^{-5} M metiamide	15.6 ± 2.3	16.9 ± 2.5	12.6 ± 2.2

[a]Cell incubations contained 3×10^{-5} M ICI 63,197 and other drugs as indicated: 7.6×10^{-6} cells (23% parietal cells); 7.4×10^{-6} cells (25% parietal cells); 7.7×10^{-6} cells (23% parietal cells) were added respectively in the experiments with 10^{-6} M histamine, 10^{-5} M 4-Me histamine, and 10^{-4} M 2-Me histamine.

lysis of red cells in response to mild osmotic shock also inhibit this system. However, agents such as ethanol which may increase membrane fluidity increase the cAMP response to histamine (Walters and Scholes, unpublished observations). We are, therefore, of the opinion that the inhibitory action of promethazine is a result of a nonspecific membrane effect. These experiments establish that dog gastric mucosa contains a histamine H_2-receptor adenylate cyclase system.

As discussed previously, prostaglandins have been shown to stimulate adenylate cyclase in membrane preparations from gastric mucosa of several species. Fig. 1 shows that PGE_1 is a good stimulant of cAMP formation in mixed cells from dog gastric mucosa and that $PGF_{2\alpha}$ is a weak stimulant. In keeping with observations in other species (Wollin *et al.*, 1976; Perrier and Griessen, 1976), in dog this effect is not confined to cells lining the fundic area of the stomach and it seemed probable that it was not a property of the parietal cell. However, in view of the disagreements in the literature concerning a role for cAMP in gastric acid secretion it seemed important to establish this poir* and determine the cellular location of the histamine H_2-receptor adenylate cyclase system.

As described in the Methods section we have fractionated the mixed cells from dog gastric mucosa. The experiment illustrated in Fig. 2 shows the response of cell fractions, with varying parietal cell content, to histamine and PGE_1. Fraction 1 containing 85% parietal cells gives a greater response to histamine, compared with the mixed cell suspension from which it was prepared, but a greatly reduced prostaglandin response. Cells with a low sedimentation rate containing few parietal cells give a greater response to prostaglandin than to histamine while fraction 2 containing 46% parietal cells gives an intermediate response. This experiment, which is typical of many

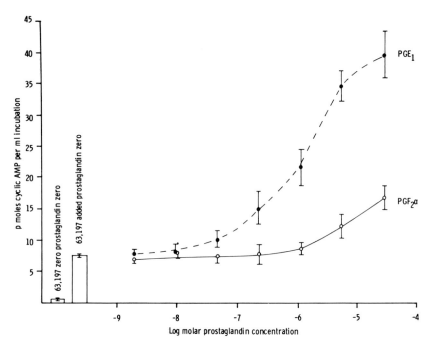

FIG. 1. The elevation of cAMP in cells from dog gastric mucosa in response to PGE_1(●) and $PGF_2\alpha$(○) in the presence of ICI 63,197 (5×10^{-5} M). 7.5×10^6 cells, of which 21% were parietal cells, were incubated (total volume 1 ml) under the standard conditions described in the Methods section. Values are mean ± SD of 4 incubations.

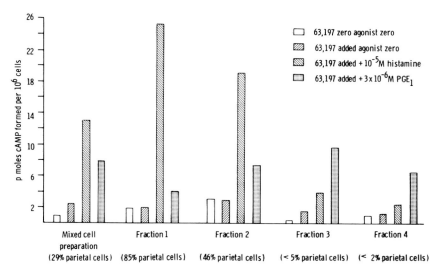

FIG. 2. The effect of histamine and PGE_1 on the elevation of cAMP concentrations in cell fractions from dog gastric mucosa containing different proportions of parietal cells. Values are the average of two incubations.

292

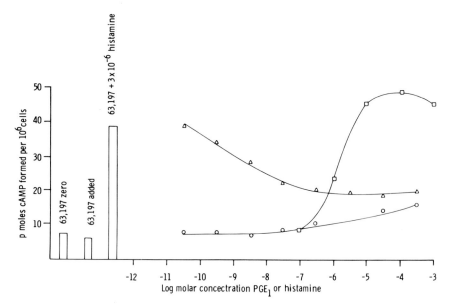

FIG. 3.   The effect of increasing concentrations of PGE$_1$ on the histamine-stimulated increase in cAMP concentrations in a parietal cell-rich fraction from dog gastric mucosa. Histamine dose-response (□), PGE$_1$ dose-response (○), inhibition of response to 3×10^{-6} M histamine by increasing concentrations of PGE$_1$ (△), in the presence of 5×10^{-5} M ICI 63,197. 0.66×10^6 *cells, of which 80% were parietal cells, were incubated (total volume 1 ml) under standard conditions described in the Methods section. Values are average of two incubations.*

others, clearly demonstrates that a histamine adenylate cyclase system, but not the prostaglandin system, is associated with the parietal cell.

Figure 3 shows that over the concentration range 10^{-10} M to 10^{-7} M PGE$_1$ inhibits the cAMP response to 3×10^{-6} M histamine in a parietal cell-rich fraction. The histamine and the PGE$_1$ dose-dependent stimulation of cAMP are also included. The small elevation of cAMP concentration caused by PGE$_1$ occurs within a higher concentration range than the inhibition of the histamine response.

Figure 4 shows that this action of PGE$_1$ is also shared by PGE$_2$ and 16,16 dimethyl PGE$_2$, which are good inhibitors of gastric acid secretion. PGF$_2\alpha$ which does not inhibit acid secretion *in vivo* also inhibits the histamine induced elevation of cAMP but its potency is only 1% that of the E type prostaglandins.

DISCUSSION

In experiments of the type illustrated in Fig. 2 we have shown that a histamine adenylate cyclase system is associated with the parietal cell rich fraction but it could be argued that this system is associated with a minor cell

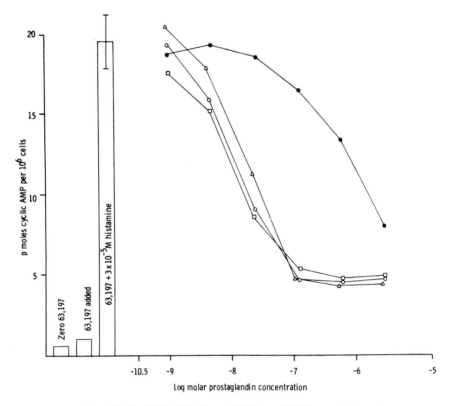

FIG. 4.   The effect of PGE_1, PGE_2, 16,16 dimethyl PGE_2, and $PGF_2\alpha$ on the histamine response of a parietal cell rich fraction from dog gastric mucosa. The effect of PGE_1 (○), PGE_2 (□), 16,16 dimethyl PGE_2 (△), and $PGF_2\alpha$ (●). 1.25×10^{-6} cells, of which 65% were parietal cells, were incubated (final volume 1 ml) under the standard conditions described in the Methods section. Values are means of two incubations except histamine stimulated value is mean ± SD of four incubations.

component. Although we have not isolated fractions consisting entirely of parietal cells, fractions containing up to 95% parietal cells have been obtained which respond strongly to histamine but weakly to prostaglandin. Furthermore, the contaminating cells are chief cells and mucus neck cells, and they give a weak response to histamine. The relative activity of histamine analogues and the apparent K_B values for metiamide and burimamide strongly suggest that the histamine induced elevation of cAMP concentration is mediated by an H_2-receptor system. Taken together these findings strongly support the view that histamine stimulation of acid secretory processes in the parietal cell is mediated via an adenylate cyclase system sensitive to H_2-receptor excitation.

Some authors (Rosenfeld et al., 1976; Amer, 1972) have suggested that the PGE_1 stimulation of adenylate cyclase in gastric mucosa is the cellular mechanism responsible for the inhibitory effects of prostaglandins on gastric acid secretion. The isolation of the prostaglandin response in a nonparietal cell fraction indicates that this viewpoint is untenable. It seems possible, by analogy with the effect of E type prostaglandins on the epithelial cells of the small intestine, that elevation of cAMP by PGE_1 in nonparietal fractions may be an effect in the mucus neck cells.

PGE_1, PGE_2, and 16,16 dimethyl PGE_2 are potent inhibitors of the histamine H_2-stimulated elevation of cAMP in dog parietal cells. They cause 50% inhibition in concentration range $10^{-8} M$–$5 \times 10^{-8} M$. The high potency of E type prostaglandins in this system suggests that these agents inhibit gastric acid secretion by inhibiting the formation of cAMP in response to histamine as proposed by Way and Durbin (1969). Experiments *in vivo* show that 16,16 dimethyl PGE_2 is more potent than the natural analogues in inhibiting gastric acid secretion. Our finding, that the potencies are reversed in this *in vitro* system, may indicate that metabolic breakdown is not an important factor in determining potency *in vitro*. The finding that $PGF_2\alpha$ shows approximately 1% the potency of PGE_1 and PGE_2 in inhibiting the histamine H_2 stimulation of cAMP concentration is in accord with its inactivity against gastric acid secretion (Robert *et al.,* 1967).

The effects we have reported for prostaglandins in gastric mucosa are similar to the dual effects of these agents in fat tissue. Thus, in adipocytes, prostaglandins inhibit cAMP formation and lypolysis induced by a number of agents, and the stimulation of cAMP in fat tissue by prostaglandins occurs in cells other than adipocytes (Butcher and Baird, 1968).

REFERENCES

Amer, M.S. (1971). Effects of aspirin, and other analgesics, histamine and some antihistamines on 3'5'-cyclic adenosine monophosphate (cAMP) phosphodiesterase (PDE) activity from rabbit liver. *Acad. Pharmaceut. Sciences* 1, 120.
Amer, M.S. (1972). Cyclic AMP and gastric secretion. *Am. J. Dig. Dis.* 17, 945-953.
Amer, M.S., and McKinney, G.R. (1972) Studies with cholecystokinin *in vitro:* IV Effects of cholecystokinin and related peptides on phosphodiesterase. *J. Pharmacol. Exper. Ther.* 183, 535-548.
Black, J.W., Duncan, W.A.M., Durant, C.J., Ganellin, C.R., and Parsons, E.M. (1972). Definition and Antagonism of Histamine H_2-receptors. *Nature (London)* 236, 385-390.
Black, J.W., Duncan, W.A.M., Emmet, J.C., Ganellin, C.R., Hasselbo, T., Parsons, M.E., and Wyllie, J.H. (1973). Metiamide—An orally-active histamine H_2-receptor Antagonist. *Agents Actions* 3, 133-137.
Brown, B.L., Albano, J.D.M., Edkins, R.P., Sgherzi, A.M., and Tampion, W. (1971). A simple and sensitive saturation assay method for the measurement of adenosine 3',5'-cyclic monophosphate. *Biochem. J.* 121, 561-562.
Butcher, R.W., and Baird, C.E. (1968). The effects of prostaglandins on adenosine 3'5'-monophosphate levels in fat and other tissues. *J. Biol. Chem.* 243, 1713.
Code, C.F. (1965). Histamine and gastric secretion: a later book, 1955-1965. *Fed. Proc.* 24, 1311-1321.

Dousa, T.P., and Code, C.F. (1974). Effect of histamine and its methyl derivatives on cyclic AMP metabolism in gastric mucosa and its blockade by an H_2-receptor antagonist. *J. Clin. Invest.* **53**, 334-337.

Dozois, R.R., Wollin, A., Rettmann, R.D., and Dousa, T.P. (1977). Effect of histamine on canine gastric mucosal adenylate cyclase. *Am. J. Physiol.* **232**(1), 35-38.

Grossman, M.I., and Konturek, S.J. (1974). Inhibition of acid secretion in dog by metiamide, a histamine antagonist acting on H_2 receptors. *Gastroenterology* **66**, 517-521.

Johnson, L.R. (1971). Control of gastric secretion: no room for histamine. *Gastroenterology* **61**, 106-118.

Kimberg, D.V. (1974). Cyclic nucleotides and their role in gastrointestinal secretion. *Gastroenterology* **67**, 1023-1064.

Mao,C.C., Shanbour, L.L., Hodgins, D.S., and Jacobsen, E.D. (1972). Adenosine 3',5'-monophosphate (cyclic AMP) and secretion in canine stomach. *Gastroenterology* **63**, 427-438.

Mao, C.C., Jacobsen, E.D., and Shanbour, L.L. (1973). Mucosal cyclic AMP and secretion in the dog stomach. *Am. J. Physiol.* **224**, 158-164.

McNeill, J.H., and Verma, S.C. (1974). Stimulation of rat gastric adenylate cyclase by histamine and histamine analogues and blockade by burimamide. *Brit. J. Pharmacol.* **52**, 104-106.

Parsons, M.E. (1973). The evidence that inhibition of histamine stimulated gastric secretion is a result of the blockade of histamine H_2-receptors. In: "International Symposium on Histamine H_2-Receptor Antagonists" (C.J. Wood and M.A. Simkins, eds.),pp. 207-215. Smith Kline and French Laboratories Ltd., Welwyn Garden City.

Parsons, M.E., Owen, D.A.A., Ganellin, C.R., and Durant, G.J. (1977). Dimaprit-[S-[3-(N,N-dimethylamino)propyl]isothiourea]-a highly specific H_2-receptor agonist. *Agent Actions* **7**, 31-37.

Perrier, C.V., and Griessen, M. (1976). Action of H_1 and H_2 inhibitors on the response of histamine sensitive adenyl cyclase from guinea pig mucosa. *Eur. J. Clin. Invest.* **6**, 113-120.

Perrier, C.V., and Laster, L. (1970). Adenyl cyclase activity of guinea-pig mucosa: stimulation by histamine and prostaglandin. *J. Clin. Invest.* **49**, 73a.

Robert, A., Nezamis, J.E., and Phillips, J.P. (1967). Inhibition of gastric secretion by prostaglandins. *Am. J. Dig. Dis.* **12**, 1073-1076.

Rosenfeld, G.C., Jacobson, B.D., and Thompson, N.J. (1976). Re-evaluation of the role of cyclic AMP in histamine-induced gastric acid secretion. *Gastroenterology.* **70**, 823-835.

Ruoff, H.J., and Sewing, K.F. (1976). Adenylate cyclase of the dog gastric mucosa: stimulation by histamine and inhibition by metiamide. *Naunyn Schmiedbergs Arch. Pharmacol.* **294**(2), 207-208.

Scholes, P., Cooper, A., Jones, D., Major, J., Walters, M., and Wilde, C. (1976). Characterization of an adenylate cyclase system sensitive to histamine H_2-receptor excitation in cells from dog gastric mucosa. *Agents Actions* **6**, 677-682.

Somerville, A.R. (1973). Adenosine 3',5'-cyclic monophosphate and affecting disorders. *Biochem. Soc. Spec. Publ.* **1**, 127-132.

Sung, C.P., Jenkins, B.C., Racey-Burns, L., Hackney, V., Spenney, J.C., Sachs, G., and Weibelhaus, V.D. (1973). Adenyl and guanyl cyclase in rabbit gastric mucosa. *Am. J. Physiol.* **225**, 1359-1363.

Tao, P., Holian, O., and Wilson, D.C. (1976). Histamine and prostaglandin interactions with cyclic AMP systems during canine gastric secretion. *Gastroenterology* **70**, 941.

Thompson, W.J., Rosenfeld, G.C., Ray, T.K., and Jacobson, E.D. (1976). Activation of adenylyl cyclase from isolated rat parietal cells by gastric acid secretagogues. *Clin. Res* **24**, 537A.

Thurston, D., Tao, P., and Wilson, D.E. (1976). Relationship between cyclic nucleotides and prostaglandin action on canine gastric secretion. *Clin. Res.* **24**, 538A.

Tulp, A., and Bont, W.S. (1975). An improved method for the separation of cells by sedimentation at unit gravity. *Anal. Biochem.* **67,** 11-21.

Way, L., and Durbin, R.P. (1969). Inhibition of gastric secretion *in vitro* by prostaglandin E_1. *Nature (London)* **221,** 871-875.

Wollin, A., Code, C.F., and Dousa, T.P. (1976). Interaction of prostglandins and histamine with enzymes of cyclic AMP metabolism from guinea-pig gastric mucosa. *J. Clin. Invest.* **57,** 1548-1553.

Wyllie, J.H., Wendy, D., Ealding, P., Hesselbro, T., and Black, J.W. (1973). Inhibition of gastric secretion in man by metiamide: A new orally active histamine H_2-receptor antagonist. *Gut.* **14,** 424.

18

Accumulation of Cyclic AMP in Brain Tissue: Role of H_1- and H_2- Histamine Receptors

John W. Daly, Elizabeth T. McNeal, and Cyrus R. Creveling
National Institute of Arthritis, Metabolism, and Digestive Diseases
National Institute of Health
Bethesda, Maryland

INTRODUCTION

The role of histamine in the central nervous system remains poorly defined in spite of more than a half century of extensive investigation. Histamine has been considered as a central neurotransmitter (Green, 1970; Snyder and Taylor, 1972; Dismukes and Snyder, 1974a; Schwartz, 1975; Schwartz *et al.*, 1976) and indeed histamine systems in brain are, in many respects, quite analogous to the established neurotransmitter systems, in particular those involving other biogenic amines–norepinephrine, dopamine, and serotonin.

Formation, Disposition, and Metabolism of Histamine in Brain.

Histamine is formed in brain by the action of a histidine decarboxylase and is inactivated primarily by the action of an imidazole-N-methyltransferase. Amine oxidases for histamine and 1-methylhistamine occur in brain. Histamine and histidine decarboxylase are present in very high levels in hypothalamus, with lower levels in cortex, hippocampus, brain stem, and in cerebellum (Schwartz *et al.*, 1970; Taylor and Snyder, 1971a). Histamine-N-methyltransferase is more uniformly distributed. Fluorescent histochemical assays, so valuable for the elucidation of noradrenergic, dopaminergic, and serotoninergic neuronal pathways, have not as yet been successfully applied to histaminergic systems. In homogenates of brain tissue histamine, histidine decarboxylase, and histamine-N-methyltransferase are associated with synaptosome fractions (Carlini and Green, 1963; Kataoka and DeRobertis,

1967; Kuhar et al., 1971; Baudry et al., 1973; Snyder et al., 1974). Histamine appears to be stored in synaptic vesicles. Histidine decarboxylase levels increase markedly during development in rat brain concurrent with synaptogenesis (Martres et al., 1975). Specific synaptosomal uptake systems–typical of other biogenic amine-transmitters–have not been firmly established for histamine (cf., Robinson et al., 1965; Snyder et al., 1966; Snyder and Taylor, 1972; Tuomisto et al., 1975). The rate of turnover of histamine in brain is extremely high, consonant with neurotransmitter function (Pollard et al., 1974; Dismukes and Snyder, 1974a, b). However, there is evidence for an additional relatively inactive metabolic pool of histamine in brain, which has been proposed to be associated with mast cells (Schwartz, 1975). Histamine is released from brain slices by potassium-induced depolarization, by reserpine, and by theophylline (Atack and Carlsson, 1972; Taylor and Snyder, 1973; Verdiere et al., 1975). All of these agents cause enhanced turnover or release of other biogenic amines more firmly established as central neurotransmitters. In vivo, histamine levels can be altered in manners reminiscent of control of other biogenic amines: Histamine levels are increased by administration of the precursor, histidine, or by inhibitors of histamine metabolism and are decreased by histidine decarboxylase inhibitors, reserpine, stress, and by certain central depressants (Atack, 1971; Taylor and Snyder, 1971a,b, 1972; Snyder and Taylor, 1972; Abou et al., 1973; Schayer and Reilly, 1973; Pollard et al., 1973a,b, 1974; Schwartz et al., 1976). Lesions of the ascending medial forebrain bundle result in profound reductions in levels of histidine decarboxylase in rat cortex, hippocampus, striatum, anterior hypothalamus, and thalamus (Garbarg et al., 1974). Histamine levels are only slightly reduced. Isolation of cerebral cortex or hippocampus by lesions results in profound reductions in histidine decarboxylase and histamine (Barbin et al., 1975, 1976). Thus, data from brain-lesioned animals strongly supports the existence of ascending histaminergic pathways. Transient increases in histamine in cerebral cortex after lesions of these pathways have been interpreted as due to the cessation of histaminergic nerve impulses (Schwartz et al., 1976)., Isolation of the hypothalamus results in a prolonged and marked elevation in histamine levels, perhaps due to proliferation of projections from histaminergic cell bodies (Dismukes et al., 1974). Histidine decarboxylase levels are also increased in isolated hypothalamus (Krishnamoorthy et al., 1973).

Central Actions of Histamine

Histamine has a variety of actions in the central nervous system consonant with neurotransmitter functions. Thus, administration of histamine intraventricularly or to specific brain loci causes a variety of behavioral and vegetative effects, including central arousal (Sawyer, 1955; Monnier and

Hatt, 1969; Monnier *et al.,* 1970; Wolf and Monnier, 1973; Schwartz, 1975), sleep (Feldberg and Sherwood, 1954; White, 1961), self stimulation (Cohn *et al.,* 1973), hypothermia (Brezenoff and Lomax, 1970; Shaw, 1971; Costentin *et al.,* 1973; Green *et al.,* 1976), enhanced water intake (Gerald and Maickel, 1972; Leibowitz, 1973), and increased respiration and vomiting (Feldberg and Sherwood, 1954; White, 1961; Bhargava and Dixit, 1968). Alterations in histamine-sensitivity have even been implicated in schizophrenia (Weckowicz and Hall, 1957 and ref. therein).

Histamine has either inhibitory or stimulatory effects on spontaneous or evoked electrical activity of central neurons. The nature of the neuronal response to histamine–inhibitory versus stimulatory–appears dependent on the type of neuron. Cerebral cortical neurons (Krnjevic and Phillis, 1963; Galindo *et al.,* 1967; Phillis *et al.,* 1968b, 1975; Haas and Bucher, 1975; Sastry and Phillis, 1976a), cerebellar Purkinje cells (Siggins *et al.,* 1971), and brain stem and spinal neurons (Bradley, 1968; Phillis *et al.,* 1968a; Hosli and Haas, 1971; Haas *et al.,* 1973) are usually inhibited by histamine, while hypothalamic neurons (Haas, 1974; Haas *et al.,* 1975) are usually excited by histamine. In one study, histamine had no effect on thalamic neurons (Curtis and Davis, 1962). Both H_1- and H_2-histaminergic agonists inhibit firing of cerebral cortical neurons (Haas and Bucher, 1975; Sastry and Phillis, 1976a). Histamine responses on cerebral neurons appear to be blocked by both H_1 and H_2 antagonists but the H_1 antagonists appear to be rather nonspecific (Phillis *et al.,* 1968b). The spontaneous firing of certain cerebral neurons is inhibited by stimulation of the rat medial forebrain bundle (Sastry and Phillis, 1976b). This inhibition is prevented by metiamide, an agent which in electrophysiological studies of central neurons appear to be a fairly specific histaminergic-antagonist (Phillis *et al.,* 1975; Haas and Bucher, 1975).

Histamine and Cyclic AMP (cAMP) Systems in Brain

Histamine, like norepinephrine, dopamine, and serotonin activates adenylate cyclase in brain homogenates (Hegstrand *et al.,* 1976) and causes accumulations of cAMP in brain slices (Daly, 1975 and ref. therein). Histamine does not, however, cause release of cAMP in ventricles of rat in contrast to the enchanced release elicited by norepinephrine, dopamine, or adenosine (Korf *et al.,* 1976). Histamine, like other biogenic amines, enhances phosphorylation of proteins in brain slices (Williams *et al.,* 1974; Williams 1976 and ref. therein). The relationship between histamine-elicited formation of cAMP and the resultant cAMP-dependent phosphorylation of proteins to the excitatory and/or inhibitory effects of histamine on central neurons is not clear. It is tempting to speculate that, like norepinephrine, histamine serves as an inhibitory neurotransmitter *via* activation of postsynaptic adenylate cyclase systems. However, a ubiquitous role for cAMP in the histamine-elicited inhibition of central neurons is not indicated. Thus, although both norepinephrine and histamine inhibit firing of cerebellar Purkinje cells (Siggins et al., 1971), only norepinephrine elicits an increase in levels of cAMP in these cerebellar neurons, as assessed by immunofluorescent assay (Siggins et al., 1973). Presynaptic adenylate cyclase systems, which are either inhibitory (Dismukes and Mulder, 1976) or facilitory (Cubeddu et al., 1974, 1975) to the release of neurotransmitters, have been proposed. Dopamine-sensitive adenylate cyclases are apparently associated with synaptic terminals innervating dopaminergic cells of the substantia nigra (Kebabian and Saavedra, 1976; Premont et al., 1976; Gale et al., 1977). Activation of presynaptic adenylate cyclases, could, for example, by reducing inhibitory inputs, be responsible for the excitation of certain central neurons by iontophoretic biogenic amines, including histamine.

Lesions of the rat medial forebrain bundle, proposed to transect ascending histaminergic pathways (cf., Garbarg et al., 1974), result in the development in hyperresponsiveness of cerebral cAMP-systems to histamine (Dismukes et al., 1975). This enhanced responsiveness to histamine is reminiscent of denervation "supersensitivity" of norepinephrine-responsive cAMP systems which develops in brain after lesions or after 6-hydroxydopamine-induced destruction of central noradrenergic systems (Dismukes and Daly, 1976b). Thus, the evidence strongly implicates a cerebral cAMP system as the post synaptic receptor for an ascending histaminergic pathway in rat. In guinea pig, lesions of the medial forebrain bundle had no effect on responsiveness of histamine-sensitive cAMP-generating systems in cerebral cortex (Dismukes et al., 1976a).

Further investigations on the relationship of histamine-elicited cAMP formation to (1) the electrophysiological responses of central neurons to histamine and (2) the central behavioral effects of histamine will certainly define the nature of the histaminergic receptors involved in the responses. At present, H_1- and H_2-histaminergic receptors appear to be important to both the inhibition of central neurons by histamine and to the histamine-elicited formation of cAMP in brain preparations.

H_1- AND H_2-HISTAMINERGIC RECEPTORS REGULATING CYCLIC AMP FORMATION IN SLICES OF BRAIN TISSUE

Histamine-elicited accumulations of cAMP in brain slice preparations were first reported in 1968 (Kakiuchi and Rall, 1968a,b). The very large accumulation of cAMP elicited by histamine in rabbit brain slices was effectively antagonized by a high concentration of an H_1 antagonist, such as tripelennamine or diphenhydramine (Kakiuchi and Rall 1968,b; Palmer *et al.,* 1972). Histaminergic agonists such as betazole and ω-N,N-dimethylhistamine elicited accumulations of cAMP in rabbit cerebral cortical slices (Shimizu *et al.,* 1970b). Subsequently, histamine responses were studied in slices from a variety of species, in particular, guinea pig where histamine is a rather effective stimulant of cAMP-generating systems. The magnitude of the response of cAMP systems to histamine in guinea pig brain slices was fourfold in cerebral cortex, eightfold in hippocampus, fivefold in thalamus, and twofold in striatum (Chasin *et al.,* 1973; Rogers *et al.,* 1975). A marginal or no response pertained in slices from cerebellum, amygdala, hypothalamus, medulla-pons, diencephalon, and brain stem. Early studies indicated that H_1 antagonists blocked histamine responses in cortical slices but caused only a partial blockade in hippocampal slices (Chasin *et al.,* 1971, 1973). Betazole and ω-N,N-dimethylhistamine were effective stimulants of cAMP-generating systems in guinea pig cerebral cortical slices (Shimizu *et al.,* 1970b). Synergistic responses of cAMP-generating systems to adenosine–histamine and to norepinephrine–histamine combinations in guinea pig cerebral cortical slices were at least partially antagonized by H_1 antagonists (Huang and Daly, 1972; Schultz and Daly, 1973a).

Histamine has little effect on cAMP levels in brain slices from rat, mouse, cat, pig, or primates. Thus, in rat cerebral cortical, hippocampal, and striatal slices, histamine had minimal effects on cAMP levels, while no effect was observed in slices from cerebellum, hypothalamus, thalamus, or midbrain (Krishna *et al.,* 1970; Forn and Krishna, 1971; Palmer *et al.,* 1973; Schultz and Daly, 1973b, Dismukes *et al.,* 1975; Dismukes and Daly, 1976a). In rat cerebral cortical slices, responses of cAMP-generating systems in the presence of a phosphodiesterase inhibitor were reduced by H_1 antagonists (Schultz and Daly, 1973b). Histamine elicited only marginal accumulations of cAMP in slices from mouse cerebral cortex or cerebellum (Krishna *et al.,* 1970; Forn and Krishna, 1971; Schultz and Daly, 1973b; Ferrendelli *et al.,* 1975; Skolnick and Daly, 1975a; Nahorski and Rogers, 1976). Marginal or no response to histamine has been reported in brain slices from monkey (Forn and Krishna, 1971; Skolnick *et al.,* 1973), human (Fumagalli *et al.,* 1971; Shimizu *et al.,* 1971; Kodama *et al.,* 1975) cat (Forn and Krishna, 1971), and pig (Sato *et al.,* 1974). Histamine was reported to elicit a significant accumulation of cAMP in pig hypothalamic slices. The hypothalamus contains the highest regional levels of histamine, but in most species histamine has no effect on cAMP levels in hypothalamic tissue. It is noteworthy that histamine has excitatory effects on hypothalamic neurons, while being inhibitory to most other central neurons.

The early studies on histamine and cAMP in brain tissue were conducted in large part before the development of specific H_1 and H_2 agonists and antagonists. In many instances relatively high concentrations of the classical

H_1 antagonists were used. Nonetheless, the results were indicative of at least partial control of central histamine-sensitive cAMP-generating systems by receptors with H_1 character. This was in marked contrast to histamine-sensitive cAMP systems in the periphery where activation involves primarily, if not wholly, H_2 receptors. Studies on the effects of relatively specific H_1 agonists, such as 2-methylhistamine and 2-aminoethylthiazole, H_2 agonists, such as 4-methylhistamine, and H_1 antagonists and H_2-antagonists on cAMP systems in brain slices have now been initiated.

In guinea pig cerebral cortical slices, responses to histamine were blocked partially by H_1 antagonists and by H_2 antagonist, metiamide, while combinations of an H_1 antagonist and metiamide cuased a complete blockade of the histamine response (Baudry et al., 1975; Rogers et al., 1975). H_1 antagonists caused a maximal inhibition of the histamine response in guinea pig cerebral cortical slices of from 60 to 80% while metiamide caused a maximal inhibition of from 50-60%. The accumulations of cAMP elicited in guinea pig cerebral cortical slices by an H_1 agonist such as 2-aminoethylthiazole or by the H_2 agonist, 4-methylhistamine, were significantly less than those elicited by histamine (Baudry et al., 1975; Dismukes et al., 1976b). Clonidine has recently been reported to be a H_2 agonist in guinea pig cerebral cortical slices (Audiger et al., 1976). In view of lack of potency of clonidine as an H_2 agonist, this histaminergic activity probably has little relevance to the central hypotensive action of this drug. Involvement of H_2 receptors in the hypotensive action of clonidine has been proposed (Karppanen et al., 1976). Intraventricular metiamide did not, however, prevent the hypotensive effect of clonidine in cats (Finch and Hicks, 1976).

In guinea pig hippocampal slices the response of cAMP-generating systems to histamine was antagonized by only about 50% with either brompheniramine or metiamide but was completely blocked by a combination of both antagonists (Fig. 1; cf., Chasin et al., 1973). 4-Methylhistamine and 2-aminoethylthiazole elicited fourfold and twofold accumulations of cAMP as compared to the tenfold accumulation elicited by histamine. The response to 4-methylhistamine was selectively blocked by metiamide, while the response to 2-aminoethylthiazole was inhibited by both H_1 and H_2 antagonists. Antagonism of the 2-aminoethylthiazole-response by metiamide did not pertain in hippocampal slices in the presence of adenosine (see p. 305).

Adenosine–histamine combinations have much greater than additive effects on levels of cAMP in guinea pig cerebral cortical and hippocampal slices (Sattin and Rall, 1970; Huang et al., 1971; Dismukes et al., 1976b). In hippocampal slices the response to histamine in the presence of adenosine was blocked much more effectively by brompheniramine than by metiamide (Fig. 1) in contrast to the nearly equal effectiveness of these antagonists in the absence of adenosine. The response to 2-aminoethylthiazole was potentiated to a much greater extent than the response to 4-methylhistamine by the

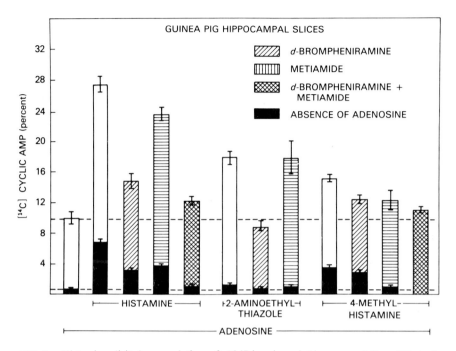

FIG. 1.   Histamine-elicited accumulations of cAMP in guinea pig hippocampal slices. Effects of H_1- and H_2-histaminergic agonists and antagonists. Accumulations of radioactive cAMP in adenine-labeled slices were measured after 8-minute incubations with histaminergic agonists (100 μM) either alone or in combination with adenosine (100 μM). Antagonists (10 μM) were added 2 minutes prior to agonists. The data—reported as percent of total radioactive adenine nucleotides present as cAMP—are from Dismukes et al., 1976b.

presence of adenosine. The 2-aminoethylthiazole response was in the presence of adenosine blocked by brompheniramine and unaffected by metiamide, unlike the results in the absence of adenosine where both H_1 and H_2 antagonists reduced the response to 2-aminoethylthiazole. The response to 4-methylhistamine was in the presence of adenosine partially blocked by both H_1 and H_2 antagonists and completely blocked only by a combination of antagonists. The results suggest that in the presence of adenosine, the H_1 contribution to histaminergic responses is greatly potentiated and that even the character of the receptor is altered so that a relatively pure H_2 agonist, 4-methylhistamine, now activates H_1 receptors. Marked increases in the apparent affinity of 4-methylhistamine and 2-aminoethylthiazole for the H_1 receptor were observed in the presence of adenosine, while the affinity for histamine was only marginally increased (Dismukes et al., 1976b). Since endogenous adenosine will contribute to greater or lesser degrees— dependent in part on differences in brain slice preparation and incubation— in the potentiation and alteration of amine responses it is obvious that the apparent contributions of H_1- and H_2-receptor mechanisms to histamine-elicited accumulations of cAMP will vary widely with a larger H_1 component manifest in slices wherein endogenous adenosine levels are high.

The relative contributions of H_1- and H_2-histaminergic mechanisms have not been studied in detail in other species. The small response to histamine in rat cerebral cortical slices was blocked by metiamide and only partially antagonized by brompheniramine (Fig. 2). Isobutylmethylxanthine was present as a phosphodiesterase inhibitor. However, antagonism of the effects of endogenous adenosine by isobutylmethylxanthine (cf., Mah and Daly, 1976) would, in these experiments, have tended to minimize the magnitude of H_1 contributions to the histamine response. In an earlier study with isobutylmethylxanthine present and with pheniramine and diphenhydramine as antagonists, an H_1 component in rat cerebral cortical slices was clearly

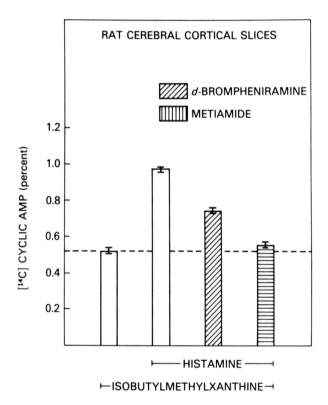

FIG. 2.   Histamine-elicited accumulations of cAMP in rat cerebral cortical slices. Effect of H_1- and H_2-histaminergic antagonists. Accumulations of radioactive cAMP in adenine-labeled slices were measured after 10-minutes incubations with histamine (100 μM). The phosphodiesterase inhibitor isobutylmethylxanthine (500 μM) was added 2 minutes prior to histamine as were the antagonists (10 μM). Data are from Dismukes et al., 1975.

evident (Schultz et al., 1973b). In chick cerebral slices, the response of cAMP-generating systems to histamine was effectively blocked by metiamide, while an H_1 antagonist had little effect (Nahorski et al., 1974). It is worthy of note that adenosine has little effect on cAMP-systems in chick cerebral slices (Edwards et al., 1974).

The apparent presence of H_1 and H_2 receptors which activate cAMP-generating systems in brain has now been established. This is analogous to the apparent presence of α- and β-adrenergic receptors which activate cAMP-generating systems in brain (cf., Daly, 1975). The H_1 response, like the α-adrenergic response, was unexpected based on data with peripheral systems where only H_2-histaminergic and β-adrenergic receptors appear to activate cAMP-generating systems. The H_1 response, like the α-adrenergic response (cf., Skolnick and Daly, 1975b; Sattin et al., 1975), appears, in brain slices, to be potentiated and perhaps altered by the presence of adenosine. Recent data have indicated that the α-adrenergic component of norepinephrine-stimulated accumulation of cAMP in rat brain slices is completely dependent on calcium ions (Schwabe and Daly, 1977). Adenosine, however, appeared to reduce the calcium-dependence of the α-adrenergic response (Schwabe et al., 1977). The apparent presence of two types of histaminergic receptors and of two types of adrenergic receptors which activate cAMP-generating systems in brain slices can be interpreted in two alternative manners as follows: (1) Coexistence of separate H_1 and H_2 receptors and of separate α- and β-adrenergic receptors. Such separate receptors could be associated with the same or different morphological compartments, i.e., presynaptic versus postsynaptic sites or neurons versus glia. (2) The interconversion of H_1 and H_2 receptors and of α- and β-adrenergic receptors, controlled perhaps by levels of adenosine, calcium ions, and perhaps other metabolic factors. The β-adrenergic receptor which activates cAMP formation in rat atrium has, indeed, been recently shown to show marked α character in atria from hypothyroid animals (Kunos et al., 1976).

Further studies of cAMP in brain slices have been designed to delineate adenosine and calcium dependency of H_1 and H_2 components of the histamine response. In addition, phosphodiesterase inhibitors have been studied to determine whether both H_1 and H_2 responses might be potentiated to different extents by inhibition of phosphodiesterases associated with the histamine-responsive compartments. Theophylline, a very weak phospho-diesterase inhibitor in brain preparations, was used primarily as an adenosine antagonist (Sattin and Rall, 1970; Mah and Daly, 1976). Isobutylmethyl-xanthine was used as a potent inhibitor of central cAMP- and cGMP-phosphodiesterases (DuMoulin and Schultz, 1975; Fredholm et al., 1976), but this compound is, in addition, an active adenosine antagonist (Mah and Daly, 1976). 4-(3-Cyclopentyloxy-4-methoxyphenyl)-pyrrolidone (ZK 62771) was used as a potent inhibitor of cAMP-phosphodiesterases. It has little effect on cGMP-phosphodiesterases (Schwabe *et al.*, 1976). A combination of ZK 62771 and theophylline provided a paradigm more comparable to that with isobutylmethylxanthine, i.e., concomitant inhibition of phosphodiesterases and reduction of the contributions of endogenous adenosine. Dipyridamole was used to activate adenosine mechanisms since at low concentrations it probably has little effect on phosphodiesterase activity but does markedly increase levels of endogenous adenosine by blocking reuptake of the riboside (Huang and Daly, 1974). Ethylene glycol-bis-(β-aminoethyl ether)-N,N'-tetraacetic acid (EGTA) was used to reduce extracellular calcium to near zero in order to probe the calcium dependency of H_1 and H_2 components (cf. Schwabe and Daly, 1977; Schwabe *et al.*, 1978).

Guinea pig cerebral cortical slices were used for these studies since earlier work had established (1) a relatively large and reproducible stimulation of cAMP formation by histamine, (2) marked synergism between histamine and adenosine, and (3) apparent contributions from both H_1- and H_2-histaminergic receptors. Adenine-labeled slices were used, since earlier studies with this technique had provided tentative evidence for the presence of two compartments of adenine nucleotides associated with histamine-sensitive cAMP-generating systems (Schultz and Daly, 1973c). The adenine-labeling technique consists of labeling intracellular adenine nucleotides during a prior incubation with radioactive adenine and then determining the effect of stimulatory agents on the percent of the total radioactive adenine nucleotide present as cAMP (Shimizu *et al.*, 1969). In brain slices radioactive adenine appears to be rather selectively incorporated into adenine nucleotide compartments associated with cAMP-generating systems (Shimizu *et al.*, 1970a; Schultz and Daly, 1973c; Shimizu and Okayama, 1973). The adenine-labeling technique has, with brain slices, given results consonant with those obtained by measurements of endogenous levels of cAMP (Schultz and Daly, 1973c and ref. therein).

The present experimental protocol differs to some extent from prior studies and is briefly as follows: Two male Hartley guinea pigs were decapitated and the brains placed immediately in cold Krebs–Ringer bicarbonate medium. All media were aerated with 95% O_2–5% CO_2. The cerebral cortices were removed as small slabs and then sliced at a 260 mμ setting with a McIlwain chopper. The slices were incubated in 15 ml of Krebs–Ringer medium at 37° for 15 minutes then labeled for 40 minutes with 20 μCi of 20 μM [^{14}C]adenine. The slices were then washed twice, incubated for 15 minutes, collected in nylon mesh, and divided into twenty portions, each of which was incubated separately for 5 minutes in 10 ml of Krebs–Ringer medium before addition of agonists. Phosphodiesterase inhibitors and antagonists were added 5 minutes and 2 minutes, respectively, prior to addition of agonists. Final incubations with agonists were for 10 minutes. Slices were then collected on nylon mesh and homogenized in 1 ml 6% trichloroacetic acid containing 0.25 μM cAMP. After centrifugation the radioactivity of 50 μl of the supernatant was measured to determine total incorporation of [^{14}C]adenine into adenine nucleotides. Cyclic AMP was isolated from the remainder of the supernatant

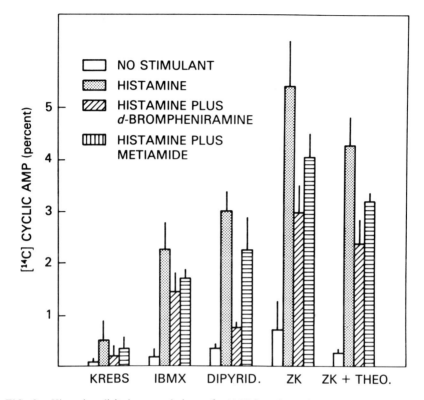

FIG. 3.   Histamine-elicited accumulations of cAMP in guinea pig cerebral cortical slices. Effects of H_1- and H_2-histaminergic antagonists. Accumulations of radioactive cAMP in adenine-labeled slices were measured after 10-minute incubations with histamine (100 μM). Antagonists (10 μM) and phosphodiesterase inhibitors were added 2 and 5 minutes, respectively, before histamine: No inhibitor (KREBS), isobutylmethylxanthine (200 μM, IBMX), dipyridamole (20 μM, DIPYRID), ZK 62771 (50 μM, ZK), theophylline (200 μM, THEO). Values are means $\pm$ S.D. of 4 to 10 experiments.

by Dowex and alumina chromatography (cf., Salomon et al., 1974). Recovery was determined by ultraviolet spectroscopy and radioactivity by scintillation spectrometry (cf., Shimizu et al., 1969). The radioactive cAMP content of the tissue has been expressed as percent of total radioactive adenine nucleotides present as cAMP.

Histamine elicited a sixfold increase in levels of radioactive cAMP in adenine-labeled guinea pig cerebral cortical slices (Fig. 3, Table I). Maximal accumulations of cAMP were elicited at 100 μM histamine with an EC_{50} of about 30 μM (data not shown). The EC_{50} for histamine-elicited accumulations of cAMP in brain slices has ranged from 7 to 50 μM in studies from a number of laboratories (Kakiuchi and Rall, 1968b; Shimizu et al., 1969; Huang et al., 1971; Chasin et al., 1973; Palmer et al., 1972; Baudry et al., 1975;

Table I

Histamine-Elicited Accumulations of Cyclic AMP in Guinea Pig Cerebral Cortical Slices and the Effect of "Phosphodiesterase Inhibitors"[a]

Agents	Conc. μM	[¹⁴C]Cyclic AMP percent – histamine	[¹⁴C]Cyclic AMP percent + histamine	Fold increase
None	—	$0.10 \pm .03$ (6)	$0.59 \pm .08$ (6)	5.9
Isobutylmethylxanthine	200	$0.19 \pm .01$ (10)	$2.4 \pm .2$ (5)	12.6
Dipyridamole	20	$0.38 \pm .04$ (5)	$3.7 \pm .6$ (5)	9.7
ZK 62771	50	$0.70 \pm .07$ (9)	$5.4 \pm .3$ (9)	7.7
ZK 62771 + theophylline	200	$0.25 \pm .02$ (4)	$4.5 \pm .3$ (4)	18.0
Theophylline	200	0.14, 0.08	0.50, 0.69	5.5

[a]Values are means $\pm$ S.E.M. with the number of experiments in parentheses or are individual values. The fold increase represents the ratio of the value with histamine (100 μM) to the basal value without histamine.

Dismukes *et al.,* 1976b). The time course for accumulations of radioactive cAMP elicited by histamine reached a maximum at about 5 minutes followed by a marked decline during the following 5 minutes (Fig. 4). Such a time course might reflect different rates of desensitization of histamine receptors in different compartments (cf., Schultz and Daly, 1973c) but this has not been investigated further. The present studies on histaminergic responses were conducted with 100 μM histamine or histaminergic agonists and with a 10-

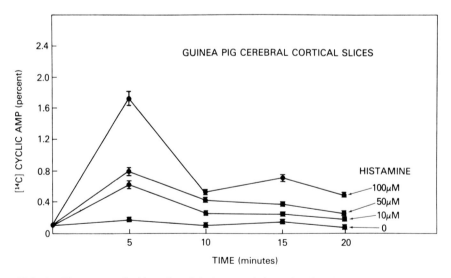

FIG. 4.   Time courses for histamine-elicited accumulations of radioactive cAMP in guinea pig cerebral cortical slices. Values are means $\pm$ S.D. for 3 to 5 experiments.

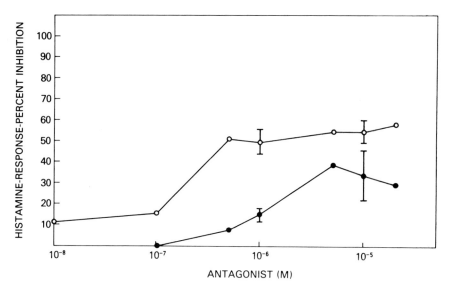

FIG. 5.   Antagonism of histamine-elicited accumulations of radioactive cAMP in guinea pig cerebral cortical slices. A phosphodiesterase inhibitor, ZK 62711 (50 μM) was added 5 minutes and d-brompheniramine (open circles) or metiamide (closed circles) 2 minutes prior to 100 μM histamine. Incubations with histamine were for 10 minutes. Values are means $\pm$ S.D. for 3 experiments or are averages for 2 experiments.

minute incubation period. Antagonists were added 2 minutes prior to agonists. Dose-response curves for the inhibition of responses of cAMP-generating systems to histamine by an H_1 antagonist, d-brompheniramine, and by an H_2 antagonist, metiamide, are shown in Fig. 5. Brompheniramine ($IC_{50} \sim 0.3 \mu M$) caused a maximal inhibition of the histamine response of about 60%, while metiamide ($IC_{50} \sim 2 \mu M$) caused a maximal inhibition of about 30%. These antagonists were employed in subsequent experiments at a 10 μM concentration. The effect of these antagonists on the response to histamine under various conditions (Fig. 3, Table II) was entirely consonant with the presence of H_1 and H_2 receptors which contribute to responses of cAMP systems to histamine in guinea pig cerebral cortical slices and with the potentiation of H_1 components by adenosine. Thus, inhibition of reuptake of endogenous adenosine by dipyridamole (Fig. 3) or addition of adenosine (Table II) greatly increased the relative contribution of the H_1 component. It would appear likely that, in the present study, endogenous adenosine had only minimal effects on the relative proprotions of H_1 and H_2 components except when reuptake of adenosine was blocked by dipyridamole. Indeed, the presence of theophylline reduced basal levels of cAMP with ZK 62771 present much more than histamine-stimulated levels of the cyclic nucleotide (Fig. 3).

The phosphodiesterase inhibitors, isobutylmethylxanthine and ZK 62771 did not appear to cause a selective potentiation of either the H_1 or H_2

Table II
Histamine-Elicited Accumulations of Cyclic AMP in Guinea Pig
Cerebral Cortical Slices and the Effect of Adenosine[a]

| Agents | [^{14}C]Cyclic AMP (percent) | |
	– adenosine	+ adenosine
None	0.10 ± .03 (6)	5.4, 5.7
Histamine	0.59 ± .08 (6)	26.5, 23.6
Histamine + brompheniramine	0.23 ± .04 (4)	7.5, 10.1
(percent inhibition)	(72 ± 3)	(72, 57)
Histamine + metiamide	0.36 ± .04 (3)	29.5, 22.1
(percent inhibition)	(54 ± 7)	(0, 6)

[a]Histamine and adenosine concentrations were 100 μM and antagonists were 10 μM. Values are means ± S.E.M. with the number of experiments in parentheses or are individual values. Percent inhibitions of the histamine-response by the antagonists are presented on separate lines in parentheses.

component of the histamine response (Fig. 3). Thus, the data with these inhibitors provide no evidence for the existence of separate compartments associated with H_1- and H_2-sensitive cAMP-generating systems in guinea pig cerebral cortical slices.

The response of histamine-sensitive cAMP systems to H_1 and H_2 agonists under a variety of conditions is shown in Fig. 6. Both 2-aminoethylthiazole and 4-methylhistamine were studied at 100 μM. The potency of these agonists is quite low. Thus, the EC_{50} of 2-aminoethylthiazole in hippocampal slices ranged from 30 to 280 μM in the presence and absence, respectively, of exogenous adenosine (Dismukes et al., 1976b), while the EC_{50} for 4-methylhistamine has been reported from 50 to 100 μM in guinea pig brain slices (Audiger et al., 1976; Dismukes et al., 1976b). The present results indicate that isobutylmethylxanthine potentiated responses to histamine, 2-aminoethylthiazole, and 4-methylhistamine nearly equally by about six- to sevenfold (Fig. 6). ZK 62711 and ZK 62711–theophylline combinations tended to potentiate the response to 4-methylhistamine to a greater extent than the responses to histamine or 2-aminoethylthiazole. Dipyridamole potentiates the response to histamine by about sevenfold, the response to 2-aminoethylthizaole by fivefold, and the response to 4-methylhistamine by about threefold. It had been expected that dipyridamole by increasing endogenous adenosine would potentiate histamine and 2-aminoethylthiazole responses to a greater extent than 4-methylhistamine responses. Adenosine does greatly potentiate the histamine and 2-aminoethylthizaole responses while having lesser effects on the response to 4-methylhistamine in

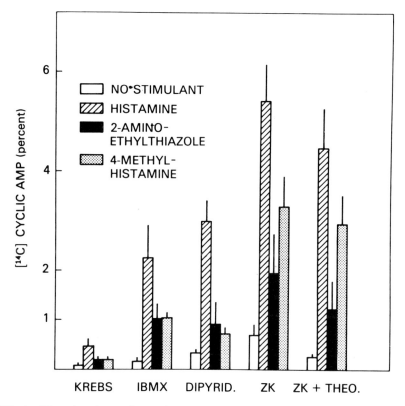

FIG. 6. Histaminergic agonists and cAMP-levels in guinea pig cerebral cortical slices. Accumulations of radioactive cAMP in adenine-labeled slices were measured after 10-minute incubations with 100 μM histaminergic agonists. Phosphodiesterase inhibitors were added 5 minutes before the agonist: No inhibitor (KREBS), isobutylmethlxanthine (200 μM, IBMX), dipyridamole (20 μM DIPYRID), ZK 62771 (50 μM, ZK), theophylline (200 μM, THEO). Values are means ± S.D. for 5 to 10 experiments.

guinea pig cerebral cortical and hippocampal slices (Fig. 1, and Rogers *et al.*, 1975).

Chelation of extracellular calcium with EGTA prior to addition of histamine had little effect on the apparent proportion of H_1 and H_2 components (Table III). However, EGTA had apparently greatly increased the release of endogenous adenosine since basal levels of cAMP were markedly increased by EGTA in a theophylline-sensitive manner. Adenosine has been reported to partially overcome the dependency of the α-adrenergic response on calcium ions (Schwabe *et al.*, 1978; Schwabe and Daly, 1977). Thus, enhanced release of adenosine under calcium-free conditions (cf., McIlwain, 1972) would be expected to complicate interpretation of the

Table III

Histamine-Elicited Accumulations of Cyclic AMP in Guinea Pig Cerebral Cortical Slices and the Effect of EGTA and Theophylline[a]

Agents	[^{14}C]Cyclic AMP percent		
	Krebs–Ringer	+EGTA	+EGTA +Theophylline
None	0.10 ± .03 (6)	0.30 ± .04 (5)	0.15 ± .02 (5)
Histamine	0.59 ± .08 (6)	1.5 ± .2 (5)	0.49 ± .07 (5)
2-Aminoethylthiazole	0.18, 0.21	1.2 ± .3 (4)	0.22 ± .04 (4)[b]
4-Methylhistamine	0.22, 0.18	0.92 ± .2 (4)	0.31 ± .03 (4)
Histamine + brompheniramine	0.23 ± .04 (3)	0.78 ± .04 (4)	0.35 ± .01 (4)[c]
(percent inhibition)	(73 ± 3)	'(65 ± 4)	(37 ± 16)
Histamine + metiamide	0.36 ± .04 (3)	0.94 ± .09 (4)	0.25 ± .04 (4)[b]
(percent inhibition)	(54 ± 7)	(52 ± 8)	(72 ± 8)
Histamine + brompheniramine + metiamide	0.13	0.64	0.16
(percent inhibition)	(98)	(85)	(82)

[a]Histamine and agonist concentrations were 100 μM, antagonists, 10 μM, EGTA 2 mM, and theophylline 200 μM. Values are means ± S.E.M. with the number of experiments in parentheses or are individual values. Percent inhibitions of the histamine response by the antagonists are presented on separate lines in parentheses.
[b]Not significant versus no agent (None) p > 0.05.
[c]Not significant versus histamine alone p > 0.05.

present data, particularly in view of the marked potentiation of H_1 responses by adenosine. The response to the H_1 antagonist, 2-aminoethylthiazole, was indeed markedly enhanced rather than reduced under EGTA conditions. In order to reduce the adenosine component, theophylline was used in combination with EGTA. The apparent H_1 contribution to the histamine response was virtually eliminated by EGTA–theophylline, and 2-aminoethylthiazole now had no effect (Table III). Thus, the H_1 component of the histamine response would appear dependent to a large extent on either extracellular calcium or adenosine, a situation which also pertains with respect to the α-component of the norepinephrine response in brain slices (Schwabe and Daly, 1977). Further studies are required to define the mechanism of interactions of histamine, calcium, and adenosine at central H_1 receptors. Clearly, however, such interactions could provide for subtle control of cAMP-generating systems dependent on the activity of neurons and related changes in calcium fluxes and adenosine levels. Calcium enters neurons during electrical activity (Baker et al., 1971) and levels and net release of adenosine increase in neurons during electrical stimulation or depolarization (McIlwain, 1972).

H_2 AND H_2 RECEPTORS REGULATING CYCLIC AMP-FORMATION IN CELL-FREE PREPARATIONS FROM BRAIN

Histamine caused a small activation of adenylate cyclases in lysed neuronal and glial fractions from rabbit cerebrum (Palmer, 1973; Spiker *et al.,* 1976). The activation was inhibited by chlorpromazine. Recently the effects of histamine on adenylate cyclase in homogenates from guinea pig brain have been studied in some detail (Hegstrand *et al.,* 1976). Histamine activated adenylate cyclases from neocortex, hippocampus, and striatum, while having no effect on cyclases from cerebellum, hypothalamus, thalamus, midbrain, pons, or medulla. GTP was present in the incubation medium. With hippocampal preparations, histamine activated adenylate cyclases by about twofold. The response was blocked by metiamide and was not affected by an H_1 antagonist, pyrilamine. The apparent loss of the H_1 response in homogenates from brain tissue is reminiscent of the similar loss of α-adrenergic responses in homogenates from rat cerebral cortex (Von Hungen and Roberts, 1973a) and of adenosine responses in homogenates from guinea pig brain (Sattin and Rall, 1970). Histamine has either no or only marginal effects on adenylate cyclases in homogenates from rat brain (Von Hungen and Roberts, 1973a,b; DeBelleroche *et al.,* 1974; Hegstrand *et al.,* 1976). Histamine-sensitive adenylate cyclases were detected in homogenates from monkey sensorimotor and cingulate cortex but not in homogenates from median orbital cortex, hippocampus, amygdala, or nucleus accumbens (Weinryb and Michel, 1976). It should be noted that histamine activated adenylate cyclases in homogenates of brain capillary preparations and that both H_1 and H_2 antagonists inhibited the response (Joo *et al.,* 1975). Thus, histamine-responsive adenylate cyclases have been observed in homogenates from neuronal, glial, and capillary-enriched fractions of brain.

In view of the apparent loss of the H_1 component in brain homogenates (Hegstrand *et al.,* 1976) such preparations do not appear to represent a particularly useful model system for detailed investigation of histaminergic control of cAMP-generating systems in brain. However, homogenates of brain tissues prepared in Krebs–Ringer buffer rather than sucrose afford a unique vesicular preparation whose cAMP-generating systems retain many properties delineated with brain slice preparations (Chasin *et al.,* 1974). Cyclic AMP is formed in these cell-free particulate preparations from endogenous, intravesicular ATP rather than from exogenous ATP. Histamine elicits a marked accumulation of cAMP in preparations from guinea pig cerebral cortex and hippocampus but not those from cerebellum. Adenosine and α-adrenergic responses are retained. Depolarizing agents cause stimulation of cAMP-systems in Krebs–Ringer homogenate preparations apparently through an adenosine–mechanism similar to that which pertains in brain

Table IV

Histamine-Elicited Accumulation of Cyclic AMP in Cell-Free, Particulate Preparations from Guinea Pig Cortex[a]

Agents	[^{14}C]Cyclic-AMP (percent)	Fold increase[b]	Percent inhibition[c]
None	1.2	—	—
Histamine (100 μM)	3.6	3.0	—
Histamine + brompheniramine (10 μM)	1.7	1.4	80
Histamine + metiamide (10 μM)	2.8	2.3	33
Adenosine (100 μM)	3.1	2.7	—
Histamine + adenosine	7.7	6.4	—

[a] A guinea pig cerebral cortex was homogenized (1 g/4 ml) with ice-cold Krebs–Ringer bicarbonate medium containing 10 μM EDTA. The medium had been preaerated with 95% O_2–5%CO_2. After centrifugation at 1000 × g for 15 minutes at 4° the pellet was reconstituted in 15 ml of Krebs–Ringer medium and labeled with 20 μCi of 24 μM [^{14}C]adenine for 15 minutes at 37° with aeration (cf., Chasin *et al.*, 1974). After centrifugation, washing (2×) and final resuspension in 12 ml Krebs–Ringer medium, the preparation was incubated for 30 minutes with aeration and then divided into ten 1 ml portions (2 mg Lowry protein/tube). Agents were added in 1 ml of Krebs–Ringer medium for a final 10-minute incubation. The final incubation was terminated by rapid chilling to 0°. After centrifugation at 100 × g for 10 minutes, the pellet was homogenized with 1 ml 6% trichloroacetic acid containing 0.25 μM cAMP. Following centrifugation, the radioactivity of 50 μl of the supernatant was measured to determine total incorporation of [^{14}C]adenine into adenine nucleotides. Cyclic AMP was isolated from the remainder of the supernatant by Dowex and alumina chromatography (cf., Salomon *et al.*, 1974). Recovery was determined by ultraviolet spectroscopy and radioactivity by scintillation spectrometry. The radioactive cAMP content of the particulate preparation is expressed as percent of total radioactive adenine nucleotides present as cAMP. Values are results from a single representative experiment. Basal and histamine-elicited levels of cAMP were 1.4 ± 0.3 and 3.9 ± 0.9% (S.E.M.) in four experiments.
[b] Ratio of value in the presence of agent(s) to basal value with no agent (none).
[c] Percent inhibition of histamine response.

slices (Shimizu *et al.*, 1975). These Krebs–Ringer particulate preparations have been shown to contain not only synaptosomes—some with attached postsynaptic vesicular entities—but in addition, large numbers of vesicular entities with a wide range of sizes (Horn and Phillipson, 1976). The nature of the histamine response in Krebs–Ringer vesicular preparations has now been investigated. The initial data clearly indicated the presence of both H_1 and H_2 components (Table IV). Thus, this preparation provides a valuable system for further investigation of the nature, role, and localization of H_1 and H_2 receptors controlling cAMP-formation in brain tissue.

SUMMARY

Histamine elicits accumulations of cAMP in brain tissue through interaction with H_1- and H_2-histaminergic receptors. The magnitude of the response and the relative contributions of H_1 and H_2 receptors to histamine-elicited accumulation of cAMP varies with species and with brain regions and is strongly influenced by extracellular levels of adenosine and calcium ions. Adenosine potentiates the H_1 component of the histamine response, while in the absence of adenosine the H_1 component is virtually completely dependent on extracellular calcium ions. A cell-free particulate preparation from Krebs–Ringer homogenates retains H_1- and H_2-sensitive cAMP-generating systems and provides a valuable model for investigation of the mechanisms whereby adenosine and calcium ions regulate the nature and/or responsiveness of histaminergic receptor-adenylate cyclase complexes in brain tissue.

ACKNOWLEDGMENTS

The authors gratefully thank Mr. William Padgett for his excellent technical assistance.

REFERENCES

Abou, Y.Z., Adam, H.M., and Stephen, W.R.G. (1973). Concentration of histamine in different parts of the brain and hypophysis of rabbit: effect of treatment with histidine, certain other amino acids and histamine. *Brit. J. Pharmacol.* **48**, 577–589.

Atack, C. (1971). Reduction of histamine in mouse brain by N^1-(DL-seryl)-N^2-(2,3,4-trihydroxybenzyl)hydrazine and reserpine. *J. Pharm. Pharmacol.* **23**, 992–993.

Atack, C., and Carlsson, A. (1972). *In vitro* release of endogenous histamine, together with noradrenaline and 5-hydroxytryptamine, from slices of mouse cerebral hemispheres. *J. Pharm. Pharmacol.* **24**, 990–992.

Audiger, Y., Virion, A., and Schwartz, J-C. (1976). Stimulatin of cerebral histamine H_2-receptors by clonidine. *Nature (London)* **262**, 307–308.

Baker, P.F., Hodgkin, A.L., and Ridgway, E.D. (1971). Depolarization and calcium entry in squid giant axons. *J. Physiol.* **218**, 709–721.

Barbin, G., Hirsch, J.C., Garbarg, M., and Schwartz, J.C. (1975). Decrease in histamine content and decarboxylase activities in an isolated area of the cerebral cortex of the cat. *Brain Res.* **92**, 170–174.

Barbin, G., Garbar, M., Schwartz, J.C., and Storm-Mathiesen, J. (1976). Histamine synthesizing afferents to the hippocampal region. *J. Neurochem.* **26**, 259–263.

Baudry, M., Martres, M.P., and Schwartz, J.C. (1973). The subcellular localization of histidine decarboxylase in various regions of rat brain. *J. Neurochem.* **21**, 1301–1309.

Baudry, M., Martres, M.P., and Schwartz, J.C. (1975). H_1- and H_2-receptors in the histamine-induced accumulation of cyclic AMP in guinea pig brain slices. *Nature (London)* **253**, 362–363.

Bhargava, K.P., and Dixit, K. (1968). The role of the chemoreceptor trigger zone in histamine-induced emesis. *Brit. J. Pharmacol.* **34**, 505–513.

Bradley, P.B. (1968). Synaptic transmission in the central nervous system and its relevance for drug action. *Internat. Rev. Neurobiol.* **11**, 1–56.

Brezenoff, H.E., and Lomax, P. (1970). Temperature changes following microinjection of histamine into the thermoregulatory centres of the rat. *Experientia* **26**, 51–52.

Carlini, E.A., and Green, J.P. (1963). The subcellular distribution of histamine, slow reacting substance and 5-hydroxytryptamine in the brain of the rat. *Brit. J. Pharmacol.* **20**, 264–277.

Chasin, M., Rivkin, I., Mamrak, F., Samaniego, G., and Hess, S.M. (1971). α- and β-Adrenergic receptors as mediators of accumulation of cyclic adenosine 3',5'-monophosphate in specific areas of guinea pig brain. *J. Biol. Chem.* **246**, 3037-3041.

Chasin, M., Mamrak, F., Samaniego, S.G., and Hess, S.M. (1973). Characteristics of the catecholamine and histamine receptor sites mediating accumulation of cyclic adenosine 3',5'-monophosphate in guinea pig brain. *J. Neurochem.* **21**, 1415-1427.

Chasin, M., Mamrak, F., and Samaniego, S.G. (1974). Preparation and properties of a cell-free hormonally responsive adenylate cyclase from guinea pig brain. *J. Neurochem.* **22**, 1031-1038.

Cohn, C.K., Bull, G.G., and Hirsch, J. (1973). Histamine: effect on self-stimulation. *Science* **180**, 757-759.

Costentin, J., Boulu, R., and Schwartz, J.C. (1973). Pharmacological studies on the role of histamine in thermoregulation. *Agents Actions* **3**, 177.

Cubeddu, L., Barnes, E., and Weiner, N. (1974). Release of norepinephrine and dopamine-β-hydroxylase by nerve stimulation. II. Effects of papaverine. *J. Pharmacol. Exper. Ther.* **191**, 444-457.

Cubeddu, L., Barnes, E., and Weiner, N. (1975). Release of norepinephrine and dopamine hydroxylase by nerve stimulation. IV. An evaluation of a role for cyclic adenosine monophosphate. *J. Pharmacol. Exper. Ther. 193*, 105-127.

Curtis, D.R., and Davis, R. (1962). Pharmacological studies upon neurones of the lateral geniculate nucleus of the cat. *Brit. J. Pharmacol.* **18**, 217-246.

Daly, J.W. (1975). Cyclic adenosine 3',5'-monophosphate role in the physiology and pharmacology of the central nervous system. *Biochem. Pharmacol.* **24**, 159-164.

De Belleroche, J.S., Das, I., and Bradford, H.F. (1974). Absence of an effect of histamine, noradrenaline and depolarizing agents on levels of adenosine-3',5'-monophosphate in nerve endings isolated from cerebral cortex. *Biochem. Pharmacol.* **23**, 835-843.

Dismukes, R.K., and Daly, J.W. (1976a). Altered brain cyclic AMP responses in rats reared in enriched or impoverished environments. *Experientia* **32**, 730-731.

Dismukes, R.K., and Daly, J.W. (1976b). Adaptive responses of brain cyclic AMP-generating systems to alterations in synaptic input. *J. Cyclic Nucleotide Res.* **2**, 321-336.

Dismukes, R.K., and Mulder, A.H. (1976). cyclic AMP and α-receptor-mediated modulation of noradrenaline release from rat brain slices. *Eur. J. Pharmacol.* **39**, 383-388.

Dismukes, K., and Snyder, S.H. (1974a). Dynamics of brain histamine. *Advan. Neurol.* **5**, 101-109.

Dismukes, K., and Snyder, S.H. (1974b). Histamine turnover in rat brain. *Brain Res.* **78**, 467-481.

Dismukes, K., Kuhar, M.J., and Snyder, S.H. (1974). Brain histamine alterations after hypothalamic isolation. *Brain Res.* **78**, 144-151.

Dismukes, R.K., Ghosh, P., Creveling, C.R., and Daly, J.W. (1975). Altered responsiveness of adenosine 3',5'-monophosphate-generating systems in rat cortical slices after lesions of the medial forebrain bundle. *Exp. Neurol.* **49**, 725-735.

Dismukes, R.K., Ghosh, P., Creveling, C.R., and Daly, J.W. (1976a). Norepinephrine depletion and responsiveness of nroepinephrine-sensitive cortical cyclic AMP-generating systems in guinea pig. *Exp. Neurol.* **52**, 206-215.

Dismukes, K., Rogers, M., and Daly, J.W. (1976b). Cyclic adenosine 3',5'-monophosphate formation in guinea pig brain slices: effect of H_1- and H_2-histaminergic agonists. *J. Neurochem.* **26**, 785-790.

DuMoulin, A., and Schultz, J. (1975). Effect of some phosphodiesterase inhibitors on two different preparations of adenosine 3',5'-monophosphate phosphodiesterase. *Experientia* **31**, 883-884.

Fdwards, C., Nahorski, S.R., and Rogers, K.J. (1974). *In vivo* changes in cerebral cyclic adenosine 3',5'-monophosphate induced by biogenic amines: association with phosphorylase activation. *J. Neurochem.* **22**, 565-572.

Feldberg, W., and Sherwood, S.L. (1954). Injections of drugs into the lateral ventricle of the cat. *J. Physiol.* **123**, 148–167.

Ferrendelli, J.A., Kinscherf, D.A., and Chang, M-M. (1975). Comparison of the effects of biogenic amines of cyclic GMP and cyclic AMP levels in mouse cerebellum *in vitro*. *Brain Res.* **84**, 63–73.

Finch, L., and Hicks, P.E. (1976). No evidence for central histamine involvement with the hypotensive effect of clonidine in cats. *Eur. J. Pharmacol.* **40**, 365–368.

Forn, J., and Krishna, G. (1971). Effect of norepinephrine, histamine, and other drugs on cyclic 3',5'-AMP formation in brain slices of various animal species. *Pharmacology* **5**, 193–204.

Fredholm, B.B., Fuxe, K., and Agnati, L. (1976). Effect of some phosphodiesterase inhibitiors on central dopamine mechanisms. *Eur. J. Pharmacol.* **38**, 31–38.

Fumagalli, R., Bernareggi, V., Berti, F., and Trabucchi, M. (1971). Cyclic AMP formation in human brain: an *in vitro* stimulation by neurotransmitters. *Life Sci.* **10(I)**, 1111–1115.

Gale, K., Giudotti, A., and Costa, E. (1977). Dopamine-sensitive adenylate cyclase: location in substantia nigra. *Science* **195**, 503–505.

Galindo, A., Krnjevic, K., and Schwartz, S. (1967). Micro-iontophoretic studies on neurones in the cuneate nucleus. *J. Physiol.* **192**, 359–377.

Garbarg, M., Barbin, G., Ferger, J., and Schwartz, J.C. (1974). Histaminergic pathway in rat brain evidenced by lesions of the medial forebrain bundle. *Science* **186**, 833–835.

Gerald, M.C., and Maickel, R.P. (1972). Studies on the possible role of brain histamine in behaviour. *Brit. J. Pharmacol.* **44**, 462–471.

Green, J.P. (1970). Histamine in "Handbook of Neurochemistry" (A. Lajtha, ed.), Vol. 4, pp. 221–250.

Green, M.D., Cox, B., and Lomax, P. (1976). Sites and mechanisms of action of histamine in the central thermoregulatory pathways of the rat. *Neurophramacology* **15**, 321–324.

Haas, H.L. (1974). Histamine: action on single hypothalamic neurones. *Brain Res.* **76**, 363–366.

Haas, H.L., and Bucher, U.M. (1975). Histamine H_2-receptors on single central neurones. *Nature (London)* **255**, 634–635.

Haas, H.L., Anderson, E.G., and Hosli, L. (1973). Histamine and metabolites: their effect and interactions with convulsants on brain stem neurones. *Brain Res.* **51**, 269–278.

Haas, H.L., Wolf, P., and Nussbaumer, J.C. (1975). Histamine: action on supraoptic and other hypothalamic neurones of the cat. *Brain Res.* **88**, 166–170.

Hegstrand, L.R., Kanof, P.D., and Greengard, P. (1976). Histamine-sensitive adenylate cyclase in mammalian brain. *Nature (London)* **260**, 163–164.

Horn, A.S., and Phillipson, O.T. (1976). A noradrenaline-sensitive adenylate cyclase in the rat limbic forebrain; Preparation, properties, and effects of agonists, adrenolytics, and neuroleptic drugs. *Eur. J. Pharmacol.* **37**, 1–111.

Hosli, L., and Haas, H.L. (1971). Effects of histamine, histidine, and imidazole acetic acid on neurones of the medulla oblongata of the cat. *Experientia* **27**, 1311–1312.

Huang, M., and Daly, J.W. (1972). Accumulation of cyclic adenosine monophosphate in incubated slices of brain tissue. 1. Structure–activity relationships of agonists and antagonists of biogenic amines and of tricyclic tranquilizers and antidepressants. *J. Med. Chem.* **15**, 458–462.

Huang, M., and Daly, J.W. (1974). Adenosine-elicited accumulation of cyclic AMP in brain slices: potentiation by agents which inhibit uptake of adenosine. *Life Sci.* **14**, 489–503.

Huang, M., Shimizu, H., and Daly, J. (1971). Regulation of adenosine cyclic 3',5'-phosphate formation in cerebral cortical slices: interaction among norepinephrine, histamine, and serotonin. *Mol. Pharmacol.* **7**, 155–162.

Joo, F., Rakonczay, A., and Wollenmann, M. (1975). cAMP-mediated regulation of the permeability in the brain capillaries. *Experientia* **3**, 582–583.

Kakiuchi, S., and Rall, T. W. (1964a). Studies on adenosine 3',5'-phosphate in rabbit cerebral cortex. *Mol. Pharmacol.* **4**, 379–388.

Kakiuchi, S., and Rall, T.W. (1968b). The influence of chemical agents on the accumulation of adenosine 3'5'-phosphate in slices of rabbit cerebellum. *Mol. Pharmacol.* **4**, 367–378.

Karppanen, H., Paakkari, I., Paakkari, P., Huotari, R., and Orma, A-L. (1976). Possible involvement of central histamine H_2-receptors in the hypotensive effect of clonidine. *Nature (London)* **259**, 587–588.

Kataoka, K., and DeRobertis, E. (1967). Histmaine in isolated small nerve endings and synaptic vesicles of rat brain cortex. *J. Pharmacol. Exper. Ther.* **156**, 114–125.

Kebabian, J.W., and Saavedra, J.M. (1976). Dopamine-sensitive adenylate cyclase occurs in a region of the substantia nigra containing dopaminergic dendrites. *Science* **193**, 683–000.

Korf, J., Bower, P.H., and Fekkes, D. (1976). Release of cerebral cyclic AMP into push–pull perfusates in freely moving rats. *Brain Res.* **113**, 551–562.

Kodama, T., Matsukado, Y., and Shimizu, H. (1973). The cyclic AMP system of human brain. *Brain Res.* **50**, 135–146.

Krishna, G., Forn, J., Voight, K., Paul, M., and Gessa, G.L. (1970). Dynamic aspects of neurohormonal control of cyclic 3',5'-AMP synthesis in brain. *Advan. Biochem. Psychopharmacol.* **3**, 155–172.

Krishnamoorthy, M.S., Garbarg, M., Feger, J., and Schwartz, J.C. (1973). Augmentation in hypothalamic histamine induced by diencephalic lesions in rats. *Agents Actions* **3**, 181–182.

Krnjevic, K., and Phillis, J.W. (1963). Actions of certain amines on cerebral cortical neurones. *Brit. J. Pharmacol.* **20**, 471–490.

Kuhar, M.J., Taylor, K.M., and Snyder, S.H. (1971). The subcellular localization of histamine and histamine methyltransferase in rat brain. *J. Neurochem.* **18**, 1515–1527.

Kunos, G., Mucci, L., and Jaeger, V. (1976). Interconconversion of myocardial adrenoceptors: its relationship to adenylate cyclase activation. *Life Sci.* **19**, 1597–1602.

Leibowitz, S., (1973). Histamine: a stimulatory effect on drinking behavior in the rat. *Brain Res.* **63**, 440–444.

Mah, H.D., and Daly, J.W. (1976). Adenosine-dependent formation of cyclic AMP in brain slice. *Pharmacol. Res. Commun.* **8**, 65–79.

Martres, M.P., Baudry, M., and Schwartz, J.C. (1975). Histamine synthesis in the developing rat brain: evidence for a multiple compartmentation. *Brain Res.* **83**, 261–275.

McIlwain, H. (1972). Regulatory significance of the release and action of adenine derivatives in cerebral systems. *Biochem. Soc. Symp.* **36**, 69–85.

Monnier, M., and Hatt, A.M. (1969). Afferent and central activating effects of histamine in brain. *Experientia* **25**, 1297–1298.

Monnier, M., Sauer, R., and Hatt, A.M. (1970). The activating effect of histamine on the central nervous system. *Internat. Rev. Neurobiol.* **12**, 265–305.

Nahorski, S.R., and Rogers, K.J. (1976). Inhibition of 3',5'-nucleotide phosphodiesterase and the stimulation of cerebral cyclic AMP formation by biogenic amines *in vitro* and *in vivo*. *Neuropharmacology* **15**, 609–612.

Nahorski, S.R., Rogers, K.J., and Smith, B.M. (1974). Histamine H_2-receptors and cyclic AMP in brain. *Life Sci.* **15**, 1887–1894.

Palmer, G.C. (1973). Adenyl cyclase in neuronal and glial-enriched fractions from rat and rabbit brain. *Res. Commun. Chem. Pathol. Pharmacol.* **5**, 603–613.

Palmer, G.C., Schmidt, M.J., and Robison, G.A. (1972). Development and characteristics of the histamine-induced accumulation of cyclic AMP in the rabbit cerebral cortex. *J. Neurochem.* **19**, 2251–2256.

Palmer, G.C., Sulser, F., and Robison, G.A. (1973). Effects of neurohumoral and adrenergic agents on cyclic AMP levels in various areas of the rat brain *in vitro*. *Neuropharmacology* **12**, 327–337.

Phillis, J.W., Tebecis, A.K., and York, D.H. (1968a). Depression of spinal motoneurones by noradrenaline, 5-hydroxytryptamine and histamine. *Eur. J. Pharmacol.* **4**, 471–475.

Phillis, J.W., Tebecis, A.K., and York, D.H. (1968b). Histamine and some antihistamines: their actions on cerebral cortical neurones. *Brit. J. Pharmacol.* **33**, 426–440.

Phillis, J.W., Kostopoulos, G.K., and Odutala, A. (1975). On the specificity of histamine H_2-receptor antagonists in the rat cerebral cortex. *Can. J. Physiol. Pharmacol.* **53**, 1205–1208.

Pollard, H., Bischoff, S., and Schwartz, J.C. (1973a). Decreased histamine synthesis in the rat brain by hypnotics and anaesthetics. *J. Pharm. Pharmacol.* **25**, 920–921.

Pollard, H., Bischoff, S., and Schwartz, J.C. (1973b). Increased synthesis and release of ^{3}H-histamine in rat brain by reserpine. *Eur. J. Pharmacol.* **24**, 399–401.

Pollard, H., Bischoff, S., and Schwartz, J.C. (1974). Turnover of histamine in rat brain and its decrease under barbiturate anaesthesia. *J. Pharmacol. Exper. Ther.* **190**, 88–99.

Premont, J., Thierry, A.M., Tassin, J.P., Glowinski, J., Blanc, G., and Bockaert, J. (1976). Is the dopamine sensitive adenylate cyclase in the rat substantia nigra coupled with 'autoreceptors'? *FEBS Letters* **68**, 99–104.

Robinson, J..D., Anderson, J.H., and Green, J.P. (1965). The uptake of 5-hydroxytryptamine and histamine by particulate fractions of brain. *J. Pharmacol. Exper. Ther.* **147**, 236–243.

Rogers, M., Dismukes, K., and Daly, J.W. (1975). Histamine-elicited accumulations of cyclic adenosine 3',5'-monophosphate in guinea pig brain slices: effect of H_1- and H_2-antagonists. *J. Neurochem.* **25**, 531–534.

Salomon, Y., Londos, C., and Rodbell, M. (1974). A highly sensitive adenylate cyclase assay. *Anal. Biochem.* **58**, 541–548.

Sastry, B..S.R., and Phillis, J.W. (1976a). Depression of rat cerebral cortical neurones by H_1 and H_2 histamine receptor agonists. *Eur. J. Pharmacol.* **38**, 269–273.

Sastry, B.S.R., and Phillis, J.W. (1976b). Evidence for an ascending inhibitory histaminergic pathway to the cerebral cortex. *Can. J. Physiol. pharmacol.* **54**, 782–786.

Sato, A., Onaya, T., Kotani, H., Harada, A., and Yamada, T. (1974). Effects of biogenic amines on the formation of adenosine 3',5'-monophosphate in porcine cerebral cortex, hypothalamus, and anterior pituitary slices. *Endocrinology* **94**, 1311–1318.

Sattin, A., and Rall, T.W. (1970). The effect of adenosine and adenine nucleotides on the cyclic adenosine 3',5'-phosphate content of guinea pig cerebral cortex slices. *Mol. Pharmacol.* **6**, 13–23.

Sattin, A., Rall, T.W., and Zanella, J. (1975). Regulation of cyclic adenosine 3',5'monophosphate levels in guinea-pig cerebral cortex by interaction of alpha adrenergic and adenosine receptor activity. *J. Pharmacol. Exper. Ther.* **192**, 22–32.

Sawyer, C.H. (1955). Rhinencephalic involvement in pituitary activaiton by intraventricular histamine in the rabbit under nembutal anesthesia. *Am. J. Physiol.* **180**, 37–46.

Schayer, R.W., and Reilly, M.A. (1973). Effect of psychoactive drugs in *in vivo* metabolism of ^{14}C-histamine in mouse brian. *Archives Internat. Pharmacodyn. Therapie* **203**, 123–129.

Schultz, J., and Daly, J.W. (1973a). Adenosine 3',5'-monophosphate in guinea pig cerebral cortical slices; Effects of α- and β-adrenergic agents, histamine, serotonin, and adenosine. *J. Neurochem.* **21**, 573–579.

Schultz, J., and Daly, J.W. (1973b). Accumulation of cyclic adenosine 3',5'-monophosphate in cerebral cortical slices from rat and mouse stimulatory effects of α- and β-adrenergic agents and adenosine. *J. Neurochem.* **21**, 1319–1326.

Schultz, J., and Daly, J.W. (1973c). Cyclic adenosine 3',5'-monophosphate in guinea pig cerebral cortical slices. I. Formation of cyclic adenosine 3',5'-monophosphate from endogenous adenosine triphosphate and from radioactive adenosine triphosphate formed during a prior incubation with radioactive adenine. *J. Biol. Chem.* **248**, 843–852.

Schwabe, U., and Daly, J.W. (1977). The role of calcium ions in accumulations of cyclic AMP elicited by α- and β-adrenergic agonists in rat brain slices. *J. Pharmacol. Exper. Ther.* **202**, 134–143.

Schwabe, U., Miyake, M., Ohga, Y., and Daly, J.W. (1976). 4-(3-Cyclopentyloxy-4-methoxyphenyl)-2-pyrrolidone(ZK 62711): a potent inhibitor of cyclic AMP-phosphodiesterases in homogenates and tissue slices from rat brain. *Mol. pharmacol.* **12**, 900–910.

Schwabe, U., Ohga, Y., and Daly, J.W. (1978). The role of calcium in the regulation of cyclic nucleotide levels in brain slices of rat and guinea pig. *Naunyn-Schmiedebergs Arch. Pharmacol.* **302**, 141–151.

Schwartz, J-C. (1975). Histamine as a transmitter in brain. *Life Sci.* **17**, 503–518.

Schwartz, J.C., Lampart, C., and Rose, C. (1970). Properties and regional distribution of histidine decarboxylase in rat brain. *J. Neurochem.* **17**, 1527–1534.

Schwartz, J-C., Barbin, G., Garbarg, M., Pollard, W., Rose, C., and Verdiere, M. (1976). Neurochemical evidence for histamine acting as a transmitter in mammalian brain. *Advan. Biochemical Pharmacol.* **15**, 111–126.

Shaw, G.G. (1971). Hypothermia produced in mice by histamine acting on the central nervous system. *Brit. J. Pharmacol.* **20**, 1279–1283.

Shimizu, H., and Okayama, H. (1973). An ATP pool associated with adenyl cyclase of brain tissue. *J. Neurochem.* **20**, 1279–1283.

Shimizu, H., Daly, J.W., and Creveling, C.R. (1969). A radioisotopic method for measuring the formation of adenosine 3′,5′-cyclic monophosphate in incubated slices of brain. *J. Neurochem.* **16**, 1609–1619.

Shimizu, H., Creveling, C.R., and Daly, J. (1970a). Stimulated formation of adenosine 3′,5′-cyclic phosphate in cerebral cortex: Synergism between electrical activity and biogenic amines. *Proc. Nat. Acad. Sci. USA* **65**, 1033–1040.

Shimizu, H., Creveling, C.R., and Daly, J.W. (1970b). The effect of histamines and other compounds on the formation of adenosine 3′,5′-monophosphate in slices from cerebral cortex. *J. Neurochem.* **17**, 441–444.

Shimizu, H., Tanaka, S., Suzuki, T., and Matsukado, Y. (1971). The response of human cerebrum adenyl cyclase to biogenic amines. *J. Neurochem.* **18**, 1157–1161.

Shimizu, H., Ichishita, H., and Miaokami, Y. (1975). Stimulation of the cee-free adenylate cyclase from guinea pig cerebral cortex by acidic amino acids and vertridine. *J. Cyclic Nucleotide Res.* **1**, 61–67.

Siggins, G.R., Hoffer, B.J., and Bloom, F.E. (1971). Studies on norepinephrine-containing afferents to Purkinje cells of rat cerebellum. III. Evidence for mediation of norepinephrine effects by cyclic 3′,5′-adenosine monophosphate. *Brain Res.* **25**, 535–553.

Siggins, G.R., Battenberg, E.F., Hoffer, B.J., and Bloom, F.E. (1973). Noradrenergic stimulation of cyclic adenosine monophosphate in rat Purkinje neurons: an immunocytochemical study. *Science* **179**, 585–588.

Skolnick, P., and Daly, J.W. (1975a). Functional compartments of adenine nucleotides serving as precursors of adenosine 3′,5′-monophosphate in mouse cerebral cortex. *J. Neurochem.* **24**, 451–456.

Skolnick, P., and Daly, J.W. (1975b). Stimulation of adenosine 3′,5′-monophosphate formation in rat cerebral cortical slices by methoxamine: interaction with an alpha-adrenergic receptor. *J. Pharmacol. Exper. Ther.* **193**, 549–588.

Skolnick, P., Huang, M., Daly, J., and Hoffer, B. (1973). Accumulation of adenosine 3′,5′-monophosphate in incubated slices from discrete regions of squirrel monkey cerebral cortex: effect of norepinephrine, serotonin, and adenosine. *J. Neurochem.* **21**, 237–240.

Snyder, S.H., and Taylor, K.M. (1972). Histamine in the brain: a neurotransmitter? in "Perspectives in Neuropharmacology" (S.H. Snyder, ed.) pp. 43–73. Oxford Univ. Press, London.

Snyder, S.H., Glowinski, J., and Axelrod, J. (1966). The physiologic disposition of ^{3}H-histamine in rat brain. *J. Pharmacol. Exper. Ther.* **153**, 8–14.

Snyder, S.H., Brown, B., and Kuhar, M.J. (1974). The subsynaptosomal localization of histamine, histidine decarboxylase and histamine methyltransferase in rat hypothalamus. *J. Neurochem.* **23**, 37–46.

Spiker, M.D., Palmer, G.C., and Manian, A.A. (1976). Action of neuroleptic agents on histamine-sensitive adenylate cyclase in rabbit cerebral cortex. *Brain Res.* **104**, 401–406.

Taylor, K.M., and Snyder, S.H. (1971a). Histamine in rat brain: sensitive assay of endogenous levels, formation *in vivo* and lowering by inhibitors of histidine decarboxylase. *J. Pharmacol. Exper. Ther.* **173**, 619–633.

Taylor, K.M., and Snyder, S.H. (1971b). Brain histamine: rapid apparent turnover altered by restraint and cold stress. *Science,* 1037–1939.

Taylor, K.M., and Snyder, S.H. (1972). Dynamics of the regulation of histamine levels in mouse brain. *J. Neurochem.* **19**, 341–354.

Taylor, K.M., and Snyder, S.H. (1973). The release of histamine from tissue slices of rat hypothalamus. *J. Neurochem.* **21**, 1215–1223.

Tuomisto, L., Tuomisto, J., and Walaszek, E.J. (1975). Uptake of histamine by rabbit hypothalamic slices. *Medical Biology* **53**, 40–46.

Verdiere, M., Rose, C., and Schwartz, J.C. (1975). Synthesis and release of histamine studied on slices of rat hypothalamus. *Eur. J. Pharmacol.* **34**, 157–168.

Von Hungen, K., and Roberts, S. (1973a). Adenylate-cyclase receptors for adrenergic neurotransmitters in rat cerebral cortex. *Eur. J. Biochem.* **36**, 391–401.

Von Hungen, K., and Roberts, S. (1973b). Catecholamine and Ca^{2+} activation of adenylate cyclase systems in synaptosomal fractions from rat cerebral cortex. *Nature (London) New Biol.* **242**, 58–60.

Weckowicz, T.E., and Hall, R. (1957). Skin histamine test in schizophrenia. *J. Nervous Mental Disease* **125**, 452–458.

Weinryb, I., and Michel, I.M. (1976). Amine-responsive adenylate cyclase activity from brain. Comparisons between rat and rhesus monkey and demosntration of dopamine-stimulated adenylate cyclase in monkey neocortex. *Psychopharmacol. Commun.* **2**, 27–38.

White, T. (1961). Some effects of histamine and two histamine metabolites on the cat's brain. *J. Physiol.* **159**, 198–202.

Williams, M. (1976). Protein phosphorylation in rat striatal slices: effects of noradrenaline, dopamine and other putative transmitters. *Brain Res.* **109**, 190–195.

Williams, M., Pavlik, A., and Rodnight, R. (1974). Cellular localization of phosphoproteins in guinea pig cerebral cortex slices sensitive to noreadrenaline, histamine, and 5-hydroxtryptamine. *Trans. Biochem. Soc.* **2**, 259–261.

Wolf, P., and Monnier, M. (1973). Electroencephalographic, behavioral, and visceral effect so intraventricular infusion of histamine in the rabbit. *Agents Actions* **3**, 196.

19

Histamine Receptors and Cyclic Nucleotides in Adipose Tissue

Vernon R. Grund
Department of Biochemical Pharmacology
School of Pharmacy
State University of New York
Buffalo, New York

Donald B. Hunninghake
Department of Pharmacology
School of Medicine
University of Minnesota
Minneapolis, Minnesota

The influence of histamine on lipid mobilization was characterized by examining the influence of H_1, H_2, and β blockers on histamine induced free fatty acid release in humans and dogs *in vivo* and by examining the effects of histamine on lipolysis and cyclic nucleotide levels in isolated rat and dog fat cells *in vitro*. Histamine was found to have a potent lipid mobilizing effect in both humans and dogs. In dogs, the effect was entirely abolished by pretreatment with metiamide but was not inhibited by propranolol. In humans, the effect was abolished by pretreatment with propranolol. H_2 blockers were not investigated in man. In both species the lipid-mobilizing effect of histamine was potentiated by the administration of diphenhydramine, an H_1 blocker. In isolated canine fat cells, histamine stimulated lipolysis by elevating the intracellular levels of adenosine 3',5'-monophosphate (cAMP). The effect of histamine to elevate cAMP levels and cause FFA release in isolated canine fat cells was specifically inhibited by cimetidine, metiamide, or burimamide indicating the involvement of H_2 receptors. In isolated rat fat cells histamine was an inhibitor of hormone-stimulated lipolysis and cAMP accumulation. This effect was overcome by the administration of H_2 antagonists, by producing high extracellular calcium concentrations, or by lanthanum administration, suggesting a role of calcium and H_2 receptors. The influence of histamine on cGMP levels in isolated fat cells is currently under investigation. These studies reveal that histamine is an important regulator of lipid mobilization and that histamine receptors, cAMP, and calcium have definite roles in determining the ultimate effect of histamine on lipid mobilization once histamine is released into the bloodstream.

It has recently been discovered that histamine H_2 receptors are present in canine adipose tissue and that the interaction of histamine with this receptor causes an elevation of adenosine 3',5'-monophosphate levels within the fat cell resulting in the hydrolysis of fat cell triglycerides to free fatty acids and glycerol (Grund *et al.*, 1975). It was also demonstrated that histamine, infused

325

intravenously, causes an abrupt elevation in serum free fatty acid and glycerol levels in man (Grund *et al.*, 1976). The purpose of the present report will be (1) to review the mechanisms by which histamine can regulate lipid mobilization in rats, dogs, and humans, (2) to present data which suggests that both H_1 and H_2 receptors may be involved in the regulation of lipid mobilization, and (3) to discuss the clinical implications of histamine's lipid-mobilizing effects in man.

CYCLIC NUCLEOTIDES AND LIPID MOBILIZATION

Lipid mobilization is the process by which fat cell triglycerides are enzymatically converted into smaller molecular weight lipids (free fatty acids and glycerol) which can pass freely out of the fat cell and into the circulation. Free fatty acids (FFA) are considered to be the major byproduct of lipid mobilization because they can be utilized for energy by muscles, re-esterified into triglycerides in adipose tissue, or converted into cholesterol, triglycerides, and lipoproteins by the liver (Steinberg, 1967). A possible pathologic consequence of excessive lipid mobilization is an increased output of low-density lipoproteins by the liver, a phenomenon often associated with the pathogenesis of atherosclerosis (Strong and Eggen, 1970; Kannel *et al.*, 1971; U.S. DHEW, 1971).

Hormones play a critical role in the control of lipid mobilization by regulating the activity of adipose tissue triglyceride lipase, the rate limiting enzyme in the lipid mobilization process. This enzyme is activated by epinephrine, norepinephrine, and other "lipolytic" hormones but cannot be activated by these hormones in the presence of insulin, prostaglandin E_1, nicotinic acid, or other "antilipolytic" substances (Vaughan *et al.*, 1964; Steinberg, 1966; Fain, 1973).

The discovery that lipolytic hormones activated triglyeride lipase by elevating the intracellular levels of adenosine 3',5'-monophosphate (cAMP) represented a major contribution towards the development of the "second messenger concept" of hormone action proposed by Sutherland and co-workers in the late 1960's (Butcher and Sutherland, 1967; Sutherland *et al.*, 1968). According to the second messenger concept the hormone, as first messenger, interacts with a specific receptor on the fat cell membrane and induces the formation of the second messenger (cAMP) by activating the enzyme, adenylate cylase, within the membrane (Butcher *et al.*, 1965; Birnbaumer and Rodbell, 1969; Butcher, 1971). The increased intracellular levels of cAMP lead to the activation of a protein kinase within the cell which in turn activates the triglyceride lipase and initiates the lipid mobilization process (Corbin and Krebs, 1969; Corbin *et al.*, 1970, 1973).

The mechanism by which insulin and other antilipolytic hormones prevent the elevation of fat cell cAMP, thus, preventing the activation of triglyceride lipase, remains a mystery. Evidence has been presented in support of insulin as an inhibitor of adenylate cyclase (Illiano and Cuatrecasas, 1972) and as an activator of cAMP phosphodiesterase (Manganiello and Vaughan, 1973; Kono et al., 1975), but the mechanisms by which these actions might be effected in the intact cell have not been explained.

Goldberg and co-workers have suggested that an elevation of intracellular guanosine 3',5'-monophosphate (cGMP) levels by the activation of guanylate cyclase might trigger biological events which oppose those events mediated by AMP (Goldberg et al., 1975). In isolated rat fat cells, Cuatrecases and co-workers have demonstrated that insulin is capable of elevating cGMP levels (Illinao et al., 1973); but some claim that the effect of insulin to elevate cGMP levels in fat cells is not associated with the inhibition of lipolysis (Fain and Butcher, 1976). Still others believe that the mechanism of action of insulin and other antilipolytic agents may best be explained by an effect on calcium mobilization (Fassina and Contessa, 1967; Hope-Gill et al., 1974, 1975; Siddle and Hales, 1975; McDonald et al., 1976). Calcium appears to play an important role in the regulation of adenylate cyclase, guanylate cyclase, phosphodiesterase, and triglyceride lipase but, as yet, no one has clarified this role or demonstrated a sequence of events linking insulin administration to changes in calcium flux and cyclic nucleotide levels in the isolated fat cell (Kakiuchi et al., 1975; Kissebah et al., 1974; Clyman et al., 1975; Rasmussen et al., 1975; Blume and Foster, 1976; Ferrendelli et al., 1976).

In this report it will be illustrated that histamine can have diverse effects on lipid mobilization which are dependent on species and experimental design (in vivo vs. in vitro). Each effect will be discussed in detail in regards to the possible mode and site of action with emphasis on the involvement of cAMP, cGMP, and calcium.

HISTAMINE AS A REGULATOR OF LIPID MOBILIZATION

The first indication that histamine might have a role in the regulation of lipid mobilization came when Fredholm and co-workers (1968; Fredholm and Frisk-Holmberg, 1971) observed that injections of histamine or agents capable of releasing endogenous histamine prompted the release of FFA and glycerol from perfused subcutaneous adipose tissue of dogs. This effect was later confirmed by a study in our laboratory which indicated that histamine was capable of inducing lipid mobilization, not only in dogs, but also in man. A comparison of the lipid mobilizing effect of histamine in humans and dogs was made by infusing identical amounts of histamine (11 μg/minute iv) over a 15 minute period and analyzing the serum for changes in FFA levels before, during and after the infusion (Fig. 1). The remarkable similarity in responses suggested to us that histamine had a definite role as a regulator of lipid mobilization in man.

Other evidence was accumulating which supported the theory that histamine had a role in the regulation of lipid mobilization. First, histamine containing mast cells were found to be abundant in mammalian adipose tissue (Stock and Westermann, 1963; Sheldon, 1965; Bieck et al., 1967; Fredholm and Frisk-Holmberg, 1971). Second, it had been known for some time that mast cell histamine was stored and released in a complex with heparin, a known activator of lipoprotein lipase (Kahlson and Rosengren, 1968). Third, stress, which is generally associated with dramatic lipid mobilizing effects in man (Cardon and Gordon, 1959; Bogdonoff and Nichols, 1965), is a well

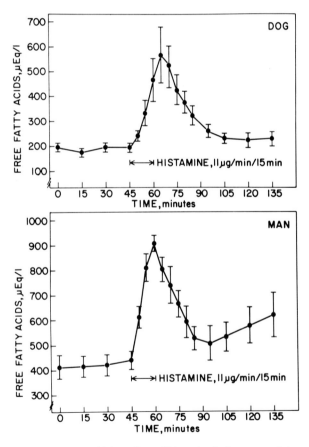

FIG. 1.   Lipid mobilizing effect of histamine in humans and dogs.

known stimulator of histamine release (Dekanski, 1945; Nasmyth, 1955; Johnson and Moran, 1969; Taylor and Snyder, 1971; Maslinski, 1975). Finally, histamine was found to be capable of elevating cAMP levels in a variety of tissues including brain (Kakiuchi and Rall, 1968), lung (Palmer, 1971), leukocytes (Bourne et al., 1971), heart (McNeill and Muschek, 1972), and gastric mucosa (Domschke et al., 1973). The ability of histamine to elevate intracellular cAMP levels was especially significant because of the well established role of cAMP as an intracellular mediator of the lipolytic response to epinephrine, glucagon, and adrenocorticotropin in isolated rat fat cells (Butcher et al., 1965, 1968).

THE ISOLATED CANINE FAT CELL MODEL

In order to study the mechanism of histamine-induced lipid mobilization, an appropriate *in vitro* model had to be established. The isolated rat fat cell model (Rodbell, 1964) had earlier been used to characterize the lipolytic response to epinephrine, norepinephrine (NE), glucagon, and adrenocorticotropin (ACTH), but this model was rejected due to the fact that rat fat cells were unresponsive to histamine. An isolated canine fat cell preparation was then developed according to a modification of Rodbell's procedure and found to be quite responsive to histamine (Fig. 2). An additional reason for choosing this model is the similarity in responsiveness of human and canine adipose tissue to lipolytic substances. Human and dog adipose tissue both respond to the lipolytic influence of catecholamines but neither species responds to glucagon and ACTH (Rudman et al., 1963; Altzuler et al., 1971; Burns et al., 1971).

The isolated canine fat cell preparation was prepared as follows: Subcutaneous adipose tissue was surgically removed from the inguinal region of the male mongrel dogs that had been anesthetized with sodium pentobarbital. The tissue was cut into small pieces and incubated at 37.5° C for 1 hour in 5 ml of Krebs–Ringer (bicarbonate or phosphate) buffer (pH 7.4) containing 1.3 mM calcium, 0.1% glucose, 2–4% bovine serum albumin, and 1.5 mg of crude collagenase (Worthington Biochemical Corp.). After the collagenase digestion, the cells were filtered in gauze and centrifuged at 400 rpm for 1 minute to float the fat cells. The infranatant liquid containing mast cells, blood cells, and other debris was removed by aspiration. The cells were then washed 3 times and resuspended in warm buffer (without collagenase) after a final filtration through 180 micron nylon mesh. Flasks containing 5 ml of the isolated fat cell suspension (approximately 200,000 cells/ml) were preincubated for 10–30 minutes prior to the addition of histamine or other lipolytic stimulators. Blocking agents, when used, were contained in the media. All incubations were conducted for specified periods at 37.5°C in a Dubnoff metabolic shaker. At the end of the incubation, FFA levels were

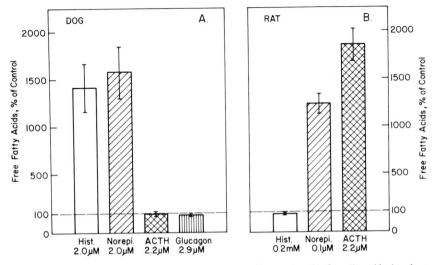

FIG. 2.   A comparison of the lipolytic responsiveness of isolated canine fat cells and isolated rat fat cells to histamine and other hormones. Fat cells were incubated for 2 hours in the presence of each substance.

determined colorimetrically by the method of Duncombe (1963) as modified by Itaya and Ui (1965). Cyclic AMP levels were determined by a modification of the protein binding method of Gilman (1970) following deproteinization of the fat cell suspension with acetone and washes with ether to remove lipids. Burimamide, metiamide, and cimetidine were supplied by Smith Kline and French Laboratories Ltd. and insulin was supplied by Eli Lilly and Company.

Role of H_2 Receptors and Cyclic AMP

In order to characterize the lipolytic effect of histamine in isolated canine fat cells we began by asking the two most obvious questions: (1) Is cAMP involved? and (2) Is a specific histamine receptor involved? The approach which was used was similar to the approach used by Butcher (1971) to establish that cAMP was involved in the lipolytic action of epinephrine in isolated rat fat cells. According to Butcher, if cAMP is involved in the lipolytic action of a hormone, then a particular set of criteria could be used to establish it. First, the effect of the hormone on FFA release should be preceded by a rise in the levels of cAMP. Second, the effect of the hormone on cAMP levels and FFA accumulation should be closely correlated over the entire dose range of the hormone used in the experiment. Third, the action of the hormone on both FFA accumulation and cAMP increases should be markedly potentiated in the presence of phosphodiesterase inhibitors which prevent the degradation of cAMP. Fourth, the action of the hormone on lipolysis should be mimicked by the administration of an exogenous cAMP derivative (N^6-2'-0-dibutyryl cAMP) assuming that this derivative could penetrate the fat cell membrane. Finally, and perhaps most important, if the lipolytic action of a substance is mediated by cAMP, then blocking agents which specifically reverse the effect of the agent on FFA accumulation should also reverse the effect on cAMP accumulation.

The time-course of histamine effects on FFA release and cAMP accumulation in isolated canine fat cells is presented in Fig. 3. The levels of cAMP began to rise immediately after the administration of histamine (1.7 μM) and peaked within 2–5 minutes. Increases in FFA levels were first detected 5 minutes after the addition of histamine but these levels continued to rise for at least 2 hours. By the end of a 60-minute incubation the FFA levels had increased nearly 700%. Cyclic AMP levels, on the other hand, only increased 80–100% and then rapidly diminished unless theophylline was present in the media to prevent degredation by phosphodiesterase. In the presence of theophylline (1 mM) cAMP levels could also be increased by 700% or more.

The concentration range over which histamine stimulated FFA release was 10^{-7} –10^{-5} M with an ED_{50} of 8×10^{-7} M. This was closely correlated with the rise in cAMP levels which was measured over the same range of histamine concentrations in the presence of theophylline. In addition, the effect of histamine (2 μM) to elevate FFA levels could be mimicked by the administration of N^6-2'-0-dibutyryl cyclic AMP (1 mM) or theophylline (1 mM) and could be inhibited by the administration of insulin (2.8 nM) or prostaglandin E_1 (2.8 μM).

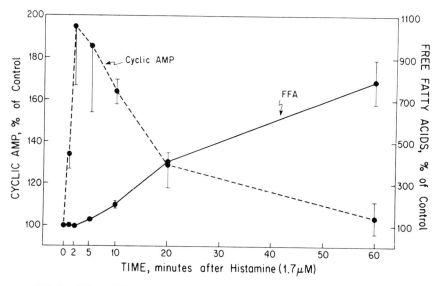

FIG. 3. Effect of histamine on cAMP and FFA levels in isolated canine fat cells.

Evidence that specific histamine-receptor blockade could prevent both the lipolytic response to histamine and the rise in cAMP which preceded it was the final criterion needed to establish histamine as a bona fide lipolytic hormone in the dog. Initial attempts to block these effects of histamine with classical H_1-type antihistamines proved unsuccessful. Tripelennamine, at concentrations of 10^{-4} M or less did not influence the lipolytic effect of histamine and concentrations of 5×10^{-4} M or greater, which caused a slight reduction in the histamine response, also reduced the response to NE.

The first agent found which would specifically reverse the lipolytic response to histamine was the H_2 blocker, burimamide (Grund et al., 1975). At a concentration of 10^{-5} M, burimamide cause a 60% inhibition of the lipolytic response to histamine (2 μM) but did not inhibit the effect of NE (2 μM). A higher concentration of burimamide (10^{-4} M) completely blocked the histamine response without reducing the response to NE. Burimamide proved to be equally effective at inhibiting the effect of histamine to elevate cAMP levels.

Influence of Cimetidine, Metiamide, and Histamine Agonists

More recent experiments using metiamide and cimetidine, the newer H_2 antagonists, have revealed that these two compounds are both effective and selective inhibitors of the effects of histamine on FFA release and cAMP accumulation in isolated canine fat cells. Both compounds cause shifts in histamine dose-response curves of a competitive nature and both compounds have pA_2 values near 6.2. Cimetidine is only slightly more potent than metiamide but is significantly more potent than burimamide. At a concentration of 10^{-5} M, cimetidine reversed the effects of histamine on lipolysis and cAMP accumulation by 95% or more but did not reverse the effect of NE (Fig. 4). In some experiments cimetidine displayed the ability to reduce basal (theophylline present) levels of cAMP (a characteristic shared with propranolol) but did not alter the basal rate of FFA release.

Further evidence for the involvement of H_2 receptors in the lipid mobilizing effect of histamine in canine adipose tissue is the lack of sensitivity of the tissue to stimulation by 2-methyl histamine, an H_1 agonist. The ED_{50} for histamine-stimulated lipolysis is 8×10^{-7} M but for 2-methyl histamine it is approximately 1×10^{-6} M.

Results from experiments with the isolated canine fat cell model are summarized in Fig. 5. It appears that histamine H_2 receptors are present on canine fat cell membranes and that specific interaction of histamine with this receptor causes an elevation in intracellular cAMP levels which ultimately leads to the hydrolysis of fat cell triglycerides to FFA and glycerol. These results are consistent with the observations that H_2-receptor activation causes a rise in cAMP levels in heart (Pöch et al., 1973; McNeill and Verma, 1974), gastric mucosa (Domschke et al., 1973), lymphocytes (Roszkowski et al., 1977), and brain (Hegstrand et al., 1976).

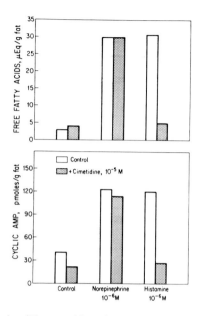

FIG. 4. Influence of cimetidine on histamine and NE induced lipolysis and cAMP accumulation in isolated canine fat cells. FFA levels were determined 1 hour after the addition of agonists and cAMP levels were determined 2 minutes after the simultaneous administration of agonists with $2 \times 10^{-4} M$ theophylline.

CANINE ADIPOCYTE

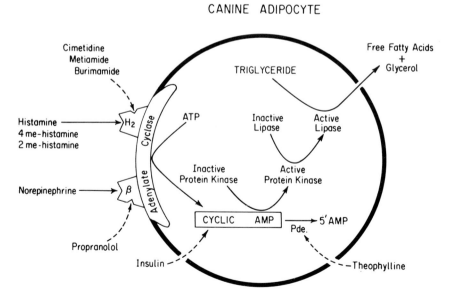

FIG. 5. Model illustrating the mechanism of histamine-induced lipid mobilization in isolated canine fat cells.

HISTAMINE-INDUCED LIPID MOBILIZATION
IN MAN

Experiments which were conducted in humans and dogs *in vivo*, (Grund *et al.*, 1976) revealed two interesting facets of histamine-induced lipid mobilization which were not evident in the isolated canine fat cell experiments. First, there is apparently more than one possible mechanism by which histamine can produce lipid mobilizing effects *in vivo*. Second, there is a distinct possibility that H_1 and H_2 receptors mediate opposing influences of histamine on lipid mobilization.

In this series of experiments the effect of identical 15-minute histamine infusions (11 μg/minute, i.v.) on serum FFA and glycerol levels was observed in humans and dogs. Dogs, in some of the experiments were pretreated with metiamide (2.2 mg/kg), diphenhydramine (2.2 mg/kg), or propranolol (0.3 mg/kg) administered intravenously over a 5-minute period beginning 10 minutes before the histamine infusion. Human subjects, in some of the experiments, were pretreated with diphenhydramine (1 mg/kg) or propranolol (75 μg/kg) in a manner similar to that used in the dog experiments. Dogs were fasted overnight then anesthetized with sodium pentobarbital for the duration of the experiment. Humans (healthy adult males) were fasted overnight and allowed to relax in a supine position for the duration of the test. Intravenous infusion catheters were inserted into each forearm (or foreleg) for the infusion of histamine or the drawing of blood samples. Tests were performed at weekly intervals. Baseline values of FFA and glycerol were determined from 4 blood samples collected at 15-minute intervals just prior to the histamine infusion. Twelve other samples were collected at specific times during and after the histamine infusion. Serum was analyzed for FFA according to the method of Duncombe (1963) as previously described, and glycerol by the enzymatic method of Garland and Randle (1962) as modified by Pinter *et al.*, (1967a).

Influence of Propranolol and Diphenhydramine

The effect of histamine on serum FFA levels in humans and dogs has already been presented (Fig. 1). A similar change in serum FFA and glycerol levels was observed in each species along with an increase in heart rate. It became evident that a major component of histamine-induced lipid mobilization in man was the result of catecholamine release since the entire effect could be blocked with propranolol. In one individual who was particularly sensitive to the lipid-mobilizing effect of histamine, there was actually a decline in FFA and glycerol levels produced by histamine in the presence of propranolol (Fig. 6). In the same individual, the lipid mobilizing effect of histamine was nearly doubled in the presence of diphenhydramine,

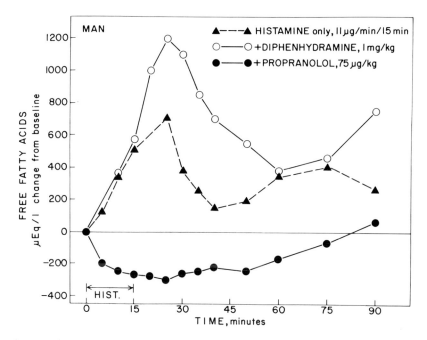

FIG. 6. Influence of diphenhydramine and propranolol on histamine-induced changes in serum FFA levels in man. These results represent 3 separate tests performed in the same individual at 2 week intervals.

an H_1 antagonist. The potentiating effect of diphenhydramine was also observed in dogs, but in this species the histamine effect was not reversed by propranolol. When diphenhydramine was used alone, it did not cause an elevation in basal FFA levels in either humans or dogs.

Influence of Metiamide

Metiamide was not available for use in human experiments but was used in the dogs. A total blockade of histamine's effect was observed in the presence of metiamide (Fig. 7) and in a few of the animals a slight, but insignificant, decrease in basal FFA levels was observed when histamine was infused in the presence of metiamide. Metiamide alone did not cause a significant change in basal FFA or glycerol levels during the 90-minute period following its administration.

These results were interpreted to mean that histamine can stimulate lipid mobilization *in vivo* by two possible mechanisms. In man, the lipid mobilizing effect of histamine is likely due to the effect of histamine to promote catecholamine release from the adrenal medulla (Robinson and Jochim, 1960; Staszewska-Barczak and Vane, 1965; Sheps and Maher, 1968),

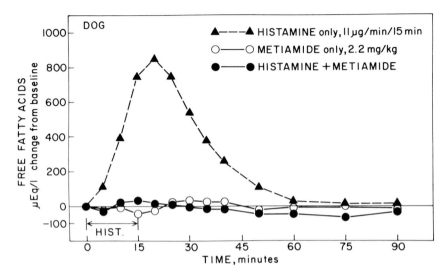

FIG. 7.   Influence of metiamide on basal and histamine-induced changes in serum FFA levels in the dog. These results represent 3 separate tests performed in the same dog at 1 week intervals.

or the result of reflex sympathetic discharge. Catecholamines are potent inducers of lipid mobilization in man and apparently only a small amount needs to be released into the circulation to cause a rise in serum FFA levels (Salvador et al., 1965; Hunninghake et al., 1967; Pinter et al., 1967b). The fact that propranolol pretreatment caused histamine to lower FFA levels in some individuals could easily be the result of α-receptor stimulation, an effect in man which opposes lipid mobilization (Burns et al., 1971; Robison et al., 1972). In the dog, the fact that the entire lipid mobilizing effect of histamine was blocked by metiamide but not by propranolol suggests that the major component of the histamine effect in dogs is due to a direct action of histamine at the H_2 receptor in canine fat cells.

Evidence for the Involvement of Both H_1 and H_2 Receptors

The effect of diphenhydramine to potentiate histamine-induced lipid mobilization in both humans and dogs remains unexplained, but suggests that both histamine receptors may serve in the regulation of lipid mobilization and that more than one site of action may be involved. Histamine not only causes the release of catecholamines from the adrenal medulla, it has also been shown to influence the release of insulin by the pancreas. This is especially significant because of the potent antilipolytic action of insulin. The effects of histamine on insulin release have never been thoroughly investigated and the reports which exist are conflicting. For example, histamine injections in dogs will cause a rise in serum insulin levels

(Lefebvre and Luyckx, 1971), but in isolated hamster islets *in vitro* histamine acts as an inhibitor of insulin release (Feldman and Lebovitz, 1971; Lebovitz and Feldman, 1973). The receptor involvement, in either case, was not characterized.

The effects of histamine to stimulate catecholamine release by the adrenal medulla also need to be clarified. According to the early studies (all performed in cats) the effect of histamine to stimulate catecholamine release by the adrenal medulla is mediated by H_1 receptors (Emmelin and Muren, 1949; Staszewska-Barczak and Vane, 1965), however, it has recently been shown that catecholamine release in other tissues may be mediated by H_2 receptors (Verma and McNeill, 1976). If the effect of histamine to stimulate catecholamine release in humans involved H_1 receptors, one would then hardly expect to see a catecholamine-mediated lipid mobilizing effect of histamine be potentiated by an H_1 blocker!

It is obvious that the mechanisms by which histamine can influence catecholamine and/or insulin release in man need to be clarified. It also remains to be established whether or not histamine receptors are actually present in human adipose tissue. It is possible that the predominant histamine receptor present in human adipose tissue is the H_1 receptor and that it mediates a negative influence of histamine on lipid mobilization. A full

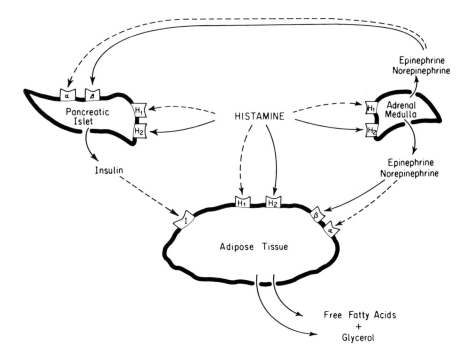

FIG. 8. Possible sites where histamine might be acting to influence lipid mobilization in man.

understanding of the mechanisms by which histamine influences lipid mobilization in man awaits a more complex study of the influence of H_1 and H_2 blockers on histamine induced changes in FFA levels and associated changes in insulin and catecholamine secretion. The possible sites which may contain histamine receptors and be involved in the regulation of lipid mobilization have been summarized in Fig. 8.

ANTILIPOLYTIC EFFECT OF HISTAMINE IN RAT FAT CELLS

The isolated rat fat cell responds to the lipolytic influence of epinephrine, NE, ACTH, and glucagon but does not respond to histamine. When histamine was added to rat fat cells in concentrations ranging from 10^{-9} M to 10^{-3} M basal levels of free fatty acids and cAMP remained unchanged or slightly decreased, even in the presence of theophylline. Similar observations had earlier been reported by Nakano and Oliver (1970). It seemed obvious that rat fat cells did not contain the same lipolytic H_2 receptor found in canine fat cells so the possibility was considered that H_1 receptors were present in rat fat cells which mediated a negative influence on lipolysis and cAMP accumulation. The further possibility that histamine might inhibit lipolysis by elevating cGMP levels was suggested by the "Yin Yang" hypothesis of biological regulation proposed by Goldberg and co-workers (1975).

To examine this possibility, isolated rat fat cells were prepared by a modification of the method of Rodbell (1964) exactly as the isolated canine fat cells had been prepared. Lipolysis was stimulated by the addition of NE (0.1 μM), theophylline (0.2 mM) or N^6-2'-0-dibutyryl cAMP (0.5 mM). Histamine or insulin were added to the suspension at various time intervals before and after the addition of the lipolytic agents to test their ability to inhibit FFA release or cAMP accumulation. In some experiments the ability of histamine and insulin to elevate cGMP was also tested. Cyclic GMP was determined in deproteinized, defatted fat cell extracts by a modification of the radioimmunoassay method of Steiner et al. (1972). Cyclic GMP was acetylated at the 2'0 position to increase assay sensitivity by a procedure similar to that described by Harper and Brooker (1975). Cyclic GMP specific antibody was furnished by Nelson D. Goldberg, University of Minnesota, Minneapolis, Minnesota.

Insulin-Like Effects on FFA and Cyclic AMP Levels

Histamine by itself did not reduce basal levels of FFA but proved to be an effective inhibitor of lipolysis which was stimulated by NE, ACTH, dibutyryl cAMP, or theophylline. Each of these agents was administered in a sufficient concentration to produce a 10–15 fold increase in FFA levels. The concentrations of histamine required to inhibit these increases in FFA ranged from 10^{-6} M to 10^{-5} M with an ED_{50} of 3×10^{-5} M. For example, when histamine (2×10^{-4} M) was added 5 minutes prior to NE or ACTH the lipolytic response was inhibited $98.4 \pm 0.9\%$ and $62.8 \pm 9.9\%$, respectively. Histamine also caused significant inhibition of the responses to dibutyryl cAMP ($79.6 \pm 4.6\%$) and theophylline ($82. \pm 0.9\%$). In each case, the degree of inhibition was nearly identical to that observed in the presence of insulin (4 μU/ml).

The effects of histamine and insulin to inhibit NE-induced FFA release and cAMP accumulation are illustrated in Fig. 9. In these experiments histamine or insulin were added to the media 30 seconds prior to NE. There appeared to

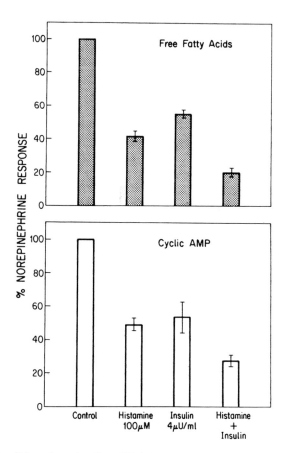

FIG. 9.   Effects of histamine or insulin on NE-induced FFA release and cAMP accumulation in isolated rat fat cells. Histamine or insulin were added 30 seconds prior to NE. FFA levels were determined 30 minutes after the addition of NE and cAMP levels were determined 10 minutes after the addition of NE in the presence of 2×10^{-4} M theophylline.

be good correlatin between inhibition of FFA release and inhibition of cAMP accumulation. The inhibition by histamine and insulin, added together, was significantly greater than the inhibition by histamine or insulin alone.

In other experiments histamine or insulin were added 10 minutes after NE in order to determine whether or not these substances could interrupt the effects of NE at a time when NE-stimulated cAMP accumulation was returning to basal levels. When FFA release was measured, either histamine $(5 \times 10^{-4}\ M)$ or insulin (8 $\mu U/ml$) completely stopped the release of FFA within 10 minutes. Preliminary evidence indicates that histamine can also interrupt the ability of NE to elevate cAMP levels (an effect which peaks within 4 minutes) when histamine is added 1 minute after NE.

The dose-related effects of histamine on NE-induced FFA release and NE-induced cAMP accumulation were parallel. When histamine was added 30 seconds prior to NE, over a concentration range of 20–500 μM, the inhibition of FFA release ranged from 17% to 86% and the inhibition of cAMP accumulation (in the presence of $2 \times 10^{-4}\ M$ theophylline) ranged from 20% to 84%.

Influence of Tripelennamine and Metiamide

The hypothesis that H_1 receptors were mediating a negative effect on lipolysis and cAMP accumulation in rat fat cells was tested by determining the dose-related influence of histamine on NE-induced FFA release in the presence and absence of tripelennamine and by determining the relative potencies of histamine, 2-methyl histamine, and 4-methyl histamine as inhibitors of NE induced lipolysis. In a series of experiments, insulin (4 $\mu U/ml$) inhibited the effect of NE (0.1 μM) on FFA release by $44.7 \pm 3.1\%$. In the same set of experiments, histamine ($10^{-4}\ M$) caused a $57.7 \pm 2.7\%$ inhibition of the response, 2-methyl histamine ($10^{-4}\ M$) caused a $54.2 \pm 5.45\%$ inhibition of the response and 4-methyl histamine caused a $36.5 \pm 3.43\%$ inhibition of the response. This seemed to suggest that H_1 receptors might be specifically involved, but dose-response experiments in the presence of H_1 or H_2 blockers proved just the opposite.

When the dose-related influence of histamine on NE-induced FFA release was studied in the presence and absence of tripelennamine or metiamide it was found that tripelennamine, the H_1 blocker, failed to reverse the antilipolytic effect of histamine indicating for the first time that H_2 receptors, Metiamide, on the other hand, caused a significant reversal of the antilipolytic effect of histamine indicating for the first time that . . . receptors, and not H_1 receptors, may be involved. The effect of metiamide by itself on the NE response was not significant.

The specificity of H_2-receptor blockade was further tested by determining the influence of metiamide and tripelennamine (at the same concentrations

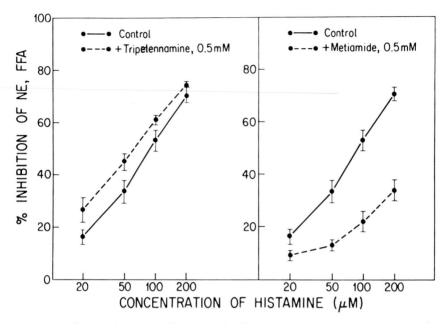

FIG. 10   Influence of tripelennamine and metiamide on the effect of histamine to inhibit NE-induced FFA release in isolated rat fat cells. Histamine was added 30 seconds prior to NE. FFA levels were determined 30 minutes after the addition of NE.

shown in Fig. 10) on the antilipolytic effect of insulin. In experiments using the same format as that illustrated in Fig. 9 it was found that metiamide selectively reversed the antilipolytic effect of histamine (by 74%) without influencing the insulin effect. Tripelennamine slightly enhanced the histamine effect (not significantly) and did not influence the effect of insulin.

These results suggested that H_2 receptors were in some way involved with the effect of histamine to inhibit NE-induced lipolysis. In preliminary experiments it has also been shown that metiamide can reverse the ability of histamine to inhibit NE-induced cAMP accumulation. The exact mechanism by which histamine (at rather high concentrations) could be reversing hormone-stimulated lipolysis by interacting with H_2 receptors was unclear. The next question which was asked was, do calcium and cGMP have a role in the antilipolytic action of histamine in rat fat cells?

Possible Role of Cyclic GMP and Ca^{2+}

An investigation of the possible role of cGMP and/or Ca^{2+} in the antilipolytic effect of histamine in isolated rat fat cells is currently underway. This investigation was prompted by the following observations:

1. Insulin, whose antilipolytic effect was mimicked by histamine, is capable of elevating GMP levels in isolated rat fat cells (Illiano et al., 1973; Fain and Butcher, 1976).

2. Histamine is known to elevate cGMP levels in various tissues including brain (Kuo et al., 1972), arteries (Sutherland et al., 1973; Clyman et al., 1975), smooth muscle (Andersson et al., 1975), and vascular endothelial cells (Buonassisi and Venter, 1976) at concentrations similar to those used to inhibit lipolysis in isolated rat fat cells.

3. Ca^{2+} plays a definite, but poorly understood, role in the antilipolytic action of insulin, prostaglandin E_1, and various other substances (Fassina and Contessa, 1976; Kissebah et al., 1974; Hope-Gill et al., 1974; 1975; Siddle and Hales, 1975; McDonald et al., 1976).

4. Ca^{2+} is a critical component of the cGMP generating system (Berridge, 1975; Rasmussen et al., 1975; Clyman et al., 1975; Ferrendelli et al., 1976).

5. Histamine is a well known regulator of membrane Ca^{2+} permeability and/or Ca^{2+} mobilization (Bohr, 1973; Douglas, 1975).

In preliminary experiments we were able to demonstrate a rise in cGMP levels of 63% and 130% by histamine (5×10^{-5}M and 5×10^{-4}M respectively) in a 5 minute incubation in the presence of the phosphodiesterase inhibitor, isobutylmethylxanthine (5×10^{-4}M). In the same experiments, cAMP levels were reduced (from the isobutylmethylxanthine control) by 62% and 60% respectively. Cyclic GMP levels were determined after purification of fat cell extracts by column chromatography on neutral alumina (WN-3) and Dowex (AG1-X8) formate columns. A more complete picture of the involvement of cGMP in the antilipolytic effect of histamine will await further experimentation.

A number of preliminary experiments suggest that Ca^{2+} may play an important role in the antilipolytic action of histamine. For example, optimal inhibition of NE-induced lipolysis by histamine occurs when the concentration of Ca^{2+} in the media is 0.5 mM. When the Ca^{2+} concentration in the media (containing 2% albumin) is increased in a stepwise fashion to 5 mM, the antilipolytic effect of histamine is completely overcome. The NE response becomes progressively greater as the concentration of Ca^{2+} is increased.

In other experiments it was revealed that lanthanum chloride (1 mM) could selectively reverse the antilipolytic effect of histamine (10^{-4} M) without decreasing the response to NE (0.1 μM) and without reversing the antilipolytic effect of insulin (4 μU/ml). This effect closely resembles the reversal of histamine's antilipolytic effect by metiamide which was discussed earlier. Lanthanum is a trivalent cation which is known to inhibit Ca^{2+} fluxes across biological membranes and therefore inhibit calcium utilizing processes (van Breeman, 1969; Weiss, 1974; Triggle and Triggle, 1976).

Another Ca^{2+} blocker, D-600, was tested for its ability to reverse histamine's antilipolytic effect. This compound is known for its ability to selectively antagonize calcium currents through specific Ca^{2+} channels (Kolhardt et al., 1972). At concentrations up to 10^{-4} M, D-600 failed to reverse the effect of either histamine or insulin. If anything, antilipolytic effects were enhanced by D-600. The reason for the difference in effects seen with lanthanum and D-600 could be explained by the fact that lanthanum can penetrate cells and reach the mitochondria while the same may not be true for D-600 (Piccinini et al., 1975). The difference , if it is a real one, would suggest that histamine might somehow be acting to mobilize intracellular Ca^{2+}. This view would be consistent with the fact that fat cells are known to contain large numbers of Ca^{2+}-containing mitochondria (Napalitano, 1965).

The current theory regarding the mechanism of antilipolytic action of histamine is that histamine interacts specifically with H_2 receptors to cause a mobilization of intracellular stores of Ca^{2+}. An increase in cytosol calcium could result in a variety of events leading to the inhibition of lipolysis. High intracellular levels of Ca^{2+} favor the inhibition of adenylate cyclase (Pohl et al., 1971; Blume and Foster, 1976), the activation of guanylate cyclase (Schultz et al., 1973; Clyman et al., 1975; Ferrendelli et al., 1976), the activation of phosphodiesterase (Kakiuchi et al., 1975; Kono et al., 1975), and the inhibition of triglyceride lipase (Kissebah, 1974). The ability of histamine to mobilize intracellular Ca^{2+} could conceivably involve the elevation of intracellular cAMP levels since H_2-receptor activation generally results in the elevation of cAMP levels (Pöch et al., 1973; McNeill and Verma, 1974; Hegstrand et al., 1976; Roszkowski et al., 1977), and cAMP is thought to be capable of releasing mitochondrial Ca^{2+} (Berridge, 1975; Rasmussen, 1975). Whether or not cGMP has a role as a mediator of the antilipolytic action of histamine remains to be determined.

CLINICAL IMPLICATIONS

Atherosclerosis is recognized as the leading cause of death in the United States and Western Europe (U. S. DHEW, 1971; Blumenthal, 1975). The influence of stress on atherosclerosis and coronary heart disease in man is widely recognized (Friedman and Rosenman, 1974) yet the mechanisms by which stress can influence the advancement of atherosclerosis are poorly understood. A good analogy may be the lack of understanding that the scientific community had just a few years ago in regards to the influence of stress on the development of gastric and duodenal ulcers.

The discovery of burimamide and other H_2 blockers has paved the way for a better understanding of the mechanisms by which stress can influence certain pathological processes in man (Black et al., 1972; Brimblecombe et al., 1973). The observations that H_2 blockers prevent not only the influence of histamine on gastric acid secretion (Wyllie et al., 1972) but also the influence of stress on gastric ulcer formation (Bodily and Fischer, 1976; Brown et al.,

1976) has led to the conclusion that histamine is an important biochemical mediator of stress-induced ulcers (Moody *et al.*, 1976).

Results obtained in the current study indicate that there may be a correlation between stress-induced histamine release and the development of atherosclerotic vascular diseases in man. Histamine was found to be a potent inducer of lipid mobilization in both humans and dogs and it became apparent that histamine can stimulate lipid mobilization not only by a direct interaction with H_2-receptors in adipose tissue but also indirectly by promoting the release of catecholamines. Lipid mobilization is one of the body's major metabolic responses to stress and the role of adrenergic mediators as a component of stress-induced lipid mobilization has been recognized for some time (Cardon and Gordon, 1959; Bogdonoff and Nichols, 1965; Rosell, 1966; Steinberg, 1966; Pinter *et al.*, 1967b). The most severe metabolic consequence of excessive lipid mobilization in man is an increased output of lipoproteins by the liver (Steinberg, 1967). A significant increase in the plasma levels of low-density lipoproteins represents a major threat to life due to the strong correlation between hyperlipoproteinaemia and atherosclerosis (Strong and Eggen, 1970; Kannel *et al.*, 1971; U. S. DHEW, 1971).

Other evidence which supports the theory that histamine may be involved in the stress related progression of atherosclerosis is the observation that chronic subcutaneous injections of histamine in cholesterol-fed rabbits, "greatly accentuated" the atherosclerotic process (Kasatkina, 1964). Supportive evidence also comes from the observations that atherosclerosis can be induced in hypercholesterolaemic baboons by immunologic injury (Howard *et al.*, 1971). Since histamine is stored in relatively high amounts in the mast cells of mamalian adipose tissue it would be constantly available for rapid release in close proximity to fat cells (Stock and Westermann, 1963; Bieck *et al.*, 1967; Fredholm and Frisk-Holmberg, 1971). It has been suggested that the role of adipose tissue mast cells is to facilitate the transport of mobilized fat into the capillary bed (Sheldon, 1965).

Histamine is apparently an important mediator of stress-induced catecholamine release from the adrenal medulla (Robinson and Jochim, 1960; Staszewska-Barczak and Vane, 1965; Sheps and Maher, 1968), and may also play an important role as a mediator stress-inhibited insulin release from the islets of Langerhans (Lefebvre and Luyckx, 1971; Feldman and Lebovitz, 1971; Lebovitz and Feldman, 1973). Because catecholamines are potent stimulators of lipid mobilization (Steinberg, 1966) while insulin is a potent inhibitor of lipid mobilization (Fain, 1973) it is obvious that histamine may influence lipid mobilization by a variety of different mechanisms.

Further studies will be necessary to completely characterize the involvement of histamine H_1 and H_2 receptors in the regulation of lipid mobilization. It is possible that cimetidine, the newest H_2 antagonist, may eventually find a clinical use as an antagonist of stress-induced lipid mobilization in man but as yet, the influence of cimetidine on histamine (or stress)-induced lipid mobilization has not been determined.

SUMMARY

1. Histamine stimulates lipid mobilization in both humans and dogs.
2. In humans, the effects of histamine were reversed by propranolol and potentiated by diphenhydramine. The influence of H_2 blockers in man was not determined.
3. In dogs, the effect was reversed by metiamide, potentiated by diphenhydramine, and unaffected by propranolol.
4. In isolated canine fat cells histamine elevated cAMP levels and stimulated lipolysis. These effects were specifically reversed by burimamide, metiamide, or cimetidine.
5. In isolated rat fat cells histamine inhibited hormone-induced lipolysis and cAMP accumulation. This effect was overcome when the cells were pretreated with metiamide, lanthanum, or high calcium concentrations.
6. These observations indicate that histamine is an important regulator of lipid mobilization by mechanisms involving H_2 receptors and cAMP. It was also revealed that histamine can influence lipid mobilization by more than one mechanism and at more than one site. The results further suggest that stress-induced metabolic responses in man may partly be due to the effects of released histamine.

ACKNOWLEDGMENTS

Supported by Grant GM 01117 from the U.S. Public Health Service and by a Research Starter Grant from the Pharmaceutical Manufacturers Association.

REFERENCES

Altszuler, N., Morrison, A., Steele, R., and Bejerknes, C. (1971). Metabolic effects of epinephrine, dibutyryl cyclic AMP, and glucagon infused intravenously into normal dogs. *Ann. N.Y. Acad. Sci.* **185**, 101-107.

Andersson, R., Nilsson, K., Wikberg, J., Johansson, S., Mohme-Lundholm, E., and Lundhold, L, (1975). Cyclic nucleotides and the contraction of smooth muscle. *Adv. Cyclic Nuc. Res.* **5**, 491-518.

Berridge, M.J. (1975). The interaction of cyclic nucleotides and calcium in the control of cellular activity. *Adv. Cyclic Nuc. Res.* **6**, 1-98.

Bieck, P., Stock, K., and Westermann, E. (1967). Über die Bedeutung des Serotonins im Fettgewebe. *Arch. Pharmacol. Exper. Pathol.* **256**, 218-236.

Birnbaumer, L., and Rodbell, M. (1969). Adenyl cyclase n fat cells II. Hormone receptors. *J. Biol. Chem.* **244**, 3477-3482.

Black, J.W., Duncan, W.A.M., Durant, D.J., Ganellin, C.R., and Parsons, E.M. (1972). Definition and antagonism of histamne H_2-receptors. *Nature (London)* **236**, 385-390.

Black, J.W., Duncan, W.A.M., Emmett, J.C., Ganellin, C.R., Hesselbo, T., Parsons, M.E., and Wyllie, J.H. (1973). Metiamide—An orally active histamine H_2-receptor antagonist. *Agents and Actions.* **3**, 133–137.

Blume, A.J., and Foster, C.T. (1976). Mouse neurobalastoma cell adenylate cyclase: regulation by 2-chloroadenosine, prostaglandin E_1 and the cations, Mg^{++}, Ca^{++}, and Mn^{++}. *J. Neurochem.* **26**, 305–311.

Blumenthal, H.T. (1975). Athero-arteriosclerosis at an aging phenomenon. in *"the Physiology and Pathology of Human Aging."* Proceedings of a Symposium on Physiology and Pathology, On Human Aging, Miami. (R. Goldman and M. Rockstein, eds.) New York, Academic Press.

Bodily, K., and Fischer, R.P. (1976). The prevention of stress ulcers by metiamide, and H_2-receptor antagonist. *J. Surg. Res.* **20**, 203–209.

Bogdonoff, M.D., and Nichols, C.R. (1965). Psychogenic effects on lipid mobilization. in *"Handbook of Physiology Section 5: Adipose Tissue."* (A.E. Renold and G.F. Cahil, Jr. eds.) pp. 613–616. Am. Phys. Soc., Washington, D.C.

Bohr, D.F. (1973). Vascular smooth muscle update. *Circ. Res.* **32**, 665–672.

Bourne, H.R., Melmon, K.L., and Lichtenstein, L.M. (1971). Histamine augments leukocyte adenosine 3′, 5′-monophosphate and blocks antigenic histamine release. *Science (Washington) 173, 743–745.*

Brimblecombe, R.W., Duncan, W.A.M., and Walker, T.F. (1973). Toxicology of metiamide. in *"international Symposium on Histamine* H_2-Receptor Antagonists" (J.C. Wood and M.A. Simkins, eds.). p.53.

Brown, P.A., Brown, T.H., and Vernikos-Danellis, J. (1976). Histamine H_2 receptor: involvement in gastric ulceration. *Life Sciences* **18**, 339–344.

Buonassisi, V., and Venter, J.C. (1976). Hormone and neurotransmitter in an established vascular endothelial cell line. *Prod. Natl. Acad. Sci., U.S.A.* **73**, 1612–1616.

Burns, T.W., Langley, P.E., and Robison, G.A. (1971). Adrenergic receptors and cyclic AMP in the regulation of human adipose tissue lipolysis. *Ann. N.Y. Acad. Sci.* **185**, 115–128.

Butcher, R.W. (1971). The second messenger concept and lipid metabolism. *Naunyn-Schmiedeberg's Arch. Pharmacol.* **269**, 358–372.

Butcher, R.W., Ho, R.J., Meng, H.C., and Sutherland, E.W. (1965). Adenosine 3′, 5′-/monophosphate in biological materials. II. The measurement of adenosine 3′, 5′-monophosphate in tissues and the role of the cyclic nucleotide in the lipolytic responses of fat to epinephrine. *J. Biol. Chem.* **240**, 4515–4523.

Butcher, R.W., Baird, C.E., and Sutherland, E.W. (1968). Effects of lipolytic and antilipolytic substances on adenosine 3′, 5′-monophosphate levels in isolated fat cells. *J. Biol. Chem.* **243**, 1705–1712.

Butcher, R.W., and Sutherland, E.W. (1967). The effect of the catecholamines, adrenergic blocking agents, prostaglandin E_1, and insulin on cyclic AMP levels in the rat epididymal fat pad *in vitro. Ann. N.Y. Acad. Sci.* **139**, 849–859.

Cardon, P. V., and Gordon, R. S. (1959) Rapid increase of plasma unesterfied fatty acids in man during rear. *J. Psychosom. Res.* **4**, 5–9.

Clyman, R. I., Blacksin, A. S., Sandler, J. A., Manganiello, V. C., and Vaughan, M. (1975). The role of calcium in regulation of cyclic nucleotide content in human umbilical artery. *J. Biol. Chem.* **250**, 4718–4721.

Corbin, J. D., and Krebs, E. G. (1969) A cyclic AMP-stimulated protein kinase in adipose tissue. *Biochem. Biophys. Res. Commun.* **36**, 328–336.

Corbin, J. D., Reimann, E. M., Walsh, D. A. and Krebs, E. G.: Activation of adipose tissue lipase by skeletal muscle cyclic adenosine 3′, 5′-monophosphate-stimulated protein kinase. *J. Biol. Chem.* **245**: 4849–4851.

Corbin, J. D., Soderling, T. R., and Park, C. R. (1973) Regulation of adenosine 3′, 5′-monophosphate-dependent protein kinase I. Preliminary characterization of the adipose tissue enzyme in crude extracts. *J. Biol. Chem.* **248**, 1813–1821.

Dekanski, J. (1945) The effect of cutaneous burns on histamine in mice. *J. Physiol. (London)* **104,** 151–160.

Domschke, W., Domschke, S., and Classen, M. (1973). Histamine and cyclic 3', 5'-AMP is gastric acid secretion. *Nature (London).* **243,** 454–455.

Douglas, W. W. (1975). Histamine and antihistamines; 5-hydroxtryptamine and antagonists in "The Pharmacological Basis of Therapeutics" (L. S. Goodman and A. Gilman eds. pp. 590–629. MacMillan Publishing Co. Inc. New York.

Duncombe, W. W. (196) The colorimetric micro-determination of long-chain fatty acids. *Biochem. J.* **88,** 7–10.

Emmelin, N., and Muren, A. (1949) Effects of antihistamine compounds on the adrenaline liberation from the suparenals. *Acta. Physiol. Scand.* **17,** 345–355.

Fain, J. N. (1973) Biochemical aspects of drug and hormone action on adipose tissue. *Pharmacological Reviews* **25,** 67–118.

Fain, J. N., and Butcher, F. R. (1976). Cyclic guanosine 3':5'-monophosphate and the regulation of lipolysis in rat fat cells. *J. Cyclic Nuc. Res.* **2,** 71–78.

Fassina, G., and Contessa, A. R. (1967) Digitoxin and prostaglandin ₁ as inhibitors of catecholamine-stimulated lipolysis and their interaction with Ca^{++} in the process. *Biochem. Pharmacol.* **16,** 1447–1453.

Feldman, J. M., and Lebovitz, H. E. (1971). The nature of the interaction of amines with the pancreatic *beta* cell to influence insulin secretion. *J. Pharmacol. Exper. Ther.* **179,** 56–65.

Ferrendelli, J. A., Rubin, E. H., and Kinscherf, D. A. (1976). Influence of divalent cations on regulation of cyclic GMP and cyclic AMP levels in brain tissue. *J. Neurochem.* **26,** 741–748.

Fredholm, B. B., and Frisk-Holmberg, M. (1971). Lipolysis in canine subcutaneous adipose tissue following release of endogenous histamine. *Eur. J. Pharmacol.* **13,** 245–259.

Fredholm, B. B., Meng, H. C., and Rosell, S. (1968). Release of free fatty acids from canine subcutaneous adipose tissue by histamine and compound 48/80. *Life Sci.* **7,** 1209–1215.

Friedman, M., and Rosenman, R. H. (1974). "Type A Behavior and Your Heart," Afred A. Knopf Inc. New York.

Garland, P. B., and Randle, P. J. (1965) A rapid enzymatic assay for glycerol. *Nature (London)* **196,** 987³988.

Gilman, A. G. (1970). A protein binding assay for adenosine 3', 5'-cyclic monophosphate. *Proc. Nat. Acad. Sci. (U.S.A.)* **67,** 305–312.

Goldberg, N. D., Haddox, M. K. Nicol, S. E., Glass, D. B., Sanford, C. H., Keuhl, F. A., and Estensen, R. 91975) Biologic regulation through opposing influences of cyclic GMP and cyclic AMP: the Yin Yang Hypothesis. *Adv. Cyclic Nuc. Res.* **5,** 307–330.

Grund, V. R., Goldberg, N. D., and Hunninghake, D. B. (1975) Histamine receptors in adipose tissue: involvement of cyclic adenosine monophosphate and the H_2-receptor in the lipolytic response to histamine in isolated canine fat cells. *J. Pharmacol. Exper. Ther.* **195,** 176–184.

Grund, V. R., Pollack, E. W., and Hunninghake, D. B. (1976) Histamine-induced lipid mobilization in humans and dogs. *J. Pharmacol. Exper. Ther.* **197,** 662–668.

Harper, J. F., and Brooker, G. (1975) Femtomole sensitive radioimmunassay for cyclic AMP and cyclic GMP after 2'0 acetylation by acetic anhydride in aqueous solution. *J. Cyclic Nuc. Res.* **1,** 207–218.

Hegstrand, I. R., Kanof, P. D., and Greengard, P. (1976) Histamine-sensitive adenylate cyclase in mammalian brain. *Nature (London)* **260,** 163–165.

Hope-Gill, H., Vydelingum, N., Kissebah, A. H., Tulloch, B. R., and Fraser, T. R. (1974). Stimulation and enhancement of the adipose tissue insulin response by procaine hydrochloride: evidence for a role of calcium in insulin action. *Horm. Metab. Res.* **6,** 457–463

Hope-Gill, H., Kissebah, A., Tulloch, B., Clarke, P., Vydelingum, N., and Fraser, T. R. (1975). The effects of insulin on adipocyte calcium flux and the interaction with the effects of dibutyryl cyclic AMP and adrenaline. *Horm. Metab. Res.* **7,** 195–196.

Howard, A. N., Patelski, J., Bowyer, D. E., and Gresham, G. A. (1971) Atherosclerosis induced in hypercholesterolaemic baboons by immunologic injury; and the effects of intravenous polyunsaturated phosphatidyl choline. *Atherosclerosis.* **14,** 17–29.

Hunninghake, D. B., Azarnoff, D. L., and Waxman, D. (1967) Drug Inhibition of catecholamine induced metabolic effects in humans. *Ann. N.Y. Acad. Sci.* **139,** 971–980.

Illiano, G., and Cuatrecasas, P. (1972). Modulation of adenylate cyclase activity in liver and fat cell membranes by insulin. *Science* **175,** 906–908.

Illiano, G., Tell, G. P. E., Siegel, M. I., and Cuatrecasas, P. (1973) Guanosine 3′, 5′-cyclic monophosphate and the action of insulin and acetylcholine. *Proc. Nat. Acad. Sci. (U.S.A.)* **70,** 2443–2447.

Itaya, K., and Ui, M. (1965). Colorimetric determination of free fatty acids in biological fluids. *J. Lipid Res.* **6,** 16–20.

Johnson, A. R., and Moran, N. C. (1969). Release of histamine from mast cells: a comparison of the effects of 40/80 and two antigen-antibody systems. *Fed. Proc.* **28,** 1716–1720.

Kahlson, G., and Rosengren, E. (1968) New approaches to the physiology of histamine. *Physiol. Rev.* **48,** 155–196.

Kakiuchi, S., and Rall, T. W. (1968). The influence of chemical agents on the accumulation of adenosine 3′, 5′-phosphate in slices of rat cerebellum. *Mol. Pharmacol.* **4,** 367–378.

Kakiuchi, S., Yamaziki, R., Teshima, Y., Uenish, K., and Miyamoto, E. (1975). Ca^{++}/Mg^{++}-Dependent cyclic nucleotide phosphodiesterase and its activator protein. *Adv. Cyclic. Nuc. Res.* **5,** 163–178.

Kannel, W. B., Castelli, W. P., Gordon, T., and McNamara, P. M. (1971). Serum cholesterol, lipoproteins, and the risk of coronary heart disease: the Framingham study. *Ann. Int. Med.* **74,** 1–12.

Kasatkina, L. V. (1964). Effects of histamine on development of experimental atherosclerosis. *Fed. Proc.* **23,** T569–571.

Kissebah, A. H., Vydelingum, N., Tulloch, B. R., Hope-Gill, and Fraser, T. R. (1974). The role of calcium in insulin action. 1. Purification and properties of enzymes regulating lipolysis in human adipose tissue: effects of cyclic AMP and calcium ions. *Horm. Metab. Res.* **6,** 247–255.

Kolhardt, M., Bauer, B., Krause, H., and Fleckenstein, A. (1972). Differentiation of the transmembrane Na and Ca channels in mammalian cardiac fibers by the use of specific inhibitors. *Pflügers. Arch. Ges. Physiol.* **335,** 309–322.

Kono, T., Robinson, F. W., and Sarver, J. A. (1975). Insulin-sensitive phosphodiesterase. Its localization, hormonal stimulation, and oxidative stabilization. *J. Biol. Chem.* **250,** 7826–7835.

Kuo, J., Lee, T., Reyes, R. L., Walton, K. G., Donnelly, T. E., and Greengard, P. (1972). Cyclic nucleotide-dependent protein kinases. X. An assay method for the measurement of guanosine 3′, 5′-monophosphate in various biological materials and a study of agents regulating its levels in heart and brain. *J. Biol. Chem.* **247,** 16–22.

Lebovitz, H. E., and Heldman, J. M. (1973). Pancreatic biogenic amines and insulin secretion in health and disease. *Fedo. Proc.* **32,** 1797–1802.

Lefebvre, P., and Luyckx, A. (1971). Effects de l'imidazole et de deux de ses dérivés sur la sécrétion d'insuline du chien anesthésié. *C. R. Acad. Sci. (Paris) Ser.* **272,** 498–504.

Manganiello, V., and Vaughan, M. (1973) An effect of insulin on cyclic adenosine 3′:5′-monophosphate phosphodiesterase activity in fat cells. *J. Biol. Chem.* **248,** 7164–7170.

Maśliński, C., (1975). Histamine and its metabolism in mammals. Part II., Catabolism of histamine and histamine liberation. *Agents Actions* **5,** 183–201.

McDonald, J. M., Bruns, D. E., and Jarett, L. (1976). Ability of insulin to increase calcium binding by adipocyte plasma membranes. *Proc. Natl. Acad. Sci. U.S.A.* **73,** 1542–1546.

McNeill, J. H., and Muschek, L. D. (1972). Histamine effects on cardiac contractility, phosphorylase, and adenyl cyclase. *J. Mol. Cell. Cardiol.* **4,** 611–624.

McNeill, J. H., and Verma, S. C. (1974). Blockade by burimamide of the effects of histamine and histamine analogs on cardiac contractility, phosphorylase activation, and cyclic adenosine monphosphate. *J. Pharmacol. Exper. Ther.* **188**, 180–188.

Moody, F. G., Cheung, L. Y., Simons, M. A., and Salewsky, C. (1976). Stress and the acute gastric mucosal lesion. *Am. J. Digestive Dis.* **21**, 148–154.

Nakano, J., and Oliver, R. D. (1970). Effect of histamine and its derivatives on lipolysis in isolated rat fat cells. *Arch. Int. Pharmacodyn. Ther.* **186**, 339–344.

Napolitano, L. (9165). The fine structure of adipose tissues In *"Handbook of Physiology Section 5, Adipose Tissue"* A. E. Renold and G. F. Cahill Jr., Eds. pp. 109–124. American Physiological Society, Washington, D. C.

Nasmyth, P. A. (1955). Histamine release and the "stress" phenomenon. *Brit. J. Pharmacol.* **10**, 51–55.

Palmer, G. C. (1971). Characteristics of the hormonal induced cyclic adenosine 3', 5'-monophosphate response in the rat and guinea pig lung *in vitro*. *Biochim. Biophys. Acta.* **252**, 561–566.

Piccinini, F., Meloni, S., Chiarra, A., and Villani, F. P. (1975). Uptake of lanthanum by mitochondria. *Pharmacol. Res. Commun.* **7**, 429–435.

Pinter, J. K., Hayashi, J. A., and Watson, J. A. (1967a). Enzymic assay of glycerol, dihydroxyacetone, and glyceraldehyde. *Arch. Biochem. Biophys.* **121**, 404–414.

Pinter, E. J., Peterfy, G., Cleghorn, J. M., and Patee, C. J. (1967b). The influence of emotional stress on fat mobilization: the role of endogenous catecholamines and the β andrenergic receptors. *Amer. M. Med. Sci.* **254**, 76–93.

Pöch, G., Kukovetz, W. R., and Scholz, N. (9173). Specific inhibition by burimamide of histamine effects on myocardial contraction and cyclic AMP. *Naunyn-Schmiedeberg's Arch. Pharmacol.* **280**, 223–228.

Pohl, S. L., Birnbaumer, L., and Rodbell, M. (1971). The glucagon-sensitive adenyl cyclase system in plasma membranes of rat liver. I. Properties. *J. Biol. Chem.* **246**, 1849–1856.

Rasmussen, H., Jensen, P., Lake, W., Freidman, N., and Goodman, D. B. P. (1975). Cyclic nucleotides and cellular calcium metabolism. *Adv. Cyclic Nuc. Res.* **5**, 375–394.

Robinson, R. L., and Jochim, K. E. (1960). Histamine and anaphylaxis on adrenal medullary secretion in dogs. *Am. J. Physiol.* **199**, 429–432.

Robison, G. A., Langley, P. E., and Burns, T. W. (1972). Adrenergic receptors in human adipocytes—Divergent effects on adenosine 3', 5'-monophosphate and lipolysis. *Biochem. Pharmacol.* **21**, 589–592.

Rodbell, M. (1964). Metabolism of isolated fat cells I. Effects of hormones on glucose etabolism and lipolysis. *J. Biol. Chem.* **239**, 375–380.

Rosell, S. (1966). Release of free fatty acids from subcutaneous adipose tissue in dogs following sympathetic nerve stimulation. *Acta. Physiol Scand.* **67**, 343–351.

Roszkowski, W., Plaut, M., and Lichtenstein, L. (1977). Selective display of histamine receptors on lymphocytes. *Science* **195**, 683–685.

Rudman, D., Brown, S. J., and Malkin, M. F. (1963). Adipokinetic actions of adrenocorticotropin, thyroid-stimulating hormone, vasopressin, α-and β-melanocyte-stimulating hormones, fraction H, epinephrine and norepinephrine in the rabbit, guinea pig, hamster, rat, pig and dog. *Endocrinology,* **72**, 527–543.

Salvador, R. A., Colville, K. I., and Burns, J. J. (1965). Adrenergic mechanisms and lipid mobilization. *Ann. N.Y. Acad. Sci.* **131**, 113–118.

Schultz, G., Hardman, J. G., Schultz, K., Baird, C. E., and Sutherland, E. W. (1973). The importance of calcium ions for the regulation of guanosine 3', 5'-monophosphate levels. *Proc. Natl. Acad. Sci. U.S.A.* **70**, 3889–3893.

Sheldon, H. (1965). Morphology of adipose tissue: a microscopic anatomy of fat in *"Handbook of Physiology"* (A. E. Ramwell and G. F. Cahill, Jr., eds.) Vol. 5). pp. 125–139. American Physiology Society, Washington, D. C.

Sheps, S. G., and Maher, F. T. (1968). Histamine and glucagon tests in diagnosis of pheochromacytoma. *J. Amer. Med. Assoc.* **205**, 895-899.

Siddle, K., and Hales, C. N. (1975). Hormonal control of adipose tissue lipolysis. *Proc. Nutr. Soc.* **34**, 233-239.

Staszewska-Barczak, J., and Vane, J. R. (1965). The release of catecholamines from the adrenal medulla by histamine. *Brit. J. Pharmacol.* **25**, 728-742.

Steinberg, D. (1966). Catecholamine stimulation of fat mobilization and its metabolic consequences. *Pharmacol. Rev.* **18**, 217-235.

Steinberg, D. (1967). The dynamics of FFA mobilization and utiization. *Progr. Biochem. Pharmacol.* **3**, 139-150.

Steiner, A. L., Parker, C. W., and Kipnis, D. M. (1972). Radioimmunoassay for cyclic nucleotides. 1. preparation of antibodies and iodinated cyclic nucleotides. *J. Biol. Chem.* **247**, 1106-1113.

Stock, K., and Westermann, E. O. (1963). Concentration of norepinephrine, serotonin, and histamine, and of amine metabolizing enzymes in mammalian adipose tissue. *J. Lipid Res.* **4**, 297-304.

Strong, J. P., and Eggen, D. A. (1970). Risk factors and atherosclerotic lesions In "Atherosclerosis," Proceedings of the Second Int. Symposium. (R. J. Jones, ed). pp. 355-364. New York, Springer-Verlag.

Sutherland, E. W., Robison, G. A., and Butcher, R. W. (1968). Some aspects of the biological role of adenosine 3', 5'-monophosphate (cyclic AMP). *Circulation* **37**, 279-306.

Sutherland, C. A., Schultz, G., Hardman, J. G., and Sutherland, E. W. (1973). Effects of vasoactive agents on cyclic nucleotide levels in pig coronary arteries. *Fed. Proc.* **32**, 773 Abs.

Taylor, K. M., and Snyder, S. H. (1971). Brain histamine: rapid apparent turnover altered by restraint and cold stress. *Science (Washington)* **172**, 1037-1039.

Triggle, C. R., and Triggle, D. J. (1976). An analysis of the action of cations of the lanthanide series on the mechanical responses of guinea-pig ileal longitudinal muscle. *J. Physiol.* **254**, 39-54.

U. S. DHEW (1971). Atherosclerosis: a report by the National Heart and Lung Institute Task Force on Arteriosclerosis (DHEW Publication No. NIH-72-219) Vol. 2. Government Printing Office, Washington, D. C.

van Breemen, C. (1969). Blockade of membrane calcium fluxes by lanthanum in relation to vascular smooth muscle contractility. *Arch. Int. Physiol.* **77**. 710-716.

Vaughan, M., Berger, J. E., and Steinberg, D. (1964). Hormone-sensitive lipase and monoglyceride lipase activities in adipose tissue. *J. Biol. Chem.* **239**, 401-409.

Verma, S. C., and McNeill, J. H. (1976). The effect of histamine isoproterenol and tyramine on rat uterine cyclic AMP. *Res. Commun. Pathol. Pharmacol.* **13**, 55-64.

Weiss, G. B. (1974). Cellular pharmacology of lanthanum. *Ann. Rev. Pharmacol.* **14**, 343-354.

Wyllie, J. H., Hesselbo, T., and Black, J. W. (1972). Effects in man of histamine H_2-receptor blockade by burimamide. *Lancet* **2**:1117-1120.

PART V
HISTAMINE RECEPTORS IN IMMUNE REACTIONS

20

Modulation of Inflammation by Histamine Receptor-Bearing Cells

Marshall Plaut and Lawrence M. Lichtenstein
Clinical Immunology Division
Department of Medicine
The Johns Hopkins University
  School of Medicine at
The Good Samaritan Hospital
Baltimore, Maryland

This chapter reviews briefly the inflammatory process and the inflammatory mechanisms, which induce release of histamine, and then discusses the diverse pro- and anti-inflammatory effects resulting from interaction of histamine with specific histamine receptors.

The response of man and many other species to "noxious" stimuli is a complex sequence of tissue changes including increased capillary permeability, infiltration of several types of leukocytes, deposition of fibrin, neovascularization, and tissue repair, collectively termed "the inflammatory response." While the initiating signal may be a nonspecific irritant, inflammation in an immune host can be triggered by specific antigens, such as cell-surface glycoproteins on invading bacteria. The initial immune event—antigen–antibody interaction—does not in itself lead to elimination of the invader, but through a series of intermediate steps (e.g., activation of the complement enzyme sequence) to generation and release of chemotactic, "activating," enzymatic, and vasoactive mediators.* These mediators collectively can assist in phagocytosis and destruction of foreign bacteria, but also may cause tissue injury (Plaut and Lichtenstein, 1978).

The classification of Coombs and Gell (1968) divides immunopathologic processes somewhat arbitrarily into four types, and in this scheme histamine is considered only in the context of "immediate hypersensitivity" reactions,

---

*A short list of mediators released from cells includes: histamine, SRS-A (slow reacting substance of anaphylaxis), ECF-A (eosinophil chemotactic factor of anaphylaxis), from basophils; beta glucuronidase and other lysosomal enzymes, from neutrophils; lysosomal enzymes from macrophages; chemotactic factors, lymphotoxin, macrophage migration inhibition factor, macrophage activating factor from lymphocytes.

C3a and C5a are two examples of components generated by activation of the complement system. Both of these molecules can trigger mast cells to release histamine and other mediators and also are chemotactic for neutrophils and other inflammatory cells (Plaut and Lichtenstein, 1978).

351

i.e., those mediated by IgE antibodies to the appropriate antigens. IgE antibodies bind avidly to receptors on the basophils and mast cells which contain most of the body stores of histamine. Interaction of antigen with mast cell-bound IgE results in secretion of histamine and other mediators. Thus, allergy to appropriate antigens can be detected by intracutaneous testing with the antigen, resulting in an immediate (within minutes) cutaneous wheal and flare which is due primarily to released histamine. Recent studies have, however, shown that immediate hypersensitivity reactions are not isolated events: the wheal and flare reaction is followed by the sequential appearance, within several hours, of neutrophils and eosinophils and later by lymphocytes and mononuclear cells, i.e., the classical features of an inflammatory response (Solley *et al.*, 1976). These observations emphasize the coordinated nature of inflammation.

Since histamine is released as one of the first events in the course of the IgE-mediated inflammatory process, it seems likely that it influences the appearance and function of the inflammatory cells which appear later. Histamine is also released *in vivo* in response to stimuli, other than antigen-IgE interaction, such as N-formylmethionyl peptides (Hook *et al.*, 1976), thought to be similar to bacterial products, and C3a and C5a (Glovsky *et al.*, 1977; Grant *et al.*, 1975) "anaphylatoxins" generated during activation of complement. Basophils are present in lymphocyte-mediated tissue infiltrates, including contact hypersensitivity reactions (Dvorak and Dvorak, 1974); they are attracted by lymphocyte-derived and other chemotactic factors (Lett-Brown *et al.*, 1976). These basophils are capable of releasing their histamine content (Askenase *et al.*, 1976), but the mechanism(s) of their activation in this tissue location is uncertain.

The released histamine can interact with receptors on vascular smooth muscle or on inflammatory cells. While the vascular effects (so-called "increased capillary permeability") of histamine have been known for years, the concept that histamine and other hormones can modulate the function of inflammatory cells is quite new. It is based on data derived from *in vitro* models in which isolated cell types of importance in the inflammatory process can be studied separately. For example, immediate hypersensitivity reactions can be analyzed by studying antigen-induced histamine release from human peripheral blood leukocytes. Washed leukocytes from allergic patients are mixed with antigen, incubated for 20 to 40 minutes at 37° C, and released histamine is assayed fluorometrically. This assay yields quantitative and reproducible dose-response curves and is readily amenable to mechanistic analysis.

This was the first assay system to be studied with respect to possible control mechanisms exercised by hormones and pharmacologic agonists. It was found that when leukocytes and antigen were incubated in the presence of catecholamines and theophylline, histamine release was markedly inhibited (Lichtenstein and Margolis, 1968). These and further observations soon led to the concept that agents which raise the level of cyclic AMP (cAMP) inhibit the release of histamine (Bourne *et al.*, 1974). This was novel inasmuch as

Sutherland *et al.* (1968) had previously shown that elevation of intracellular cAMP levels characteristically induces or facilitates secretion. It has become clear, however, that the effect of cAMP on cells depends on many factors, including baseline levels of cAMP and cyclic GMP (cGMP), state of microbular aggregation, stage of cell differentiation, and possibly subcellular compartmentalization of cAMP. A large number of studies in other *in vitro* models of inflammation have shown similar effects: the biochemical nature of inflammatory cells is such that cAMP can inhibit the intensity of their response whether it be release of histamine (basophils), release of lysosomal enzymes (neutrophils), or direct killing (cytolytically active T lymphocytes).

Several agents raise intracellular cAMP by interacting with distinct receptors linked to adenylate cyclase. Four such receptors have been described on inflammatory cells: beta adrenergic, prostaglandin (PGE's), cholera enterotoxin, and histamine. Because histamine is released by endogenous stimuli, it is likely that it can modulate inflammatory responses *in vivo* (rather than only as an *in vitro* artifact). A similarly important role can be postulated for epinephrine.

The effects of histamine on inflammation are summarized in Table I. While this discussion will focus primarily on the newly described anti-inflammatory effects of histamine, it is appreciated that histamine has other "proinflammatory" effects. Since mast cells are located adjacent to blood vessels, locally released histamine may be capable of regulating the microcirculation (Schayer, 1963), i.e., by increasing vascular permeability it assists in initiation of inflammatory responses. This response is mediated primarily through histamine-type 1 receptors. (Histamine-type 2 receptors act synergistically with histamine-type 1 receptors on vascular responses, but the type 2 receptors have tenfold less affinity for histamine; Black, 1975.) Antihistamine drugs block the immune complex deposition responsible for a type of glomerulonephritis in rabbits, suggesting that increased vascular permeability induced by vasoactive amines facilitates the deposition of these complexes (Kniker and Cochrane, 1965). Histamine release in immediate hypersensitivity reactions may also act as a "gatekeeper" to allow "useful" antibodies to reach appropriate tissue sites (Steinberg *et al.,* 1974). Migration of cells should also be facilitated by vascular changes, and it has been shown that antiserotonin drugs (in the mouse, where serotonin is the most important vasoactive amine released during IgE-mediated reactions) block delayed hypersensitivity skin reactions (Schwartz *et al.,* 1977). Presumably, vasoactive amines are necessary to facilitate mononuclear cell migration to the skin site.* Since elevated levels of histamine and histadine decarboxylase have been noted at the site of tissue growth and repair reactions (in the rat)

---

*As described below (see p. 356), high concentrations of vasoactive amines may have the opposite effect. Large amounts of histamine, by activating histamine-type 2 receptors inhibit the secretion of lymphocyte mediators. These mediators ("lymphokines") have many effects including mobilization and activation of macrophages. In their absence, delayed hypersensitivity skin tests are inhibited.

Table I

Histamine-Mediated Modulation of Inflammation[a]

Responses	Receptor		Comment
	Hist-type 1	Hist-type 2	
Vascular			
(1) Facilitation of immune complex deposition	++	+	Serotonin also important (rabbit)
(2) Facilitation of delayed hypersensitivity skin responses	(++)	(+)	Demonstrated only in mouse, where serotonin, not histamine, is the important vasoactive amine
(3) Neovascularization	(++)	(+)	Elevated levels of histamine and histidine decarboxylase are found at sites of tissue repair (rat): the role of histamine is not proven.
Inflammatory Cell			
Basophil-Mast Cell			
(1) Inhibit histamine release from basophils	–	+	
(2) Inhibit histamine release from mast cells	–	+	Monkey lung
(3) Inhibit chemotactic responsiveness	–	+	Human basophil
(4) Inhibit PCA reactions	?	?	(Rabbit)
Neutrophil			
(5) Inhibit lysosomal enzyme release	–	+	
(6) Inhibit chemotactic responsiveness	–	+	
Eosinophil			

(7) Inhibit chemotactic responsiveness	–	+	Complex observation, of uncertain significance
(8) Enhance chemotactic migration	+	–	Not mediated by histamine receptors (?)
(9) Direct chemotactic activity	–	–	
(10) Inhibit B cell maturation to plasma cell (?)	?	?	
(11) Inhibit antibody secretion from plasma cells	+?	?	
(12) Induce lymphokine production	?	?	Synergistic with serotonin in human lymphocytes
(13) Inhibit secretion of lymphokines (MIF)	–	+	Guinea pig
(14) Inhibit proliferation to T lymphocyte mitogens (concanavalin A, phytohemagglutinin)	–	+	Mouse, guinea pig
(15) Inhibit cytotoxic activity of cytolytically activ T lymphocytes	–	+	Mouse
(16) Inhibit delayed hypersensitivity skin test	–	+	Guinea pig

[a]For references, see text.

(Kahlson and Rosengren, 1968), it is also likely that histamine aids the neovascularization responses which occur late in inflammation.

In contrast to these pro-inflammatory effects, mediated principally by vascular histamine-type 1 receptors, histamine inhibits inflammatory cell effector functions by interaction with histamine-type 2 receptors. However, two recently described effects of histamine in man (discussed below)—chemotactic activity to eosinophils (Clark *et al.*, 1975; Clark *et al.*, 1977) and a synergistic action with serotonin in inducing lymphokine production by cultured lymphocytes (Foon *et al.*, 1976)—are not anti-inflammatory and probably are not mediated through either histamine-type 1 or histamine-type 2 receptors.

The quantititave nature of the *in vitro* model of antigen-induced histamine release enables detailed study of histamine effects (Bourne *et al.*, 1971; Lichtenstein and Gillespie, 1973, 1975). Histamine (10^{-7} M–10^{-5} M) inhibits antigen-induced histamine release. (While these concentrations of histamine are high, it is likely that concentrations as high as 10^{-4} M are attained locally during immediate hypersensitivity reactions.) Histamine also raises cAMP levels in human peripheral blood leukocytes. While antihistamines such as chlorpheniramine or pyrilamine do not block these effects, the histamine-type 2 antihistamines burimamide and metiamide specifically reverse these actions of histamine. By plotting dose-response curves for histamine in the presence of various concentrations of antihistamines, it is possible to calculate the potency of these antagonists. For the histamine receptor mediating inhibition of histamine release the estimated dissociation constant (K_B) for the antagonist-receptor complex is approximately 10^{-5} M for burimamide and 10^{-6} M for metiamide. The similarity of these values to those for histamine-type 2 receptors on other tissue types confirms the receptor-specific nature of this anti-inflammatory, negative feedback action.

While other model systems (except for mouse cytolytically active T lymphocytes) have not been analyzed quantitatively in such detail, the other anti-inflammatory effects of histamine that will be described are almost certainly due to interaction with histamine-type 2 receptors. It is likely that endogenous histamine release *in vivo* also can inhibit the overall amount of released mediators, since histamine inhibits *in vivo* antigen-induced passive cutaneous anaphylaxis reactions in rabbits (Kravis and Zvaifler, 1974). The kinetics of histamine release from a single cell are rapid. Therefore, histamine probably does not inhibit release from its cell of origin, but it rapidly diffuses to other mast cells and affects them. Such actions cannot be demonstrated in washed leukocytes, because the diffusion rate is too rapid, but can be measured in solid tissues such as chopped lung, where histamine diffuses faster than antigen and apparently modulates the total quantity of released histamine. In the presence of metiamide (to block the inhibitory effect of histamine) significantly greater quantities of histamine are released (Chakrin *et al.*, 1974).

Histamine, acting through histamine-type 2 receptors, inhibits at least one other function of basophils—response to chemotactic stimuli (Lett-Brown and Leonard, 1977)—and also inhibits several neutrophil functions including lysosomal enzyme release (Sosman and Busse, 1976) and responsiveness to bacterial-derived chemotactic factors (Hill *et al.*, 1975). High concentrations of histamine also inhibit the chemotactic responsiveness of eosinophils (Clark and Kaplan, 1975). However, it appears that histamine can also enhance (via histamine-type 1 receptors) the chemotactic migration of a few, rapidly migrating eosinophils (Clark *et al.*, 1977). At low concentrations histamine itself is chemotactic toward the eosinophils (this effect is not blocked either by histamine-type 1 or by histamine-type 2 antihistamines) (Clark *et al.*, 1977).

Some actions of histamine on lymphocytes are outlined in more detail in chapter 21 (by Plaut and Roszkowski). These effects have been described in animal models; a direct role for histamine in affecting human lymphocytes has not yet been convincingly demonstrated (Ballet and Merler, 1976; Verhaegen *et al.*, 1977).* Histamine apparently inhibits maturation of antigen-stimulated B cells (Fallah *et al.*, 1975) and also inhibits antibody secretion from (more mature) B cells and plasma cells (Melmon *et al.*, 1974). It inhibits proliferation due to concanavalin A and phytohemagglutinin (mitogens for T lymphocytes) in mice and guinea pigs (Rocklin, 1976; Roszkowski *et al.*, 1977b) and it inhibits MIF production by immune, antigen-challenged guinea pig lymphocytes (Rocklin, 1976). It also inhibits delayed hypersensitivity skin responses in guinea pigs (Rocklin, 1976) (see p. 353 and footnote on p. 353), presumably by its ability to inhibit secretion of MIF and other lymphokines.†

The actions of histamine have been well studied in another *in vitro* system in which a specific lymphocyte effector function is assayed. This system will be described in chapter 21 (by Plaut and Roszkowski). Briefly, when foreign (histoincompatible) tumor cells are injected into mice, the recipient mice reject the tumor cells and at the same time develop an immune response (Cerottini and Brunner, 1974). Cytolytically active T lymphocytes (i.e., lymphocytes which can kill specifically the foreign tumor cells) represent one component of the response. Histamine interacts with histamine-type 2 receptors to inhibit *in vitro* cytolytic activity of (mouse) cytolytically active T lymphocytes (Plaut *et al.*, 1973b, 1975), suggesting that histamine receptors are not randomly distributed on cells, but that functional histamine receptors appear as a consequence of the immune response. This selectivity in display of histamine receptors occurs not only in antigen-stimulated lymphocytes but also in populations from nonimmune animals. Thus, splenic T lymphocytes

---

*See Foon *et al.* (1976), who suggest that histamine acting in conjunction with serotonin can induce lymphokine release from cultured human lymphocytes. The receptor specificity of this effect has not been defined. See Supplemental Notes, A.

†It is possible that this *in vivo* effect is due to desensitization of vascular responsiveness by initial treatment with histamine. However, since 10^{-3} M burimamide was more effective than 10^{-3} M chlorpheniramine in reversing the effect, densensitization of vascular receptors is a less likely explanation unless endogenously released histamine interacts predominantly with histamine-type 2 vascular receptors in the guinea pig (Schwartz *et al.*, 1977). See Supplemental Notes, B.

and cortisone-resistant thymocytes possess histamine receptors while other lymphocytes (the majority of thymocytes, splenic B lymphocytes) do not (Roszkowsi et al., 1977a).

In summary, histamine at low concentrations activates histamine-type 1 vascular receptors to facilitate the initiation of inflammatory reactions. At high concentrations it can modulate the intensity of inflammation by activating histamine-type 2 receptors and inhibiting the effector functions of these inflammatory cells. Since lymphocyte populations (and perhaps other cell types, for example, monocytes) display markedly different sensitivities to histamine, it is likely that histamine–histamine receptor interaction exerts highly selective inhibitory effects on distinct inflammatory cell subpopulations.

SUPPLEMENTAL NOTES

A. The mechanism of action of histamine on lymphocytes is complex. Histamine appears to inhibit mouse cytotoxic T lymphocytes directly (Plaut, M., unpublished). However, its action on guinea pig MIF-producing cells is indirect: Histamine activates suppressor lymphocytes, to secrete a soluble, nondialyzable factor called "histamine-induced suppressor factor (HSF)." This factor then inhibits MIF-producing cells (Rocklin, 1977).

Several recent reports have established that histamine, at concentrations as low as 10^{-7} M, inhibits mitogen-induced proliferation of human peripheral blood lymphocytes (Strannegärd and Strannegärd, 1977; Wang and Zweiman, 1978; Plaut and Berman, 1978). Rocklin and Melmon (1978) have reported that HSF can also be generated with human lymphocytes, and that, in some individuals, as little as 10^{-9} M histamine can induce human peripheral blood lymphocytes to produce a suppressor factor that inhibits proliferation. The relatioship of these anti-inflammatory effects to the "pro-inflammatory" effect described by Foon et al (1976) is unknown.

B. Avella et al (1978) have studied the effects of the H_2 antagonist, cimetidine (vs. placebo) on delayed hypersensitivity skin tests to several antigens in patients with peptic ulcer disease. Following six weeks of treatment with cimetidine, the diameter of induration of the patients' skin tests were significantly increased. The simplest explanation is that in humans (and in contrast to results in guinea pigs) histamine is normally released during delayed hypersensitivity reactions, and acts as a negative feedback control via histamine-type 2 receptors; cimetidine inhibitis this negative feedback. However, these results have not yet been confirmed, and there are other possible interpretations. Further studies are in progress.

ACKNOWLEDGMENTS

Supported by Grants AI12810 and AI11334 from the National Institute of Allergy and Infectious Diseases, The National Institutes of Health.

Publication No. 317 of the O'Neill Research Laboratories, The Good Samaritan Hospital.

REFERENCES

Askenase, P.W., DeBernardo, R., Kashgarian, M., Douglas, J., and Tauben, D. (1976). Anaphylactic type basophil degranulation at delayed cutaneous basophil reactions. *J. Allergy Clin. Immunol.* (Abstr.). **57**, 193.

Avella, J., Madsen, J. E., Binder, H. J., and Askenase, P. W. (1978). Effect of histamine H2 receptor antagonists on delayed hypersensitivity. *Lancet* **I**, 624–626.

Ballet, J.J., and Merler, E. (1976). The separation and reactivity *in vitro* of a subpopulation of human lymphocytes which bind histamine. Correlation of histamine reactivity with cellular maturation. *Cell. Immunol.* **24**, 250–269.

Black, J.W. (1976). Histamine receptors, in "Receptors and Cellular Pharmacology." (E. Klinge, ed.) pp. 3–16. *Proc. Sixth Inter. Congr. of Pharmacology,* Helsinki, Finland.

Bourne, H.R., Melmon, K.L., and Lichtenstein, L.M. (1971). Histamine augments leukocyte cyclic AMP and blocks antigenic histamine release. *Science* **173**, 743–745.

Bourne, H.R., Lichtenstein, L.M., Henney, C.S., Melmon, K.L., Weinstein, Y., and Shearer, G.M. (1974). Modulation of inflammation and immunity by cyclic AMP. *Science* **184**, 19–28.

Cerottini, J.-C., and Brunner, K.T. (1974). Cell-mediated cytotoxicity, allograft rejection and tumor immunity. Adv. Immunol. **18**, 67–132.

Chakrin, L.W., Krell, R.D., Mengel, J., Young, D., Zaher, C., and Wardell, J.R. (1974). Effect of a histamine H_2-receptor antagonist on immunologically induced mediator release *in vitro. Agents Actions* **4**, 297–303.

Clark, R.A.F., Gallin, J.I., and Kaplan, A.P. (1975). The selective eosinophil chemotactic activity of histamine. *J. Exp. Med.* **142**, 1462–1476.

Clark, R.A.F., Sandler, J.A. Gallin, J.I., and Kaplan, A.P. (1977). Histamine modulation of eosinophil migration. *J. Immunol.* **118**, 137–145.

Coombs, R.R.A., Gell, P.G.H. (1968). Classification of allergic reactions, in "Clinical Aspects of Immunology" (R.R.A. Coombs and P.G.J.Gell, eds.), 2nd ed., pp. 575–596. Blackwell Scientific Publications, Oxford.

Dvorak, H.F., and Dvorak, A.M. (1974). Cutaneous basophil hypersensitivity, in "Progress in Immunology II" (L. Brent, and J. Holborow, eds.) Vol. 3. pp. 171–181. North Holland Publishing Company, Amsterdam.

Fallah, H.A., Maillard, J.L., and Voison, G.A. (1975). Regulatory mast cells. I. Suppressive action of their products on an *in vitro* primary immune reaction. *Annals Immunol. (Inst. Pasteur)* **126C**, 669–682.

Foon, K.A., Wahl, S.M., Oppenheim, J.J., and Rosenstreich, D.L. (1976). Serotonin-induced production of a monocyte chemotactic factor by human peripheral blood leukocytes. *J. Immunol.* **117**, 1545–1552.

Glovsky, M.M., Hugli, T.E., Ishizaka, T., and Lichtenstein, L.M. (1977). Studies on C3a$_{hu}$ on human leucocyte binding and histamine release. *Fed. Proc. (Abstr.)* **36**, 1264.

Grant, J.A, Dupree, E., Goldman, A.S., Schultz, D.K., and Jackson, A.L. (1975). Complement-induced release of histamine in human leukocytes. *J. Immunol.* **114**, 1101–1106.

Hill, H.R., Estensen, R.D., Quie, P.G., Hogan, N.A., and Goldberg, N.D. (1975). Modulation of human neutrophil chemotactic responses by cyclic 3′5′-guanosine monophosphate and cyclic 3′5′-adenosine monophosphate. *Metabolism* **24**, 447–456.

Hook, W.A., Schiffman, E., Aswanikumar, S., and Siraganian, R.P. (1976). Histamine release by chemotactic, formyl methionine-containing peptides. *J. Immunol.* **117**, 594–596.

Kahlson, G., and Rosengren, E. (1968). New approaches to the physiology of histamine. *Physiol Rev.* **48**, 155–196.

Kniker, W.T., and Cochrane, C.G. (1965). Pathogenic factors in vascular lesions of experimental serum sickness. *J. Exp. Med.* **122**, 83–97.

Kravis, T.C., and Zvaifler, N.J. (1974). Alteration of rabbit PCA reactions by drugs known to influence intracellular cyclic AMP. *J. Immunol.* **113**, 244–250.

Lett-Brown, M.A., Boetcher, D.A., and Leonard, E.J. (1976). Chemotactic response of normal human basophils to C5a and to lymphocyte-derived chemotactic factor. *J. Immunol.* **117**, 246–252.

Lett-Brown, M.A., and Leonard, E.J. (1977). Histamine-induced inhibition of normal human basophil chemotaxis to C5a. *J. Immunol.* **118**, 815–818.

Lichtenstein, L.M., and Margolis, S. (1968). Histamine release *in vitro:* inhibition by catecholamines and methylxanthines. *Science* **161**, 902–903.

Lichtenstein, L.M., and Gillespie, E. (1973). Inhibition of histamine release by histamine is controlled by an H2 receptor. *Nature (London)* **244**, 287–288.

Lichtenstein, L.M., and Gillespie, E. (1975). The effects of the H1 and H2 antihistamines on "allergic" histamine release and its inhibition by histamine. *J. Pharm. Exper. Ther.* **192**, 441–450.

Melmon, K.L., Bourne, H.R., Weinstein, Y., Shearer, G.M., Kram, J., and Bauminger, S. (1974). Hemolytic plaque formation by leukocytes *in vitro. J. Clin. Invest.* **53**, 13–21.

Plaut, M., and Berman, I.J. (1978). Histamine receptors on human and mouse lymphocytes. *J. Allergy Clin. Immunol. (Abstr.)* **61**, 132–133.

Plaut M., Lichtenstein, L.M., Gillespie, E., and Henney, C.S. (1973a). Studies on the mechanism of lymphocyte-mediated cytolysis. IV. Specificity of the histamine receptor on effector T cells. *J. Immunol.* **111**, 389–394.

Plaut, M., Lichtenstein, L.M., and Henney, C.S. (1973b). Increase in histamine receptors on thymus-derived effector lymphocytes during the primary immune response to alloantigens. *Nature (London)* **244**, 284–287.

Plaut, M., Lichtenstein, L.M., and Henney, C.S. (1975). Properties of a subpopulation of T cells bearing histamine receptors. *J. Clin. Invest.* **55**, 856–874.

Plaut, M., and Lichtenstein, L.M. (1978). Cellular and chemical basis of the allergic inflammatory response. Component parts and control mechanism, in "Allergy: Principles and Practice." (E. Middleton, Jr., C. E. Reed, and E. Ellis, eds.) pp. 115–138. C.V. Mosby Company, St. Louis, Mo.

Rocklin, R.E. (1976). Modulation of cellular immune resposes *in vivo* and *in vitro* by histamine receptor-bearing lymphocytes. *J. Clin. Invest.* **57**, 1051–1058.

Rocklin, R. E. (1977). Histamine-induced supressor factor (HSF): Effect on migration inhibitory factor production and proliferation. *J. Immunol.* **118,** 1734–1738.

Rocklin, R. E., and Melmon, K. L. (1978). Production and assay of a histamine-induced suppressor factor (HSF) by human lymphocytes. *Clin. Res. (Abstr.)* **26**, 520A.

Roszkowski, W., Plaut, M., and Lichtenstein, L.M. (1977a). Selective display of histamine receptors on lymphocytes. *Science* **195**, 683–685.

Roszkowski, W., Plaut, M., and Lichtenstein, L.M. (1977b). Histamine receptor display on lymphocyte subpopulations. *Fed. Proc. (Abstr.)* **36**, 1241.

Schayer, R.A. (1963). Induced synthesis of histamine, microcirculatory regulation and the mechanism of action of the adrenal glucocorticoid hormones, in "Progress in Allergy." (P. Kallós, and B.H. Waksman, eds.) Vol. 7, pp. 187–212. Karger, Basel.

Schwartz, A., Askenase, P.W., and Gershon, R.K. (1977). The effect of locally injected vasoactive amines on the elicitation of delayed-type hypersensitivity. *J. Immunol.* **118**, 159–165.

Solley, G.O., Gleich, G.J., Jordon, E.R., and Schroeter, A.L. (1976). The late phase of the immediate wheal and flare skin reaction. Its dependence upon IgE antibodies. *J. Clin. Invest.* **58**, 408–420.

Sosman, J., and Busse, W. (1976). Histamine inhibition of neutrophil lysosomal enzyme release: an H2 histamine receptor response. *Science* **194**, 737–738.

Steinberg, P., Ishizaka, K., and Norman, P.S. (1974). Possible role of IgE-mediated reaction in immunity. *J. Allergy Clin. Immunol.* **54**, 359–366.

Strannegärd, O. (1977). Increased sensitivity of lymphocytes from atopic individuals to histamine-induced suppression. *Scand. J. Immunol.* **6**, 1225–1231.

Sutherland, E.W., Robison, G.A., and Butcher, R.W. (1968). Some aspects of the biological role of adenosine 3',5'-monophosphate (cyclic AMP). *Circulation* **37**, 279–306.

Verhaegen, H., DeCock, W., and DeCree, J. (1977). Histamine receptor-bearing peripheral T lymphocytes in patients with allergies. *J. Allergy Clin. Immunol.* **59**, 266–270.

Wang, S. R., and Zweiman, B. (1978). Histamine suppression of human lymphocyte responses to mitogens. *Cell. Immunol.* **36,** 28-36.

21

Lymphocyte Subpopulations Bearing Histamine Receptors

Marshall Plaut and Waldemar Roszkowski†
Clinical Immunology Division
Department of Medicine
The Johns Hopkins University
  School of Medicine at
The Good Samaritan Hospital
Baltimore, Maryland

The studies we have been performing in our laboratories concern modulation of immune responses. We have concentrated on the mechanisms by which histamine can affect lymphocyte function.

Lymphocytes are heterogeneous cell-types, which can be separated into B ("bone marrow-derived") lymphocytes, which differentiate into antibody-secreting plasma cells, and T (thymus-derived lymphocytes). All T lymphocytes are supposed to originate from common precursor cells or prothymocytes, in spleen and bone marrow, which travel to the thymus to differentiate into "immature" (i.e., not antigen reactive) thymocytes. These cells differentiate into antigen-reactive cells and then migrate again, into more peripheral lymphoid tissue (i.e., into the thymic medulla and into spleen and lymph node). These differentiation stages are accompanied by changes in display of surface antigens including TL, Thy-1 (formerly called Θ), the recently described Ly antigens (Ly 1, Ly2, and Ly3), and others (Boyse and Cantor, 1977).

T lymphocytes have been further divided into at least four functional subclasses: helper cells, suppressor cells, lymphokine-producing cells (that is, cells which produce and secrete factors including migration-inhibition factor (MIF)), and cytotoxic cells. Recent studies in the mouse, especially by Boyse, Cantor, and their collaborators, are of particular interest because, on the basis of differential display of Ly antigens, they have established that these four subclasses are distinct subsets of cells which are precommitted to their functional role (Boyse and Cantor, 1977; Cantor and Boyse, 1975; Cantor *et al.*, 1976). It should be emphasized that a peripheral lymphoid organ like the spleen contains macrophages, B lymphocytes, and a heterogeneous mix of

---

†Recipient of a Fulbright-Hays Fellowship

these T lymphocyte populations, i.e., immature T cells as well as precursors of helper, suppressor, lymphokine-producing and cytotoxic lymphocytes.

Our studies on lymphocyte function have concerned principally one of these subclasses, that is, cytolytically active T lymphocytes (CTL) (Cerottini and Brunner, 1974; Henney, 1977). It is possible that histamine may affect other lymphocyte functions in a manner distinct from its effect on CTL.

Our studies on the role of histamine in lymphocyte function is supported by the evidence cited in Chapter 20, that lymphocytes possess receptors for a variety of hormones, that those agents that raise cAMP leves in inflammatory cells inhibit effector functions of these cells (Bourne et al., 1974), and also by observations that basophils are chemotactically attracted to, and are present in, cell-mediated reactions (Dvorak and Dvorak, 1974; Lett-Brown et al., 1976). Thus, histamine is present at the site of delayed hypersensitivity reactions.

In this chapter we will limit our discussion to experiments with mouse splenic lymphocytes. We will describe first, experiments defining histamine receptors in mouse spleen cells, and then evidence for variations in display of functional histamine receptors. [It should be noted that most strains of mice are insensitive to histamine (Munoz and Bergman, 1968), which suggests that they have a relatively small number of histamine-type 1 receptors. It is not known whether the insensitivity is related to our observations on changing display of histamine receptors.]

The experimental system, originally described by Brunner, takes advantage of well-defined inbred strains of mice (Brunner et al., 1968; Cerottini and Brunner, 1974). C57BL/6 (H-2^b) mice are immunized with allogeneic (i.e., histoincompatible) tumor cells, in this case P815 cells (H-2^d) derived from DBA/2 mice. Analogous to graft rejection, the immune mice reject the foreign tumor and at the same time develop cytolytically active T lymphocytes in several lymphoid organs including the spleen. At intervals typically from seven to seventeen days following immunization the mice are killed and single cell suspensions prepared from the spleen. These suspensions contain approximately 80% lymphocytes. These lymphoid populations are assayed by incubating effector cells with ^{51}Cr-labeled P815 cells. Lytic activity is detected as the release of ^{51}Cr into the supernatant, an indication of the death of the target cells. The in vitro assay is quantitative and reproducible. Killing is a linear function of time, and it is also a linear function of lymphocyte concentration. Thus, the assay lends itself to mechanistic analysis. Cytolysis in this system is due entirely to cytolytically active T lymphocytes (Cerottini and Brunner, 1974).*

---

*There are several distinct cell populations which can lyse target cells (Henney, 1977). (1) A large number of cells including macrophages, neutrophils, eosinophils, platelets, and "K" cells, all possessing Fc receptors, can lyse antibody-coated target cells, although the range of target cell types may be restricted for each effector cell (Henney, 1977; Mahmond et al., 1975; Shin et al.,

Table I
Reversibility of Inhibition of Specific Cytolysis by Histamine[a]

| Histamine | | % Specific | |
Pre	Post	cytolysis	% Inhibition
—	—	18.7	—
—	$10^{-4} M$	12.3	35
—	$10^{-5} M$	12.9	31
$10^{-4} M$	—	16.5	12
$10^{-4} M$	$10^{-4} M$	12.8	32
$10^{-5} M$	—	16.7	11
$10^{-5} M$	$10^{-5} M$	12.9	31

[a] 10^7 spleen cells obtained from C57BL/6 mice 13 days following immunization with P815 were preincubated for 1 hour in MES (minimal Eagles medium plus 10% fetal calf serum) with and/or without histamine, then centrifuged and resuspended in fresh MES with or without histamine ("post"). 10^5 ^{51}Cr-P815 cells were added, and the incubation continued an additional 3 hours.

The cytolytic assay is described in detail elsewhere (Plaut *et al.,* 1975). Briefly, effector spleen cells are obtained from 7–17 days following intraperitoneal immunization of C57BL/6 mice with 10^7 P815 in 1 ml MEM. Single cell suspensions are prepared from spleens, and are mixed in 1 ml volumes in 12 × 75 mm tubes with ^{51}Cr-labeled P815 cells. (P815 cells are carried by weekly passage as ascitic fluid in syngeneic, male DBA/2 mice). These cells are washed, suspended in MES, and incubated with ^{51}Cr for 45 minutes at 37°C. The labeled cells are then washed three times in MES. [In more recent experiments, but not in the one depicted in this table, the assay is initiated by centrifuging (200 × g, 4 minutes). This centrifugation increases the kinetics of cytolysis but does not alter the effects of histamine]. Following incubation at 37°C, a 0.5-ml aliquot of cell-free supernatant is retained for counting in a gamma-spectrometer. "Total" counts are those present in ^{51}Cr-P815 cell pellet at time zero. Cytolysis is corrected for "spontaneous leak" of ^{51}Cr from P815. This leak is the same whether P815 are incubated either alone or with spleen cells from nonimmune mice. Thus:

Percent specific cytolysis =

$$\frac{cpm\ (immune\ cells + ^{51}Cr\text{-}P815) - cpm\ (nonimmune\ cells + ^{51}Cr\text{-}P815)}{cpm\ (total\ ^{51}Cr\text{-}P815)} \times 100$$

Percent inhibition of specific cytolysis by drug =

$$\frac{Specific\ cytolysis\ (immune\ cells) - Specific\ cytolysis\ (immune\ cells + drug)}{Specific\ cytolysis\ (immune\ cells)} \times 100$$

1975). (2) A natural killer (NK) cell in the mouse can lyse a distinct spectrum of target cells, especially tumor targets (Kiessling *et al.,* 1976; Henney, 1977). (3) A "spontaneous killer" cell in human peripheral blood also lyses a broad spectrum of cells; it may or may not be comparable to mouse NK cells (West *et al.,* 1977). (4) Lymphotoxin, one product secreted by T (and B) lymphokine-producing cells, can kill certain cells (Granger and Kolb, 1968).

However, the directly cytotoxic T lymphocyte arising following alloantigenic stimulation (i.e., the cell described in the present studies) is distinguishable from antibody-dependent effector cells and NK cells, and probably does not kill by secreting a lymphotoxin.

Histamine reversibly inhibits cytolysis, since when CTL are incubated briefly with histamine and then washed, their activity is restored (Plaut *et al.*, 1973a, 1975) (Table I). The inhibition by histamine is reversed by the histamine-type 2 blockers burimamide, metiamide, and cimetidine but not by histamine-type 1 blockers such as pyrilamine and diphenhydramine. Further evidence for the role of histamine-type 2 receptors comes from studies of agonists for histamine receptors (Black *et al.*, 1972; Black, 1975). The effect of inhibiting cytolysis by histamine and congeners is as one would expect for histamine-type 2 receptors. Histamine inhibits in a dose-dependent manner with a maximal inhibition at 10^{-5} M and 50% maximal at about 10^{-6} M. 4-methylhistamine, a predominantly histamine-type 2 agonist, is nearly as potent as histamine. 2-methylhistamine, a predominantly histamine-type 1 agonist, which in other systems has less than 5% of the potency of histamine on histamine-type 2 receptors, has very little effect; approximately 5×10^{-5} M is necessary to achieve half maximal inhibition.

To analyze these receptors more quantitatively, we constructed dose-response curves for inhibition of cytolysis by histamine alone or histamine in the presence of various concentrations of antagonists (here, burimamide)

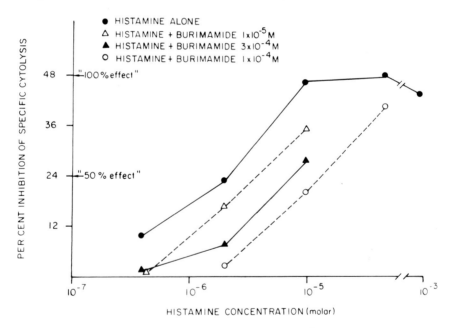

FIG. 1.   C57BL/6 mice were immunized intraperitoneally with 10^7 mastocytoma cells 14 days earlier, and spleen cell suspensions were prepared. 10^7 spleen cells were incubated with 10^{5} ^{51}Cr-P815 cells for 4 hours in the presence or absence of various concentrations of histamine and burimamide. Percent inhibition of specific cytolysis was calculated relative to cytolysis in drug-free culture tubes. Each point represents the mean of duplicate determinations, and cytolysis in drug-free mixtures is based on quadruplicate determinations. From Plant *et al.*, 1975.

Table II
K_B Values and Slopes of Schild Plots for Inhibition of Specific Cytolysis by Histamine Agonists and Antagonists[a]

Agonist	Antagonist	K_B	Slope ± S.E.
Histamine	Burimamide	$9.4 \times 10^{-6}\ M$	0.91 ± 0.15
4-methylhistamine	Burimamide	$6.9 \times 10^{-6}\ M$	0.85 ± 0.10
Histamine	Metiamide	$8.0 \times 10^{-7}\ M$	0.88 ± 0.16
4-methylhistamine	Metiamide	$2.1 \times 10^{-6}\ M$	0.89 ± 0.09

[a]Each value is based on pooled data from two separate experiments using immune mice 13 or 14 days following immunization.

(Fig. 1). As expected of a competitive antagonist burimamide shifts the dose-response curve in parallel to the right.

Similar types of curves are obtained by plotting dose-response curves in the presence of metiamide. These can be converted to Schild plots [log (dose ratio-1) versus log (antagonist)]. The Schild plot demonstrates three points (Table II): (1) As expected for competitive antagonists, the slopes are not significantly different from one. (2) K_B values (dissociation constants between histamine-type 2 antagonists and the presumptive receptors) are approximately $10^{-5}\ M$ for burimamide and $10^{-6}\ M$ for metiamide, similar to K_B values reported for histamine-type 2 receptors on other tissue types. (3) The K_B values are independent of the agonist used (i.e., histamine or 4-methylhistamine). Thus, the inhibition by histamine of cytolysis is mediated through histamine-type 2 receptors as defined by these experiments.

We have been concerned whether prolonged exposure of lymphocytes to histamine could induce desensitization, and/or whether other regulatory effects could be demonstrated. When CTL from immune mice are cultured at 4°C, cytolytic activity and inhibition by histamine are constant for at least 24 hours. However, when CTL are cultured at 37°C, while cytolytic activity remains constant, susceptibility of histamine falls within 3 hours (by an unknown mechanism). When CTL are cultured *in vitro* for 3 hours with $10^{-5}\ M$ or higher concentrations of histamine, they are "desensitized," i.e., the susceptibility to histamine falls to zero. It is interesting to note that if cells are cultured at 37°C for 24 hours, their cytolytic activity is often augmented relative to cells kept at 4°C, presumably because of the differentiation of "prekiller" cells into killer cells (Kamat and Henney, 1975). Our observations on the loss within 3 hours of functional histamine receptors are temporally related to the augmented activity after 24 hours, but the causal relationships are unknown.

Desensitization can also be demonstrated (Table III). Note that the mouse to mouse variation in lytic activity is quite high, but mouse to mouse variation in inhibition by histamine is low (e.g., 51% and 57% in the two controls here). Thus, inhibition is independent of lytic activity. The mice treated with

Table III
Effect of *in vivo* (Intraperitoneal) Administration of Histamine on Cytotoxic Activity and Inhibition by Histamine[a]

Mouse	Treatment	Percent specific cytolysis		Inhibition by histamine (%)
		No drug	Histamine	
1	None	28.2	14.0	51
2	Medium (MEM)	11.2	4.8	57
3	Histamine (3mg)	16.4	14.4	12
4	Histamine (3mg)	26.5	22.9	14

[a]C57BL/6 mice were immunized 17 days earlier with P815. At time zero, mouse 1 was untreated, mouse 2 received 1 ml of MEM intraperitoneally, and mice 3 and 4 received 3 mg histamine dihydrochloride in 1 ml MEM intraperitoneally. Two and $\frac{1}{4}$ hours later the mice were killed, and spleen suspensions were prepared and washed. These spleen cells were then used in a 4-hour cytolytic assay with 2×10^6 viable spleen cells and 4×10^4 ^{51}Cr-P815 cells, with or without histamine (10^{-5} M). Values are means of triplicates.

Viable spleen cell recoveries are respectively: no treatment: 12.4×10^7; medium: 10.2×10^7; histamine: 10.8×10^7, 6.7×10^7.

Table IV
Effects of Histamine and Antagonists on Spleen-Cell cAMP Levels[a]

Drug (M)		pmoles/10^7 cells
No drug		7.6 ± 0.6
Histamine	10^{-4}	13.7 ± 1.1
Histamine	10^{-5}	12.6 ± 1.5
Histamine	10^{-5}+ Burimamide 10^{-4}	6.0 ± 0.2
Histamine	10^{-5}+ Burimamide 10^{-5}	8.1 ± 0.9
Histamine	10^{-5}+ Metiamide 10^{-4}	7.5 ± 0.7
Histamine	10^{-5}+ Metiamide 10^{-5}	6.4 ± 1.2
Metiamide	10^{-4}	7.6 ± 0.6
Burimamide	10^{-4}	7.2 ± 0.8

[a]1.8×10^7 spleen cells from 12 day immune C57BL/6 mice were incubated in 1 ml MES with or without histamine and antagonists for 10 minutes at 37° C. The cells were centrifuged, the supernatant discarded, and the pellets resuspended in 0.5 ml 5% trichloroacetic acid. The samples were assayed for cAMP content by a method previously described in detail (Plaut *et al.*, 1975), utilizing a competitive binding assay with ^{3}H-cAMP and a binding protein from bovine adrenal gland.

Each value is the mean $\pm$ standard deviation of triplicate or quadruplicate determinations.

histamine are significantly desensitized such that inhibition is only 12% and 14%. Histamine-induced desensitization *in vivo* is consistently demonstrable between 1 and 4 hours following intraperitoneal administration of histamine and is apparently mediated through histamine-type 2 receptors. Some mice tested 24 hours after administration of histamine have lytic activity much higher than control mice, suggesting that histamine can temporarily alter an *in vivo* regulatory function; however, this augmentation is not seen consistently, and its mechanism is unknown.

These experiments have defined several properties of histamine receptors modulating CTL. To see whether histamine-type 2 receptors function by increasing cAMP levels, spleen cells were incubated with histamine, and the intracellular cAMP was determined. As shown in Table IV, histamine increases cAMP approximately twofold, and the histamine-type 2 antagonists burimamide and metiamide block the effect of histamine. Spleen cells from nonimmune mice also respond to histamine, and, even in immune mice, only 1% or fewer spleen cells are specific CTL. Thus cells in the spleen other than CTL also possess histamine receptors.

We have discussed histamine receptors in terms of inhibiting cytolysis as well as inducing cAMP elevations, and we have defined functional histamine-type 2 receptors mediating both effects. To study spleen cells directly for the presence of histamine receptors we have utiized a direct binding assay, that is, we mixed ^{3}H-histamine with cells and looked for specific "binding" of histamine to the cells. As shown in Fig. 2, binding is markedly time and temperature dependent; it is maximal in this experiment after 6 hours at 37°C. In other experiments maximal binding occurred after 2.5 hours incubation.

The binding of histamine is a linear function of cell number and also a linear function of histamine concentration up to approximately 10^{-5} *M*. Histamine inhibits binding in a dose-dependent manner, with maximal inhibition at 10^{-4} *M*. However, 2-methylhistamine, which, as already discussed is a poor activator of histamine-type 2 receptors, inhibits binding as well as histamine or 4-methylhistamine. Also, histamine-type 1 antagonists diphenhydramine and cyclizine do not inhibit binding, metiamide inhibits weakly, but burimamide is a good inhibitor. Thus, while the data is compatible with a low affinity receptor with an affinity of approximately 10^4 or 10^5, and 10^5 receptors/cell, the data with histamine agonists and antagonists define neither histamine-type 1 nor histamine-type 2 receptor specificity. This may indicate that the assay is measuring histamine uptake and metabolism as well as binding to receptors. Thus, the biological significance of the binding assay is uncertain.

The most intriguing aspects of lymphocyte histamine receptors concern differences among lymphocyte populations in susceptibility to histamine. We have made such observations concerning first, variation in histamine

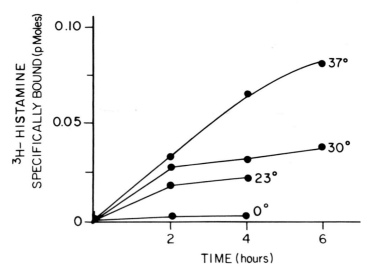

FIG. 2. Spleen cells were pooled from 5 nonimmune C57BL/6 mice and treated with 0.83% NH$_4$Cl to lyse red blood cells. 10^7 cells were incubated in 1 ml volumes with 10^{-8} M ^{3}H-histamine (i.e., 10 pmole) (specific activity 10 Ci/mM) for varying times at either 0°C, 23°C, 30°C, or 37°C. The cells were then centrifued (400 × g, 5 minutes), the pellets washed once in 3 ml cold Tris buffer, and the pellets mixed with a water soluble scintillation cocktail and counted. Specific binding in each case represents binding of cells with ^{3}H-histamine alone minus the binding of cells with ^{3}H-histamine plus 10^{-3} M unlabeled histamine. Binding in the presence of 10^{-3} M unlabeled histamine was always less than 20% of binding in the absence of excess unlabeled histamine. The "binding" of ^{3}H-histamine to glass was approximately 0.01 pmole. Each point is the mean of duplicate tubes.

receptors on CTL during the primary immune response and, second, variations in histamine receptors of lymphocyte subpopulations of nonimmune mice. We have already mentioned that histamine interacts with histamine-type 2 receptors on cytolytically active T lymphocytes to increase cAMP and inhibit cytolysis. While one might expect that all lytically active populations would be equally susceptible to inhibition by cAMP-active agents, this is not true for histamine. There is a highly significant increase in percent inhibition, from day eight to day seventeen (Plaut *et al.*, 1975; 1973b). As illustrated in Fig. 3, lytic activity first appears on day seven, reaches a peak on days ten to twelve, and then falls. When lytically active cells first appear (day eight), the inhibition by histamine is only 5%, but then progressively increases so that by day eighteen, the inhibition by histamine is about 45% and then remains relatively constant; this change in inhibition is not related to the intrinsic lytic activity. Since the inhibition is always reversed by burimamide, it is entirely due to histamine-type 2 receptor effects. We would suggest then that antigenic stimulation leads to the generation of a subpopulation of cytolytically active lymphocytes bearing histamine recep-

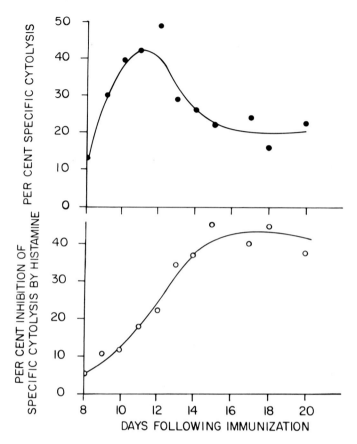

FIG. 3. C57BL/6 mice were immunized intraperitoneally with 10^7 mastocytoma cells. At intervals from 8–20 days following immunization the mice were killed and spleen cell suspensions prepared. 10^7 immune spleen cells plus 10^5 mastocytoma cells were incubated together for 4 hours. The percent specific cytolysis and percent inhibition by histamine was calculated as in Table I. The points summarize data from a total of 91 experiments. (They are the average of at least eight experiments for days 10, 11, 13, 14, and 18). From Plaut *et al.,* 1975.

tors.* Note also that the increase in histamine receptors is associated temporally with a fall in lytic activity, suggesting that histamine receptor-bearing cells may regulate CTL numbers.

Other experiments have shown that other alloantigenic mouse-strain combinations lead to similar immune response-induced increases in

---

*The altered inhibition is most likely due to changes in display of histamine receptors. It is also possible that histamine receptors are constant, and that changes in inhibition are due to changes in efficiency of linkage of receptors to the biochemical pathways leading to cytolysis. These possibiities will be distinguished only when binding assays are available, to show direct evidence of increasing histamine receptors.

histamine receptors. Also, CTL from peritoneal exudates are inhibited consistently less by histamine than splenic CTL, suggesting that locally derived CTL also differ in histamine receptor display (Plaut *et al.*, 1975).

We have attempted (unsuccessfully) to isolate histamine receptor-bearing cells. Melmon and his colleagues (Melmon *et al.*, 1972; Weinstein *et al.*, 1973) have shown that only some leukocytes (from human peripheral blood, mouse spleen, etc.) bind to histamine-coated Sepharose beads. Since this binding is inhibited by high concentrations of histamine and histamine-type 1 antihistamines, it has been presumed to be due to interaction of histamine on the beads with histamine receptors. Consequently, we first attempted to bind immune spleen populations to Sepharose beads coated, via rabbit serum albumin coupling with histamine. However, histamine receptor-bearing cells do not bind preferentially to hstamine-coated beads and, thus, cannot be purified in this manner.*

Since effector spleen cells, obtained early following immunization, are large cells, and since later in the immune response a second population of smaller cells appears (discussed in Plaut *et al.*, 1975), we attempted to relate histamine receptor-bearing cells to smaller cells. However, as shown in Fig. 4, following velocity sedimentation of spleen cells on 4% to 10% Ficoll gradients, histamine inhibition is not increased among the small cells. In fact, the small cell peak (especially fractions 7–8) has diminished inhibition by histamine. It appears from Fig. 4 that histamine receptor-bearing CTL are heterogeneously distributed among both large and small cells.

As described above, antigen-induced "maturation" results in histamine receptor display on cytolytically active T lymphocytes (Fig. 3). We asked whether lymphocyte populations that are "maturing" in terms of potential for certain types of immune function also differ in histamine receptor display. In order to study this we have looked at the cAMP responses to histamine of lymphocytes from thymus, lymph node, and spleen (Roszkowski *et al.*, 1977). As already discussed, lymphocytes from the spleen respond to histamine with a twofold to threefold increase in cAMP (Table IV). In another experiment where different lymphoid organs were compared, spleen cells had a baseline of 4.4 picomoles/10^7 cells, and histamine increased this level to 15.4 picomoles/10^7. Lymph node lymphocytes also responded with a twofold

---

*Histamine-coated beads appear to bind distinct populations of mouse cells, including suppressor T lymphocytes (Shearer *et al.*, 1972, 1974, 1977; Eichmann, 1975; Melmon *et al.*, 1976; Weinstein and Melmon, 1976). However, our data questions whether the specificity of binding is related to the histamine moiety, and other investigators (Matthyssens *et al.*, 1975) have postulated that binding is dependent on other properties such as charge. Melmon *et al.*, (1976) have noted that the cAMP responsiveness to histamine of splenic leukocytes is reduced in cells nonadherent to histamine-coated beads. However, this reduction in responsiveness is incomplete, is only partially specific, and does not occur in every experiment (Melmon *et al.*, 1974, 1976; Weinstein and Melmon, 1976), so the specificity of binding to histamine-coated beads remains unclear. See Supplemental Notes, p. 374.

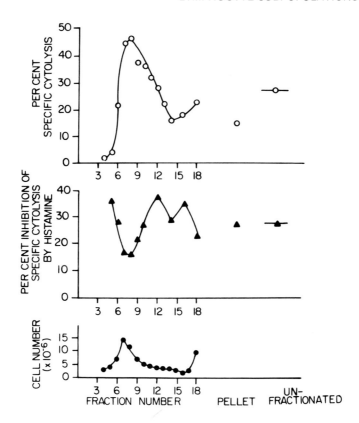

FIG. 4. Spleen cells were polled from C57BL/6 mice 13 days following immunization with 10^7 P815 cells. 3.6×10^8 cells were placed on top of a 4% to 10% Ficoll gradient as described by Green-berg (1973). Two milliliter fractions were obtained. Changes in average size [higher numbered fractions (from the bottom of the gradient) and the pellet represent larger cells] were confirmed by size distribution plotting on a Coulter counter. The cell recoveries are indicated at the bottom; the pellet contained 1.2×10^8 cells. (Total recovery = 61% of input cells.) The cytolytic assay was performed by incubating 8×10^5 effector cells with 2×10^{4} ^{51}Cr P815 for 4 1/3 hours at 37°C, with or without histamine; (also 4×10^5 effectors and 4×10^5 nonimmune spleen cells were assayed with 2×10^{4} ^{51}Cr-P815). Percent specific cytolysis and percent inhibition by histamine were calculated as described in Table I. The values for inhibition by histamine (based on 8×10^5 effectors) were confirmed because of essentially identical inhibition obtained with cytolytic assays containing 4×10^5 effectors. Values are means of duplicate or triplicate assays.

increase in cAMP, from 11.5 to 27 picomoles/10^7. In contrast thymocytes had a low baseline (e.g., 2.2), and failed to respond to histamine (up to 2.5). However, thymocytes did possess an intact adenylate cyclase since they did respond to isoproterenol. In fact, their response to isoproterenol was considerably greater (e.g., from 2.2 to 79.4) then the spleen cell response (which was only 4.4 to 16.5); so that spleen cells respond much better to histamine but much less well to isoproterenol than thymus cells.

Most thymocytes are considered immunologically immature, while thymocytes which survive *in vivo* following treatment with cortisone are considered more "mature" in that they can, for example, function as helper cells or respond to mitogens (discussed in Roszkowski *et al.*, 1977). Fig. 5 compares thymocytes from normal mice to cortisone-resistant thymocytes.

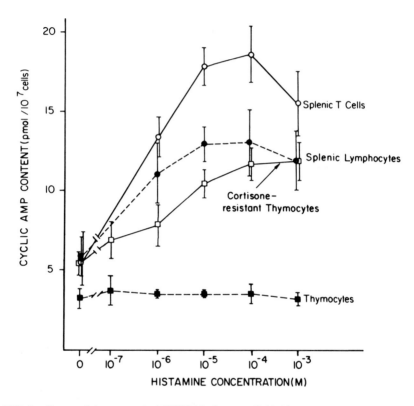

FIG. 5. Young adult age-matched C57BL/6 mice were divided into three groups. Thymocytes were obtained from untreated mice, and cortisone-resistant thymocytes were obtained 24 hours following intraperitoneal injection of 10 mg of cortisone acetate. (Thymuses from cortisone-treated mice contain only 5% of the cell number of untreated thymuses). An additional group of mice was used as a source of spleen cells. The spleen cells were treated with ammonium chloride to lyse red cells and were then filtered through glass wool to deplete adherent cells; the resultant cells are "splenic lymphocytes." Some of these cells were then incubated for 45 minutes at 37° C in nylon wool columns, and the nonadherent cells obtained ("splenic T cells"). All cell preparations were then resuspended to 2×10^7 viable cells/ml and incubated for 10 minutes with or without histamine. Intracellular cAMP was then assayed. The depletion of B cells by nylon wool passage was estimated by direct immunofluorescent staining by rhodamine conjugated goat antisera to mouse Fab fragments; unfractionated spleen cells contained 55% Ig-positive cells, while nylon wool-passed cells contained 19% Ig-positive cells. Each point represents the mean ± standard deviation of quadruplicate determinations. From Roszkowski *et al.*, 1977. Copyright 1977 by the American Association for the Advancement of Science.

Table V
**Effect of Antiserum to Thy 1.2 Antigen, in the presence of
Complement, on Histamine- or Isoproterenol-Induced Increases
in cAMP[a]**

Drug (M)		cAMP (pmole/10^7 cells)	
		Normal mouse serum	Antiserum to thy 1.2
None		4.8 ± 1.9	5.2 ± 1.1
Histamine	10^{-3}	12.3 ± 2.8	4.3 ± 1.7
Histamine	10^{-4}	13.9 ± 4.2	4.9 ± 2.0
Histamine	10^{-5}	11.9 ± 3.6	5.6 ± 2.3
Isoproterenol	10^{-5}	16.5 ± 2.6	14.3 ± 0.5

[a]Groups of ten C57BL/6 mice were killed by cervical dislocation, and spleen cells were obtained. Spleen cell suspensions (2×10^7 cells/ml) were incubated with a 1 to 10 dilution of normal mouse serum or antiserum to thy 1.2 and a 1 to 20 dilution of rabbit serum (as a source of complement) for 45 minutes at 37°C. The cells were washed, and their viability was assessed by erythrosin B exclusion. They were then resuspended (2×10^7 viable cells/ml) and incubated with or without drug; cAMP was then assayed. The results are expressed as the mean ± standard deviation of quadruplicate cultures. From Roszkowski et al., 1977. Copyright 1977 by the American Association for the Advancement of Science.

Histamine over a wide range of concentrations does not alter the cAMP level of thymocytes. However, cortisone-resistant thymocytes do respond to histamine in a dose-dependent fashion with a twofold increase in cAMP, at 10^{-4} M. Splenic lymphocytes (here depleted of macrophages on glass wool) are similar to unfractionated spleen cells described earlier (i.e., about a twofold increase in cAMP in response to histamine). However, when these spleen cells are passed through nylon wool columns to remove most B cells, the resultant population, which is enriched in splenic T lymphocytes, responds to histamine with a threefold to fourfold increase in cAMP, suggesting that there is a progressive increase in responsiveness to histamine of T cells, from thymocytes to cortisone-resistant thymocytes to splenic T lymphocytes.

If splenic T lymphocytes respond to histamine more than do unfractionated spleen cells, then B lymphocytes may have only a minimal response. This is confirmed, as shown in Table V. The cAMP response to histamine of spleen cells treated with normal mouse serum and complement is similar to untreated lymphocytes—a twofold increase. However, when cells are treated with antibody to thy 1.2 antigen (formerly called anti-θ) and complement, a treatment which eliminates T cells and leaves B cells, the cell population fails to respond to histamine. The lack of response to histamine of B cells is not because they lack adenylate cyclase or that the antibody and complement treatment has destroyed the enzyme, because B cells can respond to isoproterenol. Thus, it may be concluded that B cells lack functional histamine receptors.

In summary, we can make the following points concerning the effects of histamine on mouse lymphocyte populations. Histamine inhibits cytolysis through interaction with histamine-type 2 receptors. Prolonged *in vitro* or *in vivo* exposure to histamine of lytically active cell populations desensitizes these cells to histamine, and possibly alters some regulatory cell functions. Histamine also increases cAMP levels in several lymphoid cell populations, especially the spleen, via histamine-type 2 receptors. The "binding" of ^{3}H-histamine to spleen cells may represent binding to low affinity receptors plus uptake and/or metabolism.

Histamine receptors are not randomly distributed, but are selectively displayed on lymphocyte subpopulations: histamine receptors increase on cytolytically active T lymphocytes during the primary immune response to alloantigen. Splenic B lymphocytes possess no functional histamine receptors. Finally, the differentiation of T lymphocytes from thymocytes to cortisone-resistant thymocytes to splenic T lymphocytes is accompanied by complex hormone receptor changes including increases of functional histamine receptors and decreases of functional beta-adrenergic (i.e., isoproterenol-responsive) receptors. We suspect that these alterations of histamine receptor display indicate an important role for histamine in modulating lymphocyte function.

SUPPLEMENTAL NOTES

Rocklin (1977) has reported that histamine inhibits MIF production by antigen-sensitized guinea pig lymphocytes, indirectly: it induces suppressor cells to secrete a soluble factor, which in turn inhibits the MIF-producing cells. Rocklin et al (1978) have found that cells depleted on histamine coated beads make MIF, but that histamine does not inhibit MIF production by these depleted cells. Thus guinea pig lymphocytes may differ from mouse lymphocytes, since the guinea pig cells apparently can be depleted of histamine receptor-bearing cells on these beads. (These results might also be explained, partially, if the cells are desensitized by exposure to histamine, and do not resensitize in culture; cf. p. 365.)

ACKNOWLEDGMENTS

Many of the studies reported here were done in collaboration with Drs. Lawrence M. Lichtenstein, Elizabeth Gillespie, and Christopher S. Henney. Neil K. Dorsey, Alana Sullivan, and Linda Nordin provided expert technical assistance. Supported by Grants AI12810 and AI11334 from the National Institutes of Allergy and Infectious Diseases, the National Institutes of Health. Publication No. 318 of the O'Neill Research Laboratories, The Good Samaritan Hospital.

REFERENCES

Black, J. W. (1975). Histamine receptors, in "Receptors and Cellular Pharmacology." (E. Klinge, ed.) pp. 3–16. Proceedings of the Sixth International Congress of Pharmacology, Helsinki, Finland.

Black, J. W., Duncan, W. A. M., Durant, C. J., Ganellin, C. R., Parsons, E. M. (1972). Definition and antagonism of histamine H_2-receptors. *Nature (London)* **236**, 385–390.

Bourne, H. R., Lichtenstein, L. M., Henney, C. S., Melmon, K. L., Weinstein, Y., and Shearer, G. M. (1974). Modulation of inflammation and immunity by cyclic AMP. *Science,* **184**, 19–28.

Boyse, E. A., Cantor, H. (1977). Surface characteristics of T-lymphocyte populations. Hospital Practice 81-88, April.

Brunner, K. T., Mauel, J., Cerottini, J. -C., and Chapuis, B. (1968). Quantitative assay for the lytic action of immune lymphoid cells on ^{51}Cr-labeled allogeneic target cells *in vitro:* inhibition by isoantibody and by drugs. *Immunology,* **14**, 181–196.

Cantor, H., and Boyse, E. A. (1975). Functional subclasses of T lymphocytes bearing different Ly antigens. I. The generation of functionally distinct T-cell subclasses is a differentiative process independent of antigen. *J. Exp. Med.* **141**, 1376–1389.

Cantor, H., Shen, F. W., and Boyse, E. A. (1976). Separation of helper T cells from suppressor T cells expressing different Ly components. II. Activation by antigen: after immunization antigen-specific suppressor and helper activities are mediated by distinct T-cell subclasses. *J. Exp. Med.* **143**, 1391–1401.

Cerottini, J. -C., and Brunner, K. T. (1974). Cell-mediated cytotoxicity, allograft rejection and tumor immunity. *Adv. Immunol.* **18**, 67–132.

Dvorak, H. F., Dvorak, A. M. (1974). Cutaneous basophil hypersensitivity, in "Progress in Immunology II" (L. Brent and J. Holborow, eds.) Vol. 3, pp. 171–181. North Holland Publishing Company, Amsterdam.

Eichmann, K. (1975). Idiotype suppression. II. Amplification of a suppressor cell with anti-idiotype activity. *Eur. J. Immunol.* **5**, 511–517.

Granger, G. A., and Kolb, W. P. (1968). Lymphocyte *in vitro* cytotoxicity: mechanisms of immune and nonimmune small lymphocyte mediated target L cell destruction. *J. Immunol* **101**, 111–120.

Henney, C. S. (1977). Mechanisms of tumor cell destruction, in "Mechanisms of Tumor Immunity." (I. Green, S. Cohen, and R. T. McCluskey, eds.) pp. 55–86. John Wiley and Sons, New York.

Kamat, R., and Henney, C. S. (1975). Studies on T cell clonal expansion. I. Suppression of killer T cell production *in vivo. J. Immunol.* **115**, 1592–1598.

Kiessling, R., Petranyi, G., Kärre, K., Jondal, M., Tracey, D., and Wigzell, H. (1976). Killer cells: A functional comparison between natural immune T-cell and antibody-dependent *in vitro* systems. *J. Exp. Med.* **143**, 772–780.

Lett-Brown, M. A., Boetcher, D. A., and Leonard, E. J. (1976). Chemotactic response of normal human basophils to C5a and to lymphocyte-derived chemotactic factor. *J. Immunol.* **117**, 246–252.

Mahmoud, A. A. F., Warren, K. S., and Peters, P. S. (1975). A role for the eosinophil in acquired resistance to *Schistosoma mansoni* infection as determined by anti-eosinophil serum. *J. Exp. Med.* **142**, 805–813.

Matthyssens, G. E., Hurwitz, E., Girol, D., and Sela, M. (1975). Binding of histamine-and other ligand-conjugated macromolecules to lymphocytes. *Molec. Cellul. Biochem.* **7**, 119–126.

Melmon, K. L., Bourne, H. R., Weinstein, Y., and Sela, M. (1972). Receptors for histamine can be detected on the surface of selected leukocytes. *Science* **177**, 707–709.

Melmon, K. L., Weinstein, Y., Shearer, G. M., Bourne, H. R., and Bauminger, S. (1974). Separation of specific antibody-forming cells by their adherence to insolubilized endogenous hormones. *J. Clin. Invest.* **53**, 22-30.

Melmon, K. L., Weinstein, Y., Bourne, H. R., Shearer, G., Poon, T., Krasny, L., and Segal, S. (1976). Isolation of cells with specific receptors for amines: opportunities and problems, in "Cell Membrane Receptors for Viruses, Antigens, and Antibodies, Polypeptide Hormones, and Small Molecules." (R. F. Beers, Jr., and E. G. Bassett, eds.) pp. 117-134. Raven Press, New York.

Munoz, J., and Bergman, R. K. (1968). Histamine-sensitizing factors from microbial agents with special reference to *Bordetella pertussis. Bact. Rev.* **32**, 103-126.

Plaut, M., Lichtenstein, L. M., Gillespie, E., and Henney, C. S. (1973a). Studies on the mechanism of lymphocyte-mediated cytolysis. IV. Specificity of the histamine receptor on effector T cells. *J. Immunol.* **111**, 389-394.

Plaut, M., Lichtenstein, L. M., and Henney, C. S. (1973b). Increase in histamine receptors on thymus-derived effector lymphocytes during the primary immune response to alloantigen. *Nature (London)* **244**, 284-287.

Plaut, M., Lichtenstein, L. M., and Henney, C. S. (1975). Properties of a subpopulation of T cells bearing histamine receptors. *J. Clin. Invest.* **55**, 856-874.

Rocklin, R.E. (1977). Histamine-induced suppressor factor (HSF): Effect on migration inhibitory factor (MIF) production and proliferation. J. Immunol. *118:* 1734-1738.

Rocklin, R.E., Greineder, D., Littman, B.H., and Melmon, K.L. (1978). Modulation of cellular immune function *in vitro* by histamine receptor-bearing lymphocytes: Mechanism of action. Cell Immunol. *37:* 162-173.

Roszkowski, W., Plaut, M., and Lichtenstein, L. M. (1977). Selective display of histamine receptors on lymphocytes. *Science* **195**, 683-685.

Shearer, G. M., Melmon, K. L., Weinstein, Y., and Sela, M. (1972). Regulation of antibody response by cells expressing histamine receptors. *J. Exp. Med.* **136**, 1302-1307.

Shearer, G. M., Weinstein, Y., and Melmon, K. L. (1974). Enhancement of immune response potential of mouse lymphoid cells fractionated over insolubilized conjugated histamine columns. *J. Immunol.* **113**, 597-607.

Shearer, G. M., Simpson, E., Weinstein, Y., and Melmon, K. L. (1977). Fractionation of lymphocytes involved in the generation of cell-mediated cytotoxicity over insolubilized conjugated histamine columns. *J. Immunol.* **118**, 756-761.

Shin, H. W., Hayden, M., Langley, S., Kaliss, N., and Smith, M. R. (1975). Antibody-mediated suppression of grafted lymphomas. III. Evaluation of the role of thymic function, non-thymus-derived lymphocytes, macrophages, platelets, and polymorphonuclear leukocytes in syngeneic and allogeneic hosts. *J. Immunol.* **114**, 1255-126.

Weinstein, Y., and Melmon, K. L. (1976). Control of immune responses by cyclic AMP and lymphocytes that adhere to histamine columns. *Immunol. Comm.* **5**, 401-416.

Weinstein, Y., Melmon, K. L., Bourne, H. R., and Sela, M., (1973). Specific leukocyte receptors for small endogenous hormones. Detection by cell binding to insolubilized hormone preparations. *J. Clin. Invest.* **52**, 1349-1361.

West, W. H., Cannon, G. B., Kay, H. D., Bonnard, G. D., and Herberman, R. B. (1977). Natural cytotoxic reactivity of human lymphocytes against a myeloid cell line: characterization of effector cells. *J. Immunol.* **118**, 355-361.

PART VI
MEDICINAL CHEMISTRY

22

Chemical Development and Properties of Histamine H$_2$-Receptor Agonists and Antagonists

C. Robin Ganellin
The Research Institute
Smith Kline and French Laboratories Limited
Welwyn Garden City
Hertfordshire, England

CHEMICAL CHARACTERIZATION OF HISTAMINE

The pharmacological actions of histamine appear to be mediated by at least two distinct classes of receptor, defined as H$_1$ (Ash and Schild, 1966) and H$_2$ (Black *et al.*, 1972a); for a recent review of their distribution in different tissues, see Chand and Eyre (1975). The existence of two receptor populations raises the interesting question of whether the chemical mechanism of histamine interaction differs between the two receptor types. At present, very little is known about the structure of these receptors at the molecular level so that to attempt an answer one has to rely on studies of histamine chemistry. It is, thus, necessary to identify chemical properties of histamine which may differentiate its action at H$_1$ and H$_2$ receptors.

One approach is to characterize histamine chemically in great detail in the expectation that certain specialized properties will become evident. This method is unlikely to provide conclusive answers but it ought to be capable of posing some pertinent questions. A complementary approach is to identify chemical properties of histamine, which may be critical for its biological activity, by investigating closely related structural analogs. The procedure requires chemical comparisons to be made between such analogs and histamine in a manner which leads to correlations between chemical properties and biological activity. Structure-activity analysis is, however, complicated by the fact that histamine in aqueous solution is a mixture of various ionic species, tautomers, and conformers; which of these species may be biologically important is not self evident. Furthermore, the various species are in equilibria, i.e., they are undergoing interconversion, and indeed, these very processes may have biological significance.

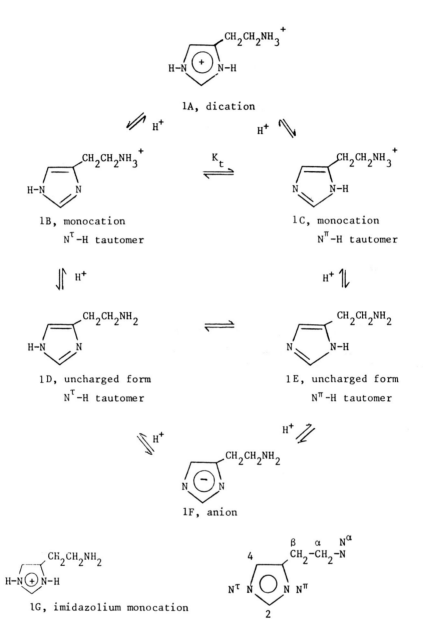

1A, dication

K_t

1B, monocation

N^τ-H tautomer

1C, monocation

N^π-H tautomer

1D, uncharged form

N^τ-H tautomer

1E, uncharged form

N^π-H tautomer

1F, anion

1G, imidazolium monocation

(2) Histamine numbering according to Black and Ganellin (1974)

FIG. 1. Ionic and tautomeric equilibria between histamine species. Side chain deprotonation of dication 1A furnishes the monocation 1G and this must also be present, although the concentration of 1G is likely to be less than 1 part in 100 relative to 1B and 1C.

378

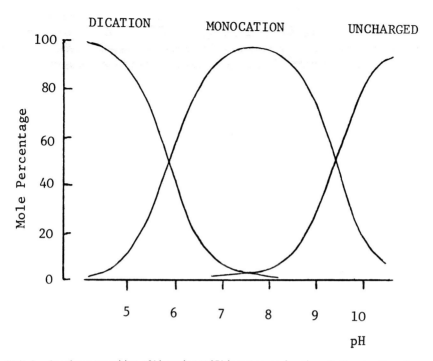

FIG. 2. Species composition of histamine at 37° in water as a function of pH, using the values pK$_{a1}$ = 5.80 and pK$_{a2}$ = 9.40.

Histamine Protonation and Tautomerism

Titration of histamine in aqueous solution gives three stoichiometric pK_a values. Fully protonated histamine is a dication (1A; Fig. 1) and the first stoichiometric ionization constant (pK_{a1} = 5.80 at 37°C) corresponds to dissociation from the ring NH to give the monocation. The second ionization constant (pK_{a2} = 9.40 at 37°C) corresponds to dissociation at the side chain $-NH_3^+$ group to give the uncharged molecule. At high pH, the ring again ionizes at NH (pK_{a2} = 14) to give an anion (Paiva *et al.,* 1970). The relative populations of the species as a function of pH are shown graphically in Fig. 2. The curve for the monocation reaches a maximum in the pH range 7–8; since this is also the physiological pH range, it suggests (but does not prove) that the physiologically important species is the monocation. At pH 7.4, 96% of histamine is present as the monocation; however, it must be remembered that the pH could be considerably lower in the vicinity of some membranes, and below pH 5.8 the dication predominates. Values for the relative populations of species at pH 7.4 and 5.4 are given in Table I. Because the imidazole ring possesses two nitrogen sites for proton dissociation, both monocation and

Table I

Population (expressed as mole percentage) of Histamine
Species in Aqueous Solution[a] at pH 7.4 and 5.4, respectively

Species		Mole percentage of species	
		At pH 7.4	At pH 5.4
Dication	1A	2.5%	71.5%
Monocation	1B + 1C	96.6%	28.5%
Uncharged	1D + 1E	1%	$3 \times 10^{-3}\%$
Anion	1F	$2.5 \times 10^{-7}\%$	$10^{-11}\%$

[a]Derived from pK_a values at 37° (Paiva *et al.*, 1970): $pK_{a1} = 5.80$; $pK_{a2} = 9.40$; $pK_{a3} = 14$.

uncharged forms are tautomeric mixtures; the full series of equilibria relating the various species is given in Fig. 1. The relative population of tautomers has been estimated for the monocation from pK_a data by comparing the corresponding N-methyl or N-benzyl derivatives (Ganellin, 1973a). The ratio of concentrations of the two monocation tautomers ([1B]/[1C]), given by the tautomeric equilibrium constant K_t was found to be approximately 4.2. Thus, according to these measurements, about 80% of histamine monocation in water is in the N^τ-H tautomeric form (for histamine numbering shown in formula 2, see Black and Ganellin 1974) and 20% in the N^π-H form. The tautomeric equilibrium constant for the uncharged molecule is unknown; an attempt has been made to calculate the relative tautomer stabilities of the isolated molecule by molecular orbital procedures but substantiation of the result by physical measurement is still required (Kang and Chou, 1975).

Histamine Conformation

Histamine is a conformationally flexible molecule. Being a 1, 2-disubstituted ethane, rotation occurs about the single bonds shown in structure 3 (Fig. 3) and the conformation can be described in terms of the three torsion angles Θ_1, Θ_2, Θ_3. For histamine itself, Θ_3, is relatively unimportant (since the NH_3^+ group is symmetrical) and the special characteristics of the molecule are determined by Θ_1, which describes the orientation of the imidazole ring, and Θ_2 which represents the orientation within the side chain. The conformational equilibria for the various ionic species have been widely studied using nuclear magnetic resonance spectroscopy (nmr) and molecular orbital calculations (Kier, 1968; Green *et al.*, 1971; Ganellin *et al.*, 1973a; Ham *et al.*, 1973; Pullman and Port, 1974; see Table II for further references).

As with other disubstituted ethanes, the most favored conformers are the trans (fully extended, $\Theta_2 = 180°$) and gauche (folded, $\Theta_2 = 60°$ or $300°$) in which the hydrogen atoms within the side chain have a staggered arrangement

(3)

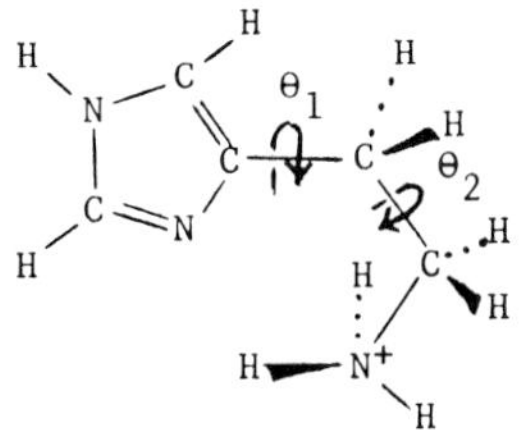

(4) Trans (extended) conformation, $\theta_2 = 180°$, (antiperiplanar)

(5) Gauche (folded) conformation, $\theta_2 = 60°$ or $300°$, (synclinal)

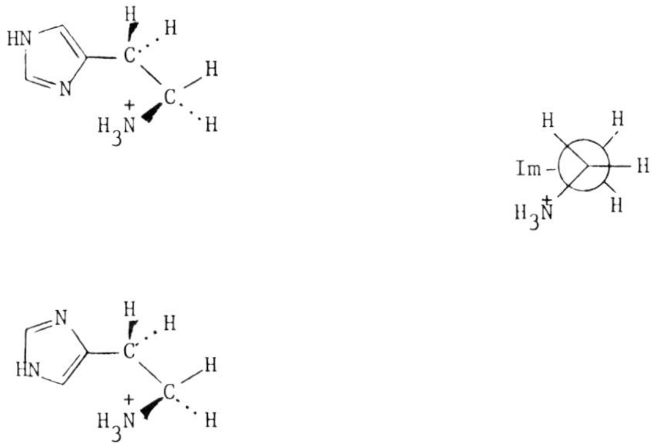

FIG. 3.   Histamine monocation (N^T-H tautomer) showing torsion angles (θ), and trans and gauche conformations; θ_1 measures the rotation of the imidazole ring, while θ_2 measures the rotation within the side chain. The form shown in (3) corresponds to $\theta_1 = 180°$, $\theta_2 = 0°$.

(Fig. 3 structures 4 and 5). However, the different methods of calculation disagree as to the relative stabilities of the conformers. The less sophisticated EHT (see Table II for key to abbreviations) or empirical treatments predict stability for both trans and gauche conformations in histamine cation and dication, with the trans conformer being slightly more stable by approximately 1 kcal/mole. These conclusions agree with experimental results derived from nuclear magnetic resonance (nmr) studies for aqueous solution. Surprisingly, the more sophisticated PCILO method gives strikingly different results and predicts conformation to be dependent upon the type of cation, viz: the dication is entirely trans but the monocation is overwhelmingly

Table II
Calculated and Observed Preferred Conformers of Histamine Species by Different Procedures[a]

Procedure	Dication	Monocation	Uncharged	Reference
Calculations on isolated molecule				
EHT		T + G		Kier, 1968
EHT	T + G	T + G		Ganellin et al., 1973a
Empirical	T + G	T + G		Kumbar, 1975
INDO		G	G	Green et al., 1971
PCILO		G	G	Coubeils et al., 1971
PCILO	T	G		Pullman and Port, 1974
CNDO/2	T	G		Ganellin et al., 1973a
STO-3G	T	G		Pullman and Port, 1974
Calculations on the modified molecule				
Hydrated PCILO	}T + (G)	T + G		Pullman and Port, 1974
F⁻ counterion CNDO	}T + G	G		Abraham and Birch, 1975
Measurement of solutions				
nmr in D₂O	T + G	T + G		Casy et al., 1970
				Ham et al., 1973
				Ganellin et al., 1973a
nmr in CDCl₃			T + G	Pepper
ir in CHCl₃			T + G	Byrn et al., 1976
Measurement of solid				
Crystal	T	T	T	see Table III

[a]The abbreviations used are: EHT, extended Hückel theory; INDO, intermediate neglect of differential overlap; PCILO, perturbative configuration interaction using localized orbitals; CNDO, complete neglect of differential overlap; nmr, nuclear magnetic resonance spectroscopy; ir, infra red spectroscopy; T, trans conformation, $\theta = 180°$, antiperiplanar; G, gauche conformation, $\theta = 60°$ or $300°$, synclinal.

guache. Calculations using the CNDO/2 and INDO methods give results similar to the PCILO calculations and these have also been confirmed by STO-3G calculations *ab initio* on the isolated molecule. The discrepancies between these calculations for the isolated molecule and the data from aqueous solution have been partly resolved by modifications that take account of a counterion or include molecules of water (the "supermolecule" approach of Pullman in which the hydration sites in histamine are bound by water of solvation); the results are summarized in Table II. However it is unlikely that the discrepancies are due solely to the presence or absence of water. Similar discrepancies are found for histamine base; the INDO and

PCILO procedures predict stability for the gauche conformer but both trans and gauche conformers of histamine base appear to be present in chloroform solution. Furthermore, in the anhydrous crystal, histamine monocation and base are present as the trans conformer, yet both species are predicted by the INDO and PCILO procedures to be overwhelmingly in gauche forms.

The preferred orientation Θ_1 of the imidazole ring also varies according to the molecular orbital calculation procedure, but the only physical measurements are crystallographic. Crystallography cannot identify relative preference under equilibrium conditions but it does indicate stable forms under a particular set of circumstances, viz., when "frozen" in the crystal lattice. So far, for the dication, monocation, and uncharged (free base) species, only the trans conformation has been obtained but various orientations of the imidazole ring have been found depending on the salt used for crystal determination. Values of Θ_1 the dihedral angle between the planes formed, respectively, by the imidazole ring and the -C-C-N side chain, are given in Table III together with the counter ions and literature references.

The molecular orbital calculations also show that there are substantial energy barriers to interconversion between trans and cis conformations but that rotation of the imidazole ring is much less restricted. These results are in keeping with the crystallographic findings viz. a single value for Θ_2 but a multiplicity of values for Θ_1.

The fact that various forms of histamine exist means that they have to be considered for possible biological significance. The best indications of their likely importance have come from structure–activity considerations of analogs (congeners), and this is discussed in the next section.

Table III
Orientations, θ_1, of the Imidazole Ring in the Various Histamine Species Found by Crystallography[a]

Salt	Dication $\theta_1°$	Monocation $\theta_1°$	Uncharged $\theta_1°$	Reference
Base			66.3	Bonnet and Ibers, 1973
Bromide		89.7		Prout et al., 1974
Bromide	30			Decou, 1964
Chloride	26.7			Bonnet et al., 1975
Phosphate	82.5			Veidis et al., 1969
Sulphate I	4.4			Yamane et al., 1973
II	9.2			
Tetrachlorocobaltate	7			Bonnet and Jeannin, 1972

[a]In each case the side chain has the trans conformation; θ_1 represents the dihedral angle between the two planes formed respectively by the imidazole ring and the –C–C–N side chain.

CHEMICAL EVIDENCE FOR THE ACTIVE FORM
OF HISTAMINE AT H_1 AND H_2 RECEPTORS

Over 30 years ago, Niemann and Hays (1942) concluded that the active form of histamine was the monocationic tautomer 1B. This conclusion followed from the original finding by Water *et al.* (1941) that 2-pyridylethylamine (6)* was a histamine-like stimulant of guinea pig smooth muscle contraction, whereas 4-pyridylethylamine (10) was not active (see Fig. 4). Neimann and Hays also noted that since 3-pyridylethylamine (9) was not

2-Pyridylethylamine monocation (6) compared with N^τ-tautomer (1B)

of histamine monocation: Formally, these have fragment (7) in common and

can chelate a proton between the nitrogen atoms as in structure (8) –

but see text:

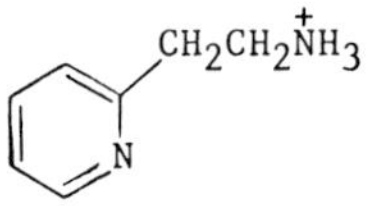

(6) 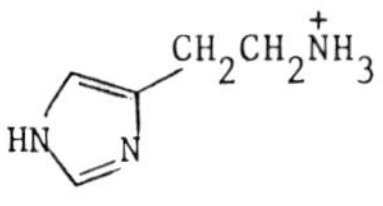   (1B)

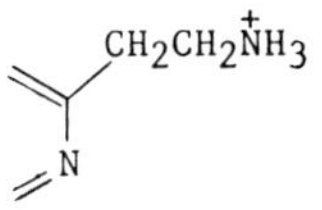

(7) 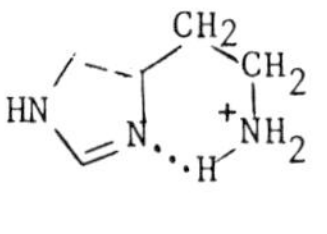   (8)

3-Pyridylethylamine (9) and 4-pyridylethylamine (10) monocations

compared with N^π-H tautomer (1C) of histamine monocation:

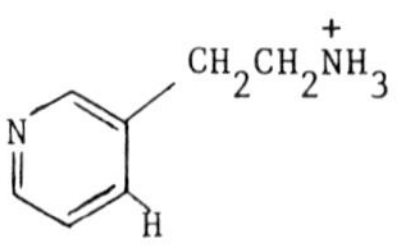

(9) 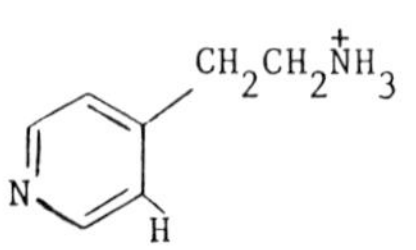   (10) 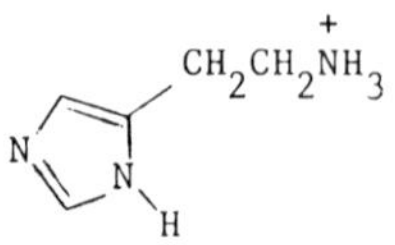   (1C)

FIG. 4.   The three isomeric pyridylethylamine structures compared with histamine tautomers.

---

*Numbers in parentheses indicate compounds in Tables.

active, then histamine tautomer 1C must also be devoid of histamine-like activity; they also suggested that tautomer 1B would be stabilised by intramolecular hydrogen bonding and asserted that for activity, chelation between the nitrogen atoms should occur in the cation (e.g., structure 8). Chemical evidence for such stabilisation has, however, been lacking and recent work on histamine argues against such structures as having particular stability, at least in aqueous solution; e.g., the pK_a studies by Paiva *et al.* (1970) on the thermodynamics of proton dissociation, the pK_a studies by Ganellin (1973a) on the relative tautomer stabilities, and the nmr investigations by Ham *et al.* (1973) and Ganellin *et al.* (1973a) on conformer stabilities.

Extensive examinations of other heterocyclic analogs of histamine have been carried out and comparison made with various actions of histamine, e.g., for stimulating contractions of the isolated guinea pig ileum (Lee and Jones, 1949) for causing a depression of the blood pressure of the anesthetized cat (Lee and Jones, 1949; Lin *et al.*, 1962), as stimulants of mammalian gastric acid secretion (Grossman *et al.*, 1952; Lin *et al.*, 1962; Ash and Schild, 1966), for inhibition of the isolated rat uterus (Ash and Schild, 1966). The findings that some compounds showed a separation in activities relative to histamine has complicated the consideration of structure–activity relationships (Barlow 1964; Jones 1966). This has become less of a problem now that the activities can be classified in terms of H_1- or H_2- receptor involvement (Ash and Schild, 1966, Black *et al.*, 1972a). Some examples of compounds showing relative selectivity as H_1- or H_2- agonists are shown in Table IV.

Evidence for the Monocation as an Active Form

At pH 7.4, the main form of histamine is the monocation, but at low pH (eg., at pH 5.4, as may occur in the vicinity of some membranes) the dication predominates (vide supra, Table 1). Thus, both monocation and dication are forms likely to be active in histamine-receptor interactions. Indications that the dication is probably not an active form come from comparing active histamine analogs which have a heterocyclic ring with a very low pK_a so that the population of dication is extremely small. Examples such as 3-(1, 2, 4-triazolyl) ethylamine (17) 2-thiazolylethylamine (12) and 4-chlorohistamine (15) are shown in Table V. These compounds have very low dication populations even at pH 5.4 (eg., 3-(1, 2, 4-triazolyl) ethylamine has only 0.01% of molecules in the dication at pH 5.4) and yet they have at least 10% of the potency of histamine at either H_1 or H_2 receptors; thus, the dication is unlikely to be an active species.

There is less evidence as to whether the uncharged (free base) form is active. All compounds so far known to be active are strongly basic amines (see Jones 1966) which exist mainly in cationic forms at physiological pH. The tertiary amine N^α, N^α-dimethylhistamine (18) is active at H_1 and H_2 receptors but the

Table IV

H$_1$- and H$_2$-Receptor Activities of Some Selective Agonists Assayed in our Laboratories

Compound name and structure	Agonist activity relative to histamine = 100 (95% confidence limits)		
	H$_1$	H$_2$	
	ileum[a]	g.s.[b]	atrium[c]
Selective H$_1$			
6A 2-Pyridylethylamine	5.6(5.0–6.3)[d]	~0.2[e]	2.5(1.5–3.6)[f]
6B N$^\alpha$-Methyl-2-pyridylethylamine (Betahistine)[g]	8.0(7.2–8.8)[h]	~0.2[h]	1.5(1.2–1.7)[i]
11A 2-Methylhistamine	16.5(15.1–18.1)[j,k]	2.0[j]	4.4(4.1–4.8)[j]
11B 2,N$^\alpha$,N$^\alpha$-Trimethylhistamine	16.8(15.8–17.7)[l]	1.4[l]	
12 2-Thiazolylethylamine	26(19.7–32.7)[m]	~0.3	2.2(2.0–2.5)
Selective H$_2$			
13 3-Pyrazolylethylamine (Betazole)[n]	0.12(0.10–0.14)[o]	~0.5[p]	2.1(1.4–2.8)

14A	4-Methylhistamine[q] $CH_3\text{-}CH_2CH_2NH_2$ (imidazole)	$0.23(0.20\text{-}0.27)^{i,q}$	$39^{i,r}$	$43(40\text{-}46)^{j}$
14B	4.N^{α}-Dimethylhistamine[s] $CH_3\text{-}CH_2CH_2NHMe$ (imidazole)	$0.16(0.1\text{-}0.2)^{i,s}$	$8.2^{i,t}$	$36(26\text{-}49)$
14C	4.N^{α},N^{α}-Trimethylhistamine $CH_3\text{-}CH_2CH_2NMe_2$ (imidazole)	0.1^{i}	$3.0^{i,u}$	$13.5(12.7\text{-}14.2)$
15	4-Chlorohistamine $Cl\text{-}CH_2CH_2NH_2$ (imidazole)	$1.7^{i,w}$	12	11^{v}
16	S-(3-Dimethylaminopropyl)isothiourea (Dimaprit)[x] $\begin{array}{c}H_2N\\HN\end{array}\!\!\text{C-S}(CH_2)_3NMe_2$	$<0.0001^{x}$	19.5^{x}	$71(61\text{-}81)^{x}$

[a] Tested for stimulating contraction of isolated guinea pig ileum in the presence of atropine (Durant *et al.*, 1975a unless otherwise indicated).

[b] Tested by rapid intravenous injection for stimulation of gastric acid secretion in the atropinized and vagotomized anesthetized rat (Durant *et al.*, 1975a, unless otherwise indicated).

[c] Tested for stimulation of rate in the spontaneously beating isolated guinea pig right atrium in the presence of propranolol (previously unreported results are from R.C. Blakemore and M.E. Parsons, Smith Kline and French Laboratories Ltd., Welwyn Garden City, England).

[d] Ash and Schild (1966) report 3%; see also Arunlakshana and Schild (1959).

[e] Ash and Schild (1966) report 0.7%.

[f] Partial agonist; only achieved 49% (±2.5% SEM; n = 8) of the maximal response to histamine, (R.C. Blakemore and M.E. Parsons).

(continued)

Table IV (continued)

[g] Serc.

[h] R.C. Blakemore and M.E. Parsons.

[i] Partial agonist; only achieved 39% ($\pm$10% SEM; $n = 4$) of the maximal response to histamine, (R.C. Blakemore and M.E. Parsons).

[j] Black et al., (1972a).

[k] Lee and Jones (1949) report 30%.

[l] Durant et al., (1976).

[m] Lee and Jones (1949) report 30%.

[n] Histalog (from Eli Lilly and Co.).

[o] Ash and Schild (1966) report 0.06%; Lin et al. (1962) report 1%; van den Brink (1969) reports 0.02%.

[p] Ash and Schild (1966) report 4.2%. Rosiere and Grossman (1951) tested this compound given subcutaneously in dogs and later (Grossman et al., 1952) reported that it had approximately 1.4% of the activity of histamine.

[q] Bertaccini et al. (1972) report 1%; they name this compound as 5-methylhistamine.

[r] Bertaccini et al. (1972) report 40%.

[s] Bertaccini et al. (1976) report 0.2%; they name this compound as 5-methyl-N-methylhistamine.

[t] Bertaccini et al. (1976) report 25%.

[u] Also studied by Impicciatore et al. (1974) in cats.

[v] R.C. Blakemore in Ganellin (1974).

[w] H_1 activity is probably an overestimate; material may have been contaminated with histamine.

[x] Parsons et al. (1977).

Table V

Histamine Congeners with Weakly Basic Rings. Ring pK_a Values, Mole Percentages at 37° of Dication at pH 7.4 and 5.4, and H_1- or H_2-agonist activities. For All Compounds Except Histamine, the Mole Percentage of Monocation is Greater than 97% at Either pH

Compound name and structure	Ring pK_a 37°	Mole percentage of dication at pH 7.4	pH 5.4	Receptor Activity[a] H_1 ileum	H_2 g.s.
Histamine $HN{\sim}N$ —CH$_2$CH$_2$NH$_2$	5.8	2.5%	71.5%	100	100
(12) 2-Thiazolylethylamine (thiazole ring, CH$_2$CH$_2$NH$_2$)	~1.5[b]	10^{-4}	10^{-2}	26	
(15) 4-Chlorohistamine (imidazole ring, Cl, CH$_2$CH$_2$NH$_2$)	3.1[c]	5×10^{-3}	0.5		12
(17) 1,2,4-Triazol-3-ylethylamine (triazole ring, CH$_2$CH$_2$NH$_2$)	1.4[d]	10^{-4}	10^{-2}	12.7[e]	13.7[e]

[a] Agonist activities as indicated in Table IV.
[b] Holmes and Jones (1960) report pK_{a1} 1.68 and pK_{a2} 9.53 at 25° for the isomeric 4-thiazolylethylamine.
[c] Ganellin (1974) reports pK_{a1} 3.23 and pK_{a2} 9.34 at 25°.
[d] E.S. Pepper in Durant et al. (1975a).
[e] Black et al. (1972a).

quaternary ammonium derivative N^α, N^α, N^α-trimethylhistamine (19) is extremely weak (Fig. 5). Therefore, a proton on the N^α-ammonium group appears to be of importance for agonist activity at both H_1 and H_2 receptors (Durant et al., 1975a). If the main function of the proton were hydrogen bonding then activity would appear to reside exclusively with the monocation, but if the proton were required to dissociate then the uncharged form would be generated, possibly as a transient species. The uncharged form might be required for access (e.g., penetration of membranes) or be involved in receptor interaction e.g. in assisting imidazole-mediated proton transfer at the receptor site (Weinstein et al., 1976).

Evidence for the Involvement of Tautomerism at H_2 Receptors

Although histamine is tautomeric it is probable that imidazole tautomerism is not functionally involved in H_1-receptor stimulation. This follows from the finding that 2-pyridylethylamine (6) (Walter et al., 1941; Hunt and

N^{α},N^{α}-Dimethylhistamine (18) is active at H_1 and H_2 receptors, but $N^{\alpha},N^{\alpha},N^{\alpha}$-trimethylhistamine (19) is extremely weak :

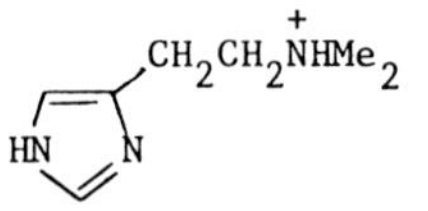

(18)

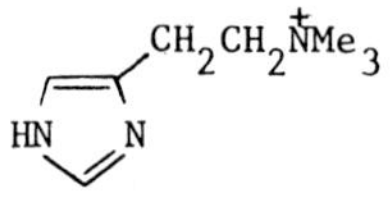

(19)

thus, agonist activity is associated with the presence of the side chain unit: $-CH_2-CH_2-\overset{+}{N}{\overset{\diagup}{\underset{\diagdown}{-}}}H$

The side chain may form a hydrogen bond to a base, B:

$$-CH_2-CH_2-\overset{+}{N}{\overset{\diagup}{\underset{\diagdown}{-}}}H...B$$

or it may dissociate, giving up its proton to a base B^- and becoming uncharged:

$$-CH_2-CH_2--\overset{+}{N}{\overset{\diagup}{\underset{\diagdown}{-}}}H \quad B \longrightarrow -CH_2-CH_2-N{\overset{\diagup}{\underset{\diagdown}{}}} + HB$$

FIG. 5.   Side chain N-methylhistamines.

Fosbinder, 1942) and 2-thiazolylethylamine (12) (Lee and Jones, 1949), which cannot tautomerise, have histamine-like activity in stimulating contractions of the guinea pig ileum (an H_1-receptor system). The activity of these compounds, taken together with the inactivity of their isomers (3-pyridylethylamine and 5-thiazolylethylamine) also indicates that the N^T-H tautomer of histamine monocation is the active form at H_1 receptors (Durant et al., 1975a), in agreement with the previous suggestions, of Niemann and Hays (1942). These nontautomeric heterocyclic ethylamines are only weakly active at H_2 receptors, however, and it appears that effective H_2-receptor agonists are compounds which can undergo a 1,3-prototropic tautomerism (Durant et al., 1975a). Further indications of the importance of a tautomerism for H_2-receptor agonist activity come from a comparison of the activities of 4-substituted histamine derivatives (Table VI). 4-Methylhistamine (14) is about half as active as histamine; replacement of methyl by electron withdrawing substituents reduces activity. Thus, 4-chloro- and 4-bromo-histamine (15 and 20) have about one-tenth and 4-nitrohistamine (21) has less than one-hundredth of the activity of histamine. Electron-withdrawing substituents in the 4-position of the imidazole ring change the relative tautomer concentrations since they alter the electron densities at the nitrogen atoms and affect proton acidities; the effect is more pronounced at the nearer nitrogen atom so that the relative stabilities of the tautomers change in comparison with histamine (Ganellin, 1974). The population of the N^T-H tautomer of 4-methylhistamine is similar to that of histamine but is reduced by one order of magnitude for 4-chlorohistamine and by two orders of magnitude for 4-nitrohistamine (Table VI). These reductions in populations of the N^T-H tautomer approximately parallel the changes in H_2-receptor agonist activities. Of course, the tautomeric effect may not be the only factor affecting receptor activity; the substituent will exert other effects, e.g., steric, polarity, and lipid-water distribution. However, the results are suggestive and one is led to the speculative deduction that either the N^T-H tautomer is the biologically active form of histamine at the H_2 receptor or that the free-energy difference between the two tautomers must be small for effective biological activity. This latter observation suggests that tautomerism

Table VI

Tautomer Concentration Ratios, K_t, Percentage Mole Fractions of N^T-H Tautomer, and H_2-Receptor Agonist Activities (relative to histamine = 100) of 4-Substituted Histamine Monocations

Compound number	R	K_t^a	% mole fraction[b] N^T-H	H_2-receptor agonist activity[c]
Histamine	H	2.4	71	100
14	CH_3	4.1	80	43[d]
15	Cl	0.13	12	11
20	Br	0.11	10	9[e]
21	NO_2	0.009	0.9	0.6

[a] $K_{t,R}$ = antilog $[3.4\,(\sigma_{m,CH2CH2NH3+} - \sigma_{m,R})]$
$\sigma_{m,CH2CH2NH3+}$ taken as + 0.11 (Ganellin, 1974).

[b] Mole fraction of monocation—not the mole fraction of total species which would be pH dependent.

[c] Activities determined in vitro on guinea pig right atrium, in the presence of propranolol, expressed relative to histamine = 100 (R.C. Blakemore in reference Ganellin, 1974).

[d] 95% fiducial limits 40–46.

[e] 95% fiducial limits 7.4–10.1.

(or proton transfer) might be involved in the H_2-receptor action of histamine (Ganellin, 1974) and that histamine could act as a proton-transfer agent. Pictorially (Fig. 6) one can envisage the imidazole ring catalyzing the transfer of a proton from site A to site B, and perhaps a catalytic mechanism of some kind may be involved in the events leading to an effective H_2-receptor response (Durant *et al.*, 1975a). Such a proton transfer mechanism is analogous to the function of imidazole in the histidyl residues of certain enzymes, e.g., the catalytic site in chymotrypsin (Blow, 1976). A similar mechanism has also been proposed by Weinstein *et al.* (1976) on theoretical grounds.

H_1 receptors

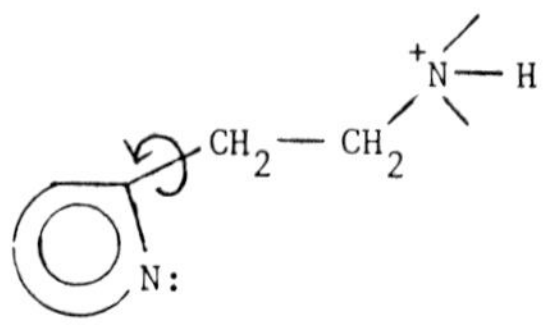

indicating (i)   side-chain cation and $\overset{+}{N}$-H

(ii)   heterocyclic ring with basic N:
       (with lone pair of electrons) in ortho position

(iii) ring rotation or possible "essential"
       conformation

H_2 receptors

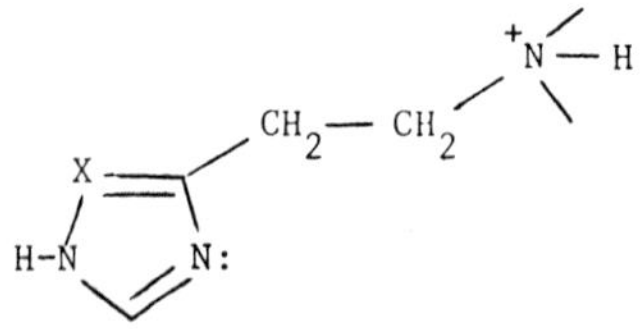

indicating (i)   side-chain cation and $\overset{+}{N}$-H

(ii) N^{τ}-H tautomer and amidine system

(iii) possible function as a proton transfer agent,

thus:

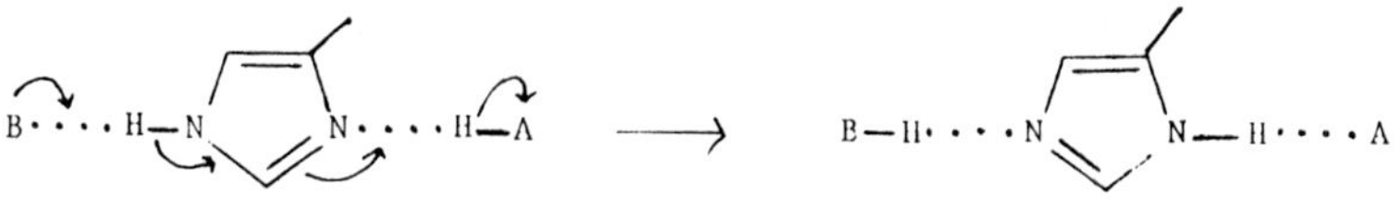

FIG. 6.   Functional chemical requirements of agonists at histamine receptors.

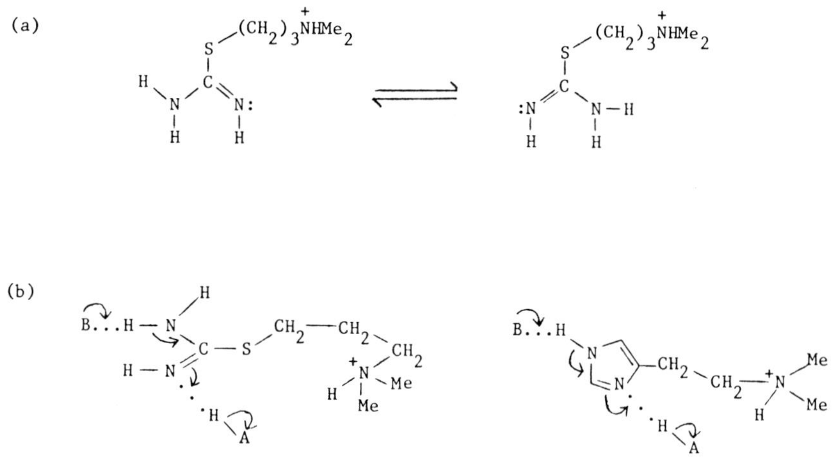

(a)

(b)

dimaprit N^α,N^α-dimethylhistamine

FIG. 7. Dimaprit formulae, illustrating (a) tautomerism of isothiourea group and (b) comparison with N^α,N^α-dimethylhistamine to show a possible similarity in function as proton transfer agents (see Durant et al., 1977c).

The recently described selective H_2-receptor agonist, dimaprit [S-(3-N,N-dimethylaminopropyl)isothiourea] (Parsons et al., 1977; Durant et al., 1977c) provides additional evidence for the involvement of tautomerism. Dimaprit has two basic centres and pK_a studies indicate that at pH 7.4 about 5% of the molecules will be present as the monocation analogous to histamine monocation. Chemical comparison suggests that the $-NHMe_2^+$ group corresponds to the $-NH_3^+$ of histamine (or more correctly, to the $-NHMe_2^+$ group of N^α,N^α-dimethylhistamine) and that the isothiourea group of dimaprit may simulate the imidazole ring of histmaine (Durant et al., 1977c). Isothioureas resemble imidazoles in that both are planar 6π-electron systems which incorporate an amidine; the latter in the uncharged form, has N-H and N(lone pair of electrons) and undergoes 1,3-protropic tautomerism. Tautomerism of dimaprit is depicted in Fig. 7 and a comparison made with N^α,N^α-dimethylhistamine showing a possible similarity in function as proton transfer agents.

Evidence for an Active Conformation

A series of methyl-substituted histamines was studied with respect to conformational properties and receptor selectivities (Ganellin et al., 1973b) and it was suggested that the dramatic receptor selectivity of 4-methylhistamine (which has 40% of the potency of histamine as an H_2-receptor stimulant but only 0.2% at H_1 receptors) could be accounted for in the difference between its conformational properties and those of histamine (Ganellin, 1973b); this permitted the definition of an "H_1-essential" conformation, (see also Farnell *et al.*, 1975), i.e., a conformation essential to drug activity which has to be adopted by histamine at some stage during productive interaction at the H_1-receptor site. This is the fully extended trans conformation, where $\theta_1 = 0°$ and $\theta_2 = 180°$, in which the carbon and nitrogen atoms are coplanar with the ring (illustrated in Fig. 8), and there is a maximum separation (interatomic distance of 5.1 A) between the charged ammonium group and the ring N^π-nitrogen atom. Furthermore, in this conformation any effect from the side chain in obscuring the lone electron pair at N^π is minimal. This would be a very satisfactory situation if the nitrogen atom were involved in donating its electron pair during productive drug-receptor interaction.

The described "H_1-essential" conformation is not a minimum energy form. Indeed, for histamine, the trans rotamer ($\theta_2 = 180°$) is predicted by EHT calculations to be at a minimum energy when $\theta_1 = 120°$, whereas the "H_1-

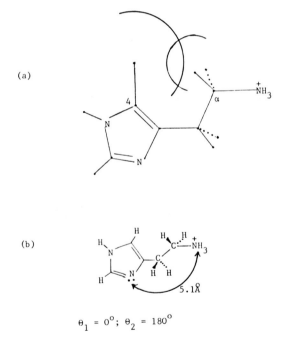

(a)

(b)

$$\theta_1 = 0°; \quad \theta_2 = 180°$$

FIG. 8.   Showing: (a) Steric interaction between the C_4-methyl and α-methylene groups in 4-methylhistamine in the coplanar ($\theta_1 = 0°$), trans ($\theta_2 = 180°$) conformation; intersecting arcs represent the overlap of van der Waals zones.
(b) Proposed H_1 receptor "essential" conformation of histamine.
(c) CPK model of histamine monocation in the proposed H_1 receptor "essential" conformation. The model illustrates the close approach between the hydrogen atoms of the side chain α-CH_2 and the ring 4-position.

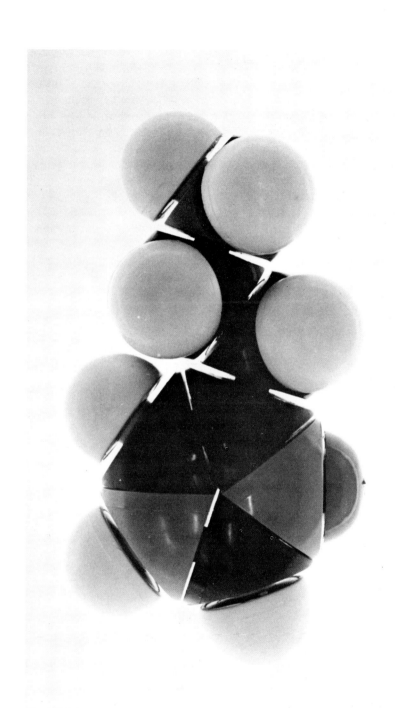

essential" conformation at $\theta_1 = 0°$ is calculated to have an energy about 3 kcal/mol above this (although the value may be an overestimate; see Richards *et al.*, 1975). This leads one to speculate that histamine may be required to undergo a conformational change during H_1-receptor stimulation. One can envisage that a histamine molecule would arrive in the neighborhood of the site of action in one of its most probable (minimum energy) conformations and that it might then either interact with the receptor and undergo a change which involves the "H_1-essential" conformation or, under a perturbing influence of the receptor, it might adopt the "H_1-essential" conformation prior to forming a drug-receptor complex. The described conformation may be only one of several forms involved during receptor stimulation or, indeed, it may be involved in only a transient manner while the agonist undergoes a required conformational change. Thus, rotation of the imidazole ring may also be involved in the action of histamine at H_1 receptors.

Since 4-methylhistamine is an effective agonist at H_2 receptors it follows that conformations inaccessible to 4-methylhistamine, such as those where θ_1 approaches $0°$, are not involved in H_2-receptor interactions.

Summary

The above indications are summarised in Fig. 6. The active form of histamine for both receptors is likely to be the N^T-H tautomer of the monocation (1B), which is also the most prevalent species in water at around neutrality, and a side chain NH appears to be needed. However, different chemical properties of histamine may be associated with interactions at the two receptor types. At the H_1 receptor, imidazole tautomerism is not a functional requirement, but the presence of the nitrogen atom ortho to the ammoniumethyl group appears to have special significance. The ring may also need to be able to freely rotate or at least to achieve coplanarity with the side chain. At the H_2 receptor, the tautomeric property of the imidazole ring of histamine appears to be of importance and histamine might be involved as a proton-transfer agent.

DISCOVERY AND DEVELOPMENT OF HISTAMINE H_2-RECEPTOR ANTAGONISTS

Three compounds have been widely studied as histamine H_2-receptor antagonists, viz: burimamide (22) (Black *et al.*, 1972a), metiamide (23) (Black *et al.*, 1973a), and cimetidine (24) (Brimblecombe *et al.*, 1975) (see Fig. 9 for structures). Like histamine, these compounds are imidazole derivatives with structurally specific side chains, but they differ chemically from histamine in

22 Burimamide[a]

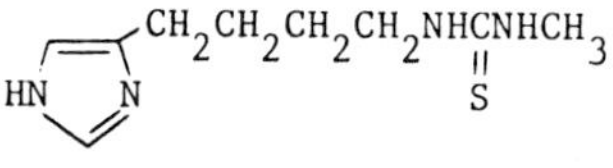

$$\text{HN} \diagdown \text{N} \diagup \text{CH}_2\text{CH}_2\text{CH}_2\text{CH}_2\text{NHCNHCH}_3 \quad (\overset{\parallel}{\text{S}})$$

23 Metiamide[b]

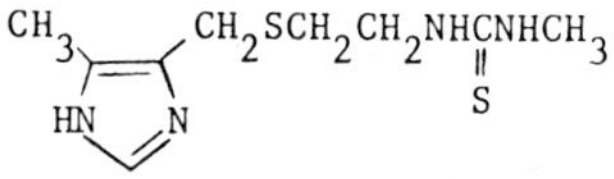

$$\text{CH}_3 \diagdown \diagup \text{CH}_2\text{SCH}_2\text{CH}_2\text{NHCNHCH}_3 \quad (\overset{\parallel}{\text{S}})$$
$$\text{HN} \diagdown \text{N}$$

24 Cimetidine[c]

$$\text{CH}_3 \diagdown \diagup \text{CH}_2\text{SCH}_2\text{CH}_2\text{NHCNHCH}_3$$
$$\text{HN} \diagdown \text{N} \qquad \overset{\text{N}}{\underset{\diagdown \text{CN}}{}}$$

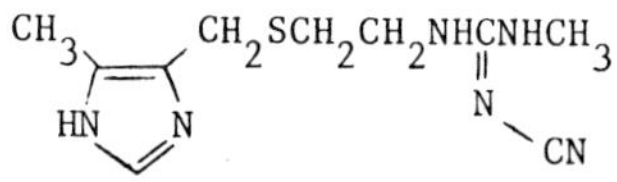

FIG. 9. Structures of H_2-receptor antagonists.

[a]Burimamide is N-methyl-N'-[4-(imidazol-4-yl)butyl]thiourea
[b]Metiamide is the USAN Council approved name for N-methyl-N'-{2-[(5-methylimidazol-4-yl)methylthio]ethyl}thiourea
[c]Cimetidine is the USAN Council approved name for N"-cyano-N-methyl-N'-{2-[(5-methylimidazol-4-yl)methylthio]ethyl}guanidine, Tagamet®.

two important respects, viz: the side chains are longer, and formally uncharged at physiological pH (cf. histamine which exists mainly in the cationic form at pH 7.4). These antagonists bear very little resemblance to the structure of the conventional antihistamine drugs, the H_1-receptor antagonists (general formula 33, in Table X). The H_2-antagonist structures were derived from extensive structure–activity studies, and the aforementioned structural features appear to be of considerable importance in determining both selectivity of drug action and antagonist potency.

To judge whether these observations have significance requires a knowledge of structure–activity relationships, but the perception of such relationships depends on the manner in which the problem has been viewed and analyzed. Our notions of what is chemically important in these structures have been conditioned by the results obtained in our search for antagonists. Therefore, to provide perspective it is essential to indicate something of their derivation.

Development of Burimamide

The initial conception was to seek compounds capable of competitively antagonizing those actions of histamine that were not blocked by the conventional antihistamine drugs; however, a chemical starting point had to be specified. Nothing was known to us about the chemical structure of the physiological site of action of histamine; our chemical knowledge was restricted to histamine and related agonists, and to the H_1-receptor antihistaminic drugs. Since we were concerned with actions not blocked by these latter, the conventional antihistamines seemed unattractive as starting points. We therefore concentrated our attention on histamine and attempted to design an antagonist by modifying the structure. We started with the simple-minded view that we were seeking a molecule that would compete with histamine for its receptor site. We thought that such a molecule would have to be recognized by the receptor, then bind more strongly than histamine, but not trigger off the usual response.

Many different approaches were tried; we drew on analogies derived from known examples of biochemical relationships between other types of receptor agonists and antagonists, or enzyme substrates and inhibitors, or antimetabolites. We modified the structure of histamine to alter deliberately its chemical properties but we generally retained some definite aspect of histamine structure or chemistry. Some of the approaches taken have been summarized previously (Durant *et al.*, 1973a; Ganellin *et al.*, 1976).

The "breakthrough" came with the discovery that the guanidine analogue of histamine, N^α-guanylhistamine (25) (Table VII) was a partial agonist which at high doses was shown to antagonize maximal histamine-induced gastric acid secretion (Durant *et al.*, 1975). The antagonist activity of this compound was barely detectable but it provided a basis for drug development. We had to consider whether it was coincidental that guanylhistamine was both an antagonist and structurally related to histamine. Structure–activity investigations indicated that guanidines, *per se*, did not act as antagonists but that the presence of the imidazole ring appeared to be a necessary feature; this suggested that the imidazole and guanidine groups probably acted co-operatively. We also had to identify the particular chemical properties that conferred antagonist activity in order to make analogues of increased potency. Thus, we had to identify the differences in chemical properties between guanylhistamine and histamine and relate these to the biological effects. One may note that, inter alia, the guanidinium group is planar (whereas the ammonium group of histamine is tetrahedral) and has the positive charge distributed over three nitrogen atoms. The intramolecular distance between the ring and side chain terminal nitrogens is potentially greater than in histamine and there are three N sites for potential interactions instead of one. These observations specify several structural variables for examination, particularly the length of the side chain and the number of N sites.

It was found that for certain structures, extension of the side chain furnished compounds which were more active as antagonists, although still being partial agonists. An example is the guanidine homolog, SK&F 91486

Table VII
Structures of Some Early Compounds and Their H_2-Receptor
Antagonist Activities[a]

Compound	Structure	K_B $\times 10^{-6}$ M
25 N^α-Guanylhistamine: the "lead"; a weakly active partial agonist	$\underset{HN \diagdown N}{\diagup}\!\!\!\!\!\diagup^{CH_2CH_2\underset{+NH_2}{\overset{NHCNH_2}{\underset{\|}{}}}}$	130
26 SK&F 91486: lengthening the side chain increases activity	$\underset{HN \diagdown N}{\diagup}\!\!\!\!\!\diagup^{CH_2CH_2CH_2\underset{+NH_2}{\overset{NHCNH_2}{\underset{\|}{}}}}$	22
27 SK&F 91581: thiourea analogue is much less active as an antagonist, but is not an agonist	$\underset{HN \diagdown N}{\diagup}\!\!\!\!\!\diagup^{CH_2CH_2CH_2\overset{NHCNHMe}{\underset{S}{\underset{\|}{}}}}$	115[b]
22 Burimamide: lengthening the side chain again, dramatically increases antagonist activity	$\underset{HN \diagdown N}{\diagup}\!\!\!\!\!\diagup^{CH_2CH_2CH_2CH_2\overset{NHCNHMe}{\underset{S}{\underset{\|}{}}}}$	7.8

[a]Dissociation constant, K_B, determined *in vitro* on guinea pig right atrium against histamine stimulation; see footnote Table IX; from Blakemore and Parsons in Durant *et al.*, 1977a.

[b]Refined data; previous value of 350 reported by Durant *et al.*, 1973.

(26) (Table VII) (Parsons *et al.*, 1975). It was also found that amidines and isothiourea groups could be used in place of guanidine to provide partial agonists (Black *et al.*, 1972b, 1973b). A common feature of these structures is that they are strong bases which at physiological pH accept a proton and become positively charged. There is, thus, a strong resemblance between these structures and histamine, viz: they incorporate an imidazole ring and a cationic side chain. It seemed possible that these features provided the necessary binding properties for a competitive antagonist, but also permitted the molecule to mimic histamine and act as an agonist. This posed a considerable dilemma, because the chemical groups which appeared to be required for antagonist activity were the very same groups that seemed to confer the agonist effects. How then, could these properties be separated?

In an attempt to separate agonist and antagonist activities, the strongly basic guanidine group was replaced by nonbasic groups which, though polar, would not be charged. Such an approach furnished the thiourea derivative SK&F 91581 (27) (Table VII); in this molecule, thione sulphur (=S) replaces the imino nitrogen (=NH) of guanidine and makes the remaining N atoms relatively nonbasic. This compound did not act as a partial agonist, but it was only weakly active as an antagonist. Further exploration revealed that with this type of structure, extending the length of the alkylene chain resulted in a marked increase in antagonist potency, exemplified by the drug, burimamide. Burimamide was found to be about 100 times more active than N^{α}-guanylhistamine as an H_2-receptor antagonist and did not act as a partial agonist (Black *et al.*, 1972a). Thus, modifying the side chain had conferred both selectivity and antagonist potency (Table VII).

Development of Metiamide

Although burimamide was sufficiently selective pharmacologically it seemed to lack adequate oral bioavailability needed for exploring its therapeutic potential, and it appeared that a more active compound was required. Various attempts were made to produce a more suitable drug. One approach was based on the realization that burimamide in aqueous solution is a mixture of many chemical species in equilibrium and attention was focussed on the imidazole ring of burimamide. In aqueous solution at physiological pH (7.4) burimamide exists as an equilibrium mixture of mainly three different imidazole species; the two uncharged tautomers B and C and the cation A (Fig. 10, R = – $(CH_2)_4NHCSNHCH_3$). If only one of these forms were active its relative population could determine the amount of drug required for a given effect. The populations of these species were estimated from the electronic influence of the side chain. A substituent R in the 4(5)-position alters the electron densities at the ring nitrogen atoms and affects proton

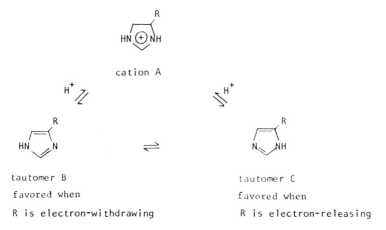

FIG. 10. Equilibria between imidazole species; substituents R in 4(5)-position of the imidazole ring alter tautomerism.

acidity. Its effect is more marked at the nearer nitrogen atom so that if R is an electron-withdrawing group, the 1, 4-tautomer B should predominate; if it is electron releasing, the 1, 5-tautomer C should predominate. The fraction present as cation A is determined by the ring pK_a and the pH of the medium. The electronic influence of the side chain can be assessed from the measured ring pK_a using the Hammett equation: $pK_{a(R)} = pK_{a(H)} + \rho\sigma_m$; (Charton, 1965a).

Measurements of ring basicity (pK_a) showed that the burimamide side chain is electronically different from that of histamine; for burimamide it is electron-releasing whereas for histamine the side chain is electron-withdrawing. The effect is to alter the basicity (pK_a) and tautomeric properties of the respective rings, resulting in a change in the relative populations of the three ring species (A, B, and C shown in Fig. 10) present in solution. The burimamide structure was therefore modified so as to increase the equilibrium concentration of imidazole species considered most likely to be active (Black *et al.*, 1974). The best results were obtained by favoring the species B, which is also the species most prevalent for histamine at pH 7.4. This was achieved by replacing a methylene group ($-CH_2-$) with an isosteric thioether ($-S-$) link in the side chain, in order to make it electron-withdrawing, and substituting an electron-releasing methyl group in the ring to favor still further the tautomer B. This approach was successful and furnished the more active compound, metiamide (23) (Black *et al.*, 1973a).

The consequences of the structural manipulation of burimamide in terms of pK_a and H_2-receptor antagonist activity are shown in Table VIII. It can be seen that modifying the side chain in burimamide by isosteric replacement of $-CH_2-$ by $-S-$ to favor tautomer B, reduces the ring pK_a, and gives a more active compound (thiaburimamide, 28). Introducing a 4(5)-methyl group gives metiamide (23) and increases further the preference for tautomer B but decreases the combined populations of the uncharged tautomers (B and C) through raising the ring pK_a. Although these are opposing effects the net result is that metiamide is more active still. By contrast, the analogous structural modification of burimamide viz: incorporation of a ring 4(5)-methyl group to give methylburimamide (29) does not increase activity. In this case the two ring substituents have nearly equal electronic effects in the same direction; the methyl group counterbalances the electronic influence of the side chain on tautomerism but it raises the ring pK_a to 7.80 so that at pH 7.4 the predominant species is the cation, A (72%). This illustrates one of the problems of attempting to manipulate the biological properties of drug molecules through altering chemical structures. The changes in chemical properties accompanying structural modifications often impose their own inherent limitations; a structural change, biologically advantageous with respect to a given chemical property, may affect some other chemical property in a biologically disadvantageous way and one has to discover the optimum balance of opposing influences. Although the methyl group was

Table VIII
Effect of Structural Manipulation of Burimamide. Apparent pK_a Values[a] at 37°, Mole Percentages of Imidazole Cation at pH 7.4, and H$_2$-Receptor Antagonist Activities[b], K_B

$$R_1 \diagdown \diagup CH_2XCH_2CH_2NHCNHMe$$
with imidazole ring (HN⊕NH) and S on the thiocarbonyl

Compound	R_1	X	pK_a'	mole % of cation A at pH 7.4	K_B (95% limits)[b] × 10^{-6} M
22 Burimamide	H	CH$_2$	7.25	40	7.8 (6.4–9.6)
28 Thiaburimamide	H	S	6.25	7	3.2 (2.5–4.5)
23 Metiamide	CH$_3$	S	6.80	20	0.92 (0.74–1.15)
29 Methylburimamide	CH$_3$	CH$_2$	7.80	72	8.95 (5.6–15)

[a] pK_a data from Black et al. 1974.
[b] Dissociation constant, K_B, determined in vitro on guinea pig right atrium against histamine stimulation; data from Black et al., 1974.

introduced to increase the tautomer ratio, it also increases the amount of cation; these are opposing influences but one does not know what the optimum will be until one tests it out experimentally. These results emphasize that the properties of the imidazole ring seem to have a special importance for H$_2$-receptor activity.

Development of Cimetidine

A wider study of the structural requirements for H$_2$-receptor antagonists led to investigation of the effect of replacing the thiourea group of metiamide. One approach taken was to examine isosteric replacement of the thiourea sulphur atom (=S) of metiamide. Replacement by carbonyl oxygen (=O) gives the urea analog (30) but this is much less active as an antagonist (Table IX). Replacement by imino nitrogen (=NH) provides the guanidine (31); interestingly, this guanidine analog differs from the previous guanidine derivatives (e.g., structures 25 and 26) in that it does not behave as a partial agonist. It has H$_2$-receptor antagonist activity but is much less potent than metiamide (Table IX), (Durant et al., 1977a).

The guanidine (31) is very basic (pK_a > 13) and exists almost exclusively in the cationic form at physiological pH. To obtain a compound with ionization properties more closely resembling those of metiamide, the guanidine group of (31) was modified by introducing a further substituent X. The basicity of guanidines is very susceptible to substituent effects and can be markedly reduced by substituting electron-withdrawing groups at the nitrogen atoms. A relationship between substituent effect and guanidinium pK_a has been demonstrated by Charton (1965b) using the inductive substituent constant σ_I in the Hammett equation: $pK_{a,X} = pK_{a,H} + \rho\sigma_{I,X}$. A plot of pK_a vs. σ_I for a series of monosubstituted guanidines is shown in Fig. 11; the ρ value of -24 indicates the extreme sensitivity of pK_a to substituent effects in guanidines. The cyano and nitro groups are sufficiently electron-withdrawing to reduce pK_a by over 14 units, to values < 0; indeed, the ionization constants of cyanoguanidine (pK_a -0.4, Hirt *et al.*, 1961) and nitroguanidine (pK_a -0.9; Bonner and Lockhardt, 1958) approach that of thiourea (pK_a -1.2; Janssen, 1962). The nitroguanidine (32) and cyanoguanidine (24) analogs of metiamide were synthesized and found to be active antagonists (Table IX), comparable with metiamide. Of these two compounds, the cyanoguanidine (cimetidine) is slightly more potent and was selected for development (Brimblecombe *et al.*, 1975).

As shown in Fig. 12, a trisubstituted guanidinium cation exists in equilibrium with three conjugate bases since proton dissociation can occur

Table IX
Structures and H$_2$-Receptor Antagonist Activities[a,b] of Metiamide, Cimetidine, and Isosteres[c]

CH$_3$ —— CH$_2$SCH$_2$CH$_2$NHCNHCH$_3$ || Y HN N

Compound	Y	in vitro[a] K_B × 10^{-6} M	(95% limits)	in vivo[b] ID$_{50}$ μmol kg^{-1}
		Antagonist Activity		
23 Metiamide (thiourea)	S	0.92	(0.74–1.15)	1.6
30 Urea isostere	O	22	(8.9–65)	27
31 Guanidine isostere	NH	16	(8.1–32)	12
32 Nitroguanidine isostere	N.NO$_2$	1.4	(0.79–2.8)	2.1
24 Cimetidine (cyanoguanidine)	N.CN	0.79	(0.68–0.92)	1.4

[a]Activities determined against histamine stimulation of guinea pig right atrium *in vitro* (R.C. Blakemore and M.E. Parsons, Smith Kline & French Laboratories, Welwyn Garden City, England). The dissociation constant (K_B) was calculated from the equation $K_B = B/(x - 1)$, where x is the respective ratio of concentrations of histamine needed to produce half-maximal responses in the presence and absence of different concentrations (B) of antagonist, and $- \log K_B = pA_2$.

[b]Activity as an antagonist of histamine stimulated gastric acid secretion in anesthetized rats using a lumen-perfused preparation (Black *et al.*, 1972a). Compounds given by rapid intravenous injection during a near maximal plateau of histamine stimulated gastric acid secretion. The ID$_{50}$ is the dose required to produce 50% of inhibition, and was estimated from the linear regression of log [1/(100–1)] on log dose where 1 = percentage inhibition (R.C. Blakemore and M.E. Parsons, Smith Kline and French Laboratories, Welwyn Garden City, England).

[c]From Durant *et al.*, 1977a.

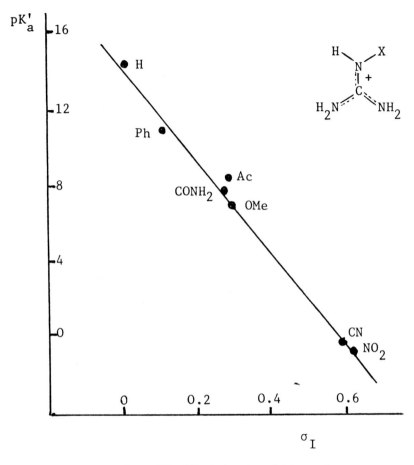

FIG. 11.   Apparent pK_a values at 25° of N-substituted guanidinium cations vs σ_I substituent constants. Data from Charton (1965b). The line corresponds to the equation $pK'_a = 14.20 - 24.1\,\sigma_I$.

from each of three nitrogen atoms. Powerful electron-withdrawing substituents X favor the imino tautomer over the amino tautomers since the proton on the adjacent nitrogen in the cation is more acidic than the protons on the more distant terminal nitrogen atoms (Charton, 1965b), and cyanoguanidines exist predominantly in the cyanoimino form. In cyanoguanidines and thioureas the cyanoimino ($=N.CN$) and thione sulphur ($=S$) functionalities have a similar effect in reducing the electron density on the amino groups in the 1,1-diaminomethylene $[H_2N)_2C=]$ system. Cyanoguanidine and thiourea have many chemical properties in common (Brimblecombe et al., 1975; Durant et al., 1977a). They are planar structures of similar geometries; they are weakly amphoteric (very weakly basic and acidic) so that in the pH range 2–12 they are unionized; they are very polar and hydrophilic. Comparing

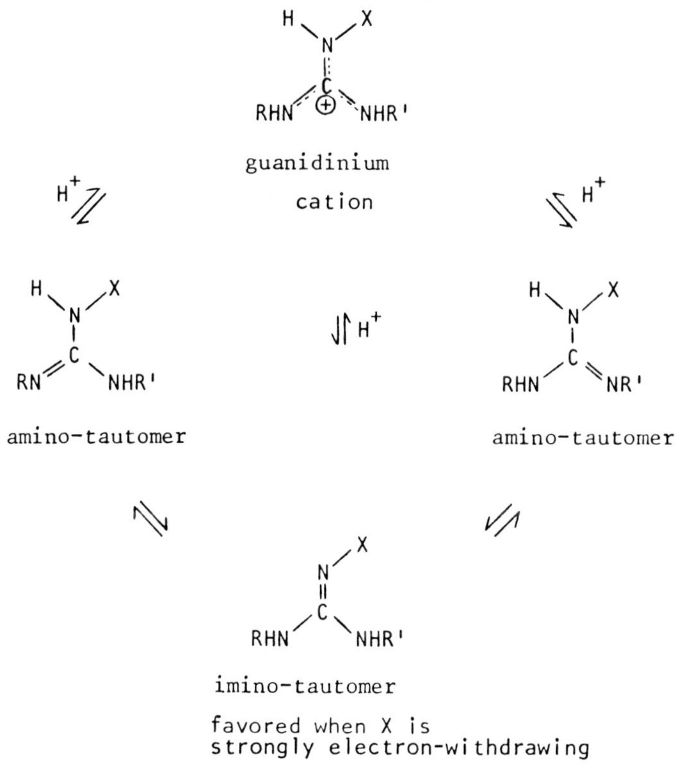

guanidinium

cation

amino-tautomer

amino-tautomer

imino-tautomer

favored when X is
strongly electron-withdrawing

FIG. 12. Equilibria between guanidinium cation and the three conjugate bases.

cimetidine with metiamide, it is seen that the cyanoimino group =N. CN replaces the thione =S sulphur atom. Many of the physicochemical properties of cimetidine and metiamide are similar and reflect the characteristics of cyanoguanidine and thiourea (Brimblecombe *et al.*, 1975; Durant *et al.*, 1977a). At H_2 receptors the cyanoguanidine and thiourea groups therefore act as bioisosteres (Durant *et al.*, 1977b).

Chemical Comparison between H_1- and H_2-Receptor Antagonists

There is a marked chemical distinction between these H_2-receptor antagonists and the conventional H_1-receptor antagonists (Table X). The H_1-antagonists possess aryl or heteroaryl rings (as in the general formula (33)) which need not have a structural relationship to the imidazole ring of histamine; the aryl groups confer considerable lipophilicity (the octanol–water partition ratio P is often greater than 1000; see Table II in Durant *et al.*, 1973) and probably act in hydrophobic binding; the H_1-receptor antagonists resemble histamine in possessing a side chain group (usually ammonium) which is positively charged at physiological pH. In marked contrast burimamide, metiamide and cimetidine are hydrophilic molecules (they have low partition ratios); they bear a structural relationship to histamine in having an imidazole ring but differ in the side chain which, though polar is uncharged. These substantial chemical differences probably account for the considerable degree of selectivity shown by the respective antagonists in distinguishing the two types of receptor. Thus, H_1-receptor recognition is determined by the ammonium group, but at H_2 receptors it is determined by the imidazole ring.

The H_2-receptor antagonists, being uncharged in the side chain, are unable to mimic the stimulant actions of histamine; they are not agonists. Finally, one may note that their low lipophilicity probably limits access to the central nervous system and avoids some of the "side-effects" normally associated with use of the H_1-receptor antihistaminic drugs; unlike the lipophilic H_1-receptor antagonists, burimamide, metiamide, and cimetidine do not produce overt signs of central nervous system action in behavioral tests and have only weak local anesthetic activity (Black and Spencer, 1973; Brimblecombe and Duncan, 1977).

Dynamic–Structure–Activity Analysis

In the above description of histamine and related agonists, and in the development of the H_2-receptor antagonists, use has been made of a particular type of structure–activity analysis. From the outset the aim has been to chemically characterize the drug molecules in terms of their chemical

Table X
Chemical Differentiation between Histamine and its Antagonists[a]

H_2 Antagonist	Histamine (Agonist)	H_1 Antagonist
Imidazole hydrophilic	Imidazole hydrophilic	Aryl Rings lipophilic
Thiourea Cyanoguanidine uncharged	Ammonium charged	Ammonium charged

[a]General formula of H_1 antagonists:

$$\begin{array}{c} Ar' \\ \diagdown \\ \quad\; X - C - C - \overset{+}{N}HRR \\ \diagup \\ Ar \end{array}$$

33

DYNAMIC STRUCTURE-ACTIVITY ANALYSIS

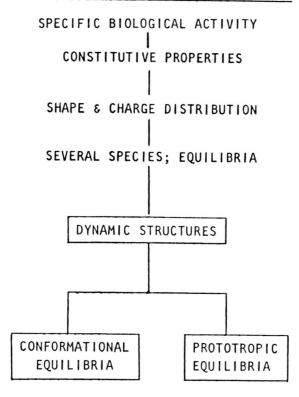

FIG. 13.

properties since these should provide the link between chemical structure and biological properties.

Drug molecules must exert their biological actions through their ability to interact at the molecular level, e.g., with enzymes or receptor structures. These molecular interactions are determined, fundamentally, by the size and shape of molecules, and by the electron density distribution and polarizabilities within molecules. However, when we have tried to characterize the molecules pertinent to histamine receptor interactions we have found that they do not have unique shapes or single charge distributions. They exist in various conformations and protonated (or differently charged) forms. Furthermore these different forms are usually interconvertible and exist in equilibrium. Thus, one has to identify the separate forms and their probable importance. One must know something about the relative populations, i.e., how likely is it that a molecule adopts a particular conformation, or a particular charge distribution? It follows that changing a drug's structure may also change the relative importance of particular forms and this may affect a specific biological activity. We identify this aspect as dynamic–structure–activity analysis (DSAA) (Fig. 13). If altering structure disfavors the biologically active form, then presumably this would reduce activity. It is also conceivable that on occasions an equilibrium between two forms is mechanistically necessary, so that displacing the equilibrium may alter activity.

We take as a starting point the chemical characterization of the drug molecule in terms of its different species, i.e., conformations and protonated (or ionized) forms, and the quantitative interrelationships between the species (eg., equilibrium constants, free energy differences, energy barriers to interconversion). We then modify structure to alter a particular equilibrium or favor (or disfavor) a particular species and investigate whether the changes correlate with an altered specific biological activity. By this means it has been possible to infer something about the chemical mechanism of drug action, and it has also indicated the way to alter drug structure in order to deliberately modify drug activity, ie., provide a method for drug design.

Chemical Controls for Use in Studies Involving Histamine Receptors

The respective classes of histamine antagonists provide valuable tools for analyzing biological actions of histamine in terms of H_1- or H_2-receptor involvement. In situations where administered histamine gives good dose-response relationships, and these are shifted in a parallel fashion in the presence of a selective antagonist, such that the Schild plot of log $(DR-1)$ upon log (concentration of antagonist) has a linear regression, of slope not significantly different from unity, the case for inferring receptor involvement is very strong.

There may be instances, however, where analysis is more complex, eg., where both H_1 and H_2 receptors are involved in mediating the response. Under these circumstances it may be worthwhile to use the highly selective agonists which are now available, as an adjunct to assist in the analysis. The selective agonists may also be useful in providing additional evidence for the involvement of histamine receptors in cases where quantitative studies on histamine prove to be difficult. Where the antagonists act in an apparently noncompetitive manner, one must also consider whether other mechanisms are interfering; for example, the antagonist might affect histamine distribution (such as access to the receptor, uptake to other tissues, metabolism) or it may interfere with the response mechanism, eg., by affecting the transport of metal ions or by altering energy regulating systems.

Table XI
Compounds for Use as Chemical Controls in Studies of Possible Histamine Receptor Involvement

Active agent	Use	Control Compound[a]
Histamine	agonist $H_1 + H_2$	Tele-methylhistamine[b]
2-Pyridylethylamine[c]	agonist H_1	4-Pyridylethylamine[d]
Dimaprit[e]	agonist H_2	SK&F 91487[f]
Burimamide[g] Metiamide[i]	antagonist H_2	SK&F 91581[h]

[a]The control compounds may still have some receptor activity, but they are much less potent.

b 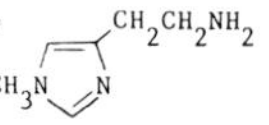
(see Ganellin *et al.*, 1973b).

c 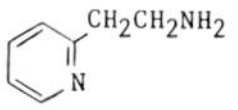
6 (Table IV).

d 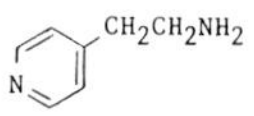
10 (Fig. 4)
(see Durant *et al.*, 1975a).

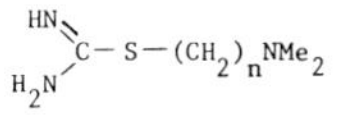

[e]n = 3, 16 in Table 4.
[f]n = 2, see Durant *et al.*, 1977c.

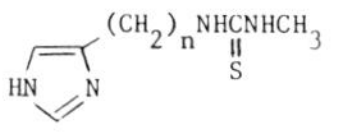

[g]n = 4, 22 in Table 7.
[h]n = 3, 27 in Table 3.
[i]23 (Table IX).

In cases where histamine is not administered but the possible involvement of endogeneous histamine is being investigated, the problems are much greater. Here one must be extremely cautious; if an antagonist interferes with a particular biological response one should not simply presume that it owes its actions to an antagonism of endogenous histamine at its receptors, but further evidence should be sought. Although the antagonists are highly selective agents, they are still chemical substances and are therefore potentially able to exert other effects.

Obviously, because a drug (whether antagonist or agonist) acts at a particular population of receptors, it does not follow that all observed effects of the drug are due to receptor interactions. In this sense it may be helpful to use chemical control substances which match many of the chemical properties of the active drugs but which lack the specific structural properties needed for effective receptor interactions. Such compounds are listed in Table XI, viz. telemethylhistamine used in conjunction with histamine or 2- or 4-methylhistamines; 4-pyridylethylamine used in conjunction with the selective H_1-receptor agonist, 2-pyridylethylamine; SK&F 91487 [2-(S-dimethylaminoethyl)isothiourea] used in conjunction with the highly selective H_2-

receptor agonist, dimaprit; SK&F 91581 [N-methyl-N'-[3-(imidazol-4-yl)propyl]thiourea] used in conjunction with the H_2-receptor antagonists, burimamide or metiamide. Many other control substances may be devised, but the compounds mentioned in Table XI have the merit of being available, synthetically. The use of such controls should be considered whenever the analysis of histamine-mediated effects appears to be complex. If, in a particular test system, both the active agent and the chemical control are found to be similarly active, one must seriously question whether the effect arises from direct interaction with histamine receptors.

REFERENCES

Abraham, R. J., and Birch, D. (1975). The use of the counter-ion in molecular orbital calculations of histamine conformations. *Molecular Pharmacol.* **11**, 663–666.

Arunlakshana, O., and Schild, H. O. (1959). Some quantitative uses of drug antagonists. *Brit. J. Pharmacol.* **14**, 48–58.

Ash, A. S. F., and Schild, H. O. (1966). Receptors mediating some actions of histamine. *Br. J. Pharmac. Chemother.* **27**, 427–439.

Barlow, R. B. (1964). Direct Actions on Tissues: Drugs Affecting Histamine Receptors, in "Introduction to Chemical Pharmacology," 2nd Ed. pp. 344–377. Methuen, London.

Bertaccini, G., Impicciatore, M., Vitali, T., and Plazzi, V. (1972) Pharmacological activities of 2-(5-methyl-4-imidazolyl)ethylamine. *Farmaco* **27**, 680–682.

Bertaccini, G., Impicciatore, M., and Vitali, T. (1976). Biological activities of a new specific stimulant of histamine. *Farmaco* **31**, 934–938.

Black, J. W., and Ganellin, C. R. (1974). Naming of substituted histamines. *Experientia* **30**, 111–113.

Black, J. W., and Spencer, K. E. V. (1973). Metiamide in systematic screening tests, in "International Symposium on histamine H_2-receptor antagonists" (C. J. Wood and M. A. Simkins, eds.), pp 23–27 Smith Kline & French Laboratories Ltd., Welwyn Garden City.

Black, J. W., Duncan, W. A. M., Durant, G. J., Ganellin, C. R., and Parsons, M. E. (1972a). Definition and antagonism of histamine H_2-receptors. *Nature (London)* **236**, 385–390.

Black, J. W., Durant, G. J., Emmett, J. C., and Ganellin, C. R. (1972b). Isothioureas and their derivatives. *Brit. Pat.* 1296544.

Black, J. W., Duncan, W. A. M., Emmett, J. C., Ganellin, C. R., Hesselbo, T., Parsons, M. E., and Wyllie, J. H. (1973a). Metiamide—an orally active histamine H_2-receptor antagonist. *Agents Actions* **3**, 133–137.

Black, J. W., Durant, G. J., Emmett, J. C., and Ganellin, C. R., (1973b). Pharmaceutical compositions comprising amidine derivatives. *Brit. Pat.* 1305546.

Black, J. W., Durant, G. J., Emmett, J. C., and Ganellin, C. R. (1974). Sulphur-methylene isosterism in the development of metiamide, a new histamine H_2-receptor antagonist. *Nature (London)* **248**, 65–67.

Blow, D. M. (1976) Structure and mechanism of chymotrypsin. *Accts. Chem. Res.* **9**, 145–152.

Bonner, T. G., and Lockhardt, J. C. (1958). The denitration of nitroguanidines in strong acids. Part II. Absorption spectra and pK_a values of certain nitroguanidines. *J. Chem. Soc.* 3858–3861.

Bonnet, J. J., and Ibers, J. A. (1973). The structure of histamine. *J. Amer. Chem. Soc.* **95**, 4829–4833.

Bonnett, J. J., and Jeannin, Y. (1972) Etude cristallographique du tetrachlorocobaltate (II) d'histamine diprotonée. *Acta Cryst.* **B28**, 1079–1085.

Bonnett, J. J., Jeannin, Y., and Laaouini, M. (1975). Structure cristalline du chlorure d'histaminedium. *Bull. Soc. Fr. Minéral.* Cristallogr. **98**, 208–213.

Brimblecombe, R. W., Duncan, W. A. M., Durant, G. J., Emmett, J. C., Ganellin, C. R., and Parsons, M. E. (1975). Cimetidine: a non-thiourea H_2-receptor antagonist. *J. Int. Med. Res.* **3**, 86–92.

Brimblecombe, R. W., and Duncan, W. A. M. (1977). The relevance to man of pre-clinical data for cimetidine. in "Cimetidine—Proceedings of the 2nd International Symposium on Histamine H_2-receptor Antagonists" (W. L. Burland and M. A. Simkins, eds.) pp 54–66. Excerpta Medica, Amsterdam-Oxford.

Byrn, S. R., Graber, C. W., and Midland, S. L. (1976). Comparison of the solid and solution conformations of methapyriline, tripelennamine, diphenhydramine, histamine and choline The infared-X-ray method for determination of solution conformations. *J. Org. Chem.* **41**, 2283–2288.

Casy, A. F., Ison, R. R., and Ham, N. S. (1970). The conformation of histamine in solution: ^{1}H nuclear magnetic resonance study. *Chem. Commun.* 1343–1344.

Chand, N., and Eyre, P. (1975). Classification and biological distribution of histamine receptor sub-types. *Agents Actions* **5**, 277–295.

Charton, M. (1965a). Electrical effects of ortho substituents in imidazoles and benzimidazoles. *J. Org. Chem.* **30**, 3346–3350.

Charton, M. (1965b). The application of the Hammett equation to amidines. *J. Org. Chem.* **30**, 969–973.

Coubeils, J. L., Courrière, P., and Pullman, B. (1971). Recherches quantiques sur la conformation et la structure électronique de l'histamine. *C. R. Acad. Sci. (Paris), Ser. D.* **272**, 1813–1816.

Decou, D. F. (1964). X-ray investigations of crystalline histamine free base and histamine dihydrobromide. Dissertation No. 64-9987, Univ. Microfilms Inc., Ann. Arbor, Michigan.

Durant, G. J., Emmett, J. C., and Ganellin, C. R. (1973). Some chemical aspects of histamine H_2-receptor antagonists. in "International Symposium on histamine H_2-receptor antagonists" (C. J. Wood and M. A. Simkins, eds.) pp 13–22. Smith Kline & French Laboratories Ltd., Welwyn Garden City.

Durant, G. J., Ganellin, C. R., and Parsons, M. E. (1975a). Chemical differentiation of histamine H_1- and H_2-receptor agonists. *J. Med. Chem.* **18**, 905–909.

Durant, G. J., Parsons, M. E., and Black, J. W. (1975b). Potential histamine H_2-receptor antagonists. 2. N^α-Guanylhistamine. *J. Med. Chem.* **18**, 830–833.

Durant, G. J., Emmett, J. C., Ganellin, C. R., Roe, A. M., and Slater, R. A. (1976). Potential histamine H_2-receptor antagonists. 3. Methylhistamines. *J. Med. Chem.* **19**, 923–928.

Durant, G. J., Emmett, J. C., and Ganellin, C. R. (1977a). The chemical origin and properties of histamine H_2-receptor antagonists, in "Cimetidine-Proceedings of the 2nd International Symposium on Histamine H_2-Receptor Antagonists" (W. L. Burland and M. A. Simkins, eds.) pp 1–12. Excerpta Medica, Amsterdam-Oxford.

Durant, G. J., Emmett, J. C., Ganellin, C. R., Miles, P. D., Prain, H. D., Parsons, M. E., and White, G. R. (1977b). Cyanoguanidine-thiourea equivalence in the development of the histamine H_2-receptor antagonist, cimetidine. *J. Med. Chem.* **20**, 901–906.

Durant, G. J., Ganellin, C. R., and Parsons, M. E. (1977c). Dimaprit-[S-3[3-(N,N-dimethylamino)propyl]isothiourea]—A highly specific histamine H_2-receptor agonist. Part 2. Structure-activity considerations. *Agents Actions* **7**, 39–43.

Farnell, L., Richards, W. G., and Ganellin, C. R. (1975). Conformation of histamine derivatives. 5. Molecular orbital calculations of the H_1-receptor "essential" conformation of histamine. *J. Med. Chem.* **18**, 662–666.

Ganellin, C. R. (1973a). The tautomer ratio of histamine. *J. Pharm. Pharmac.* **25**, 787–792.

Ganellin, C. R. (1973b). Conformation of histamine derivatives. 3. A relationship between conformation and pharmacological activity. *J. Med. Chem.* **16**, 620–623.

Ganellin, C. R. (1974). Imidazole tautomerism of histamine derivatives, in "Molecular and Quantum Pharmacology" (E. D. Bergmann and B. Pullman, eds.), pp 43–53. D. Reidel Publishing Company, Dordrecht-Holland.

Ganellin, C. R., Pepper, E. S., Port, G. N. J., and Richards, W. G. (1973a). Conformation of histamine derivatives. 1. Application of molecular orbital calculations and nuclear magnetic resonance spectroscopy. *J. Med. Chem.* **16**, 610–616.

Ganellin, C. R., Port, G. N. J., and Richards, W. G. (1973b). Conformation of histamine derivatives. 2. Molecular orbital calculations of preferred conformations in relation to dual receptor activity. *J. Med. Chem.* **16**, 616–620.

Ganellin, C. R., Durant, G. J., and Emmett, J. C. (1976). Some chemical aspects of histamine H_2-receptor antagonists. *Fed. Proc.* **35**, 1924–1930.

Green, J. P., Kang, S., and Margolis, S. (1971). Molecular characteristics of histamine and 5-hydroxytryptamine pertinent to binding. *Mem. Soc. Endocrin.* No. 19., 727–741.

Grossman, M. I., Robertson, C., and Rosiere, C. E. (1952) The effect of some compounds related to histamine on gastric acid secretion. *J. Pharmacol. Exper. Ther.* **104**, 277–283.

Ham, N. S., Casy, A. F., and Ison, R. R. (1973). Solution conformations of histamine and some related derivatives. *J. Med. Chem.* **16**, 470–475.

Hirt, R. C., Schmitt, R. G., Strauss, H. L., and Koren, J. G. (1961) Spectrophotometrically determined ionization constants of derivatives of symmetric triazine. *J. Chem. Eng. Data* **6**, 610–612.

Holmes, F., and Jones, F. (1960). Metal complexes of histamine and some structural analogues. Part 1. *J. Chem. Soc.* 2398–2401.

Hunt, W. H., and Fosbinder, R. J. (1942). A study of some beta-2, and 4, pyridylalkylamines. *J. Pharmacol. Exper. Ther.* **75**, 299–307.

Impicciatore, M., Mossini, F., Plazzi, V., Chiavarini, M., and Bertaccini, G. (1974). Azione della dimetil 2[5-metil-4-imidazoli)]etilamina [5-Med] sulla secrezione gastrica del gatto. *Atteneo Parmense, Acta Bio-Med.* **45**, 145–148.

Janssen, M. J. (1962). Physical properties of organic thiones. Part IV. The basicity of the thiocarbonyl group in various thiones. *Rec. Trav. Chim. Pays-Bas Belg.* **81**, 650–660.

Jones, R. G. (1966). Chemistry of histamine and analogs. Relationship between structure and pharmacological activity, in "Hand. Exp. Pharm. XVIII/1 Histamine and Anti-histaminics," (M. Rocha e Silva, ed.) pp. 1–43. Berlin, Springer-Verlag.

Kang, S., and Chou, D. (1975). Tautomerism of histamine. *Chem. Phys. Letters* **34**, 537–541.

Kier, L. B. (1968) Molecular orbital calculations of the preferred conformations of histamine and a theory on its dual activity. *J. Med. Chem.* **11**, 441–445.

Kumbar, M. (1975). Stable conformations of histamine by empirical method. *J. Theor. Biol.* **53**, 333–340.

Lee, H. M., and Jones, R. G. (1949). The histamine activity of some β-aminoethyl heterocyclic nitrogen compounds. *J. Pharmacol. Exper. Ther.* **95**, 71–78.

Lin, T. M., Alphin, R. S., Henderson, F. G., Benslay, D. N., and Chen, K. K. (1962). The role of histamine in gastric hydrochloric acid secretion. *Ann. N. Y. Acad. Sci.* **99**, 30–44.

Niemann, C., and Hays, J. T. (1942). The relation between structure and histamine-like activity. *J. Amer. Chem. Soc.* **64**, 2288–2289.

Paiva, T. B., Tominaga, M., and Paiva, A. C. M. (1970). Ionization of histamine, N-acetylhistamine and their iodinated derivatives. *J. Med. Chem.* **13**, 689–692.

Parsons, M. E., Blakemore, R. C., Durant, G. J., Ganellin, C. R., and Rasmussen, A. C. (1975). 3-[4(5)-Imidazolyl]propylguanidine (SK&F 91486)—a partial agonist at histamine H_2-receptors. *Agents Actions* **5**, 464.

Parsons, M. E., Owen, D. A. A., Ganellin, C. R., and Durant, G. J. (1977). Dimaprit-[S-[3-(N,N-dimethylamino)propyl]isothiourea]-A highly specific histamine H_2-receptor agonist. Part 1. Pharmacology. *Agents Actions* **7**, 31–37.

Prout, K., Critchley, S. R., and Ganellin, C. R. (1974). 2-(4-Imidazolyl)ethylammonium bromide (histamine monohydrobromide). *Acta Cryst.* **B30**, 2884–2886.

Pullman, B., and Port, J. (1974). Molecular orbital study of the conformation of histamine: the isolated molecule and solvent effect. *Molecular Pharmacol.* **10**, 360–372.

Richards, W. G., Hammond, J., and Aschman, D. G. (1975). Barriers to internal rotation in histamine and 4-methylhistamine. *J. Theor. Biol.* **51**, 237–239.

Rosiere, C. E., and Grossman, M. I. (1951). An analog of histamine that stimulates gastric acid secretion without other actions of histamine. *Science* **113**, 651.

van den Brink, F. G., (1969). Histamine and Antihistamines. Molecular Pharmacology, Structure-Activity Relations, Gastric Acid Secretion, Drukkerij Gebr. Janssen N. V. Nijmegen, pp. 179–180.

Veidis, M. V., Palenik, G. J., Schaffrin, R., and Trotter, J. (1969) Crystal structure of histamine diphosphate monohydrate. *J. Chem. Soc.* **A**, 2659–2666.

Walter, L. A., Hunt, W. H., and Fosbinder, R. J. (1941). β-(2-and 4-Pyridylalkyl)-amines. *J. Amer. Chem. Soc.* **62**, 2771–2773.

Weinstein, H., Chou, D., Johnson, C. L., Kang, S., and Green, J. P. (1976). Tautomerism and the receptor action of histamine: a mechanistic model. *Molecular Pharmacol.* **12**, 738–745.

Yamane, T., Ashida, T., and Kakudo, M. (1973). The crystal structure of histamine sulphate monohydrate. *Acta Cryst.* **B29**, 2884–2891.

Index

A 23187, 29
Acetylcholine, 58, 64, 66, 68
Adenylate cyclase, 48, 53, 79, 94, 185, 186, 187, 188, 189, 190, 192, 196, 198, 199, 204, 205, 256, 272, 286, 291, 293, 294, 315, 317, 353
ADH, 246, 247
Adipose tissue, 325, 337
Amine precursor uptake and distribution system (APUD), 6
2-Aminoethylthiazole, 304, 305, 312, 313, 314
3-(2-aminoethyl 1,2,4-triazole), 145, 148, 150 156, 272
3-(2-aminoethyl) pyrazole-2-HCL, 145, 148, 150, 156
Anaphylatoxin, 2, 352
Angiotensin-histamine interaction, 109
Antidiuresis, 236, 237, 238, 239, 240, 241, 242, 243, 244
Antigen-induced histamine release, 356
APUD system, 6
Aromatic L-amino acid decarboxylase, 4

Basal secretion, 58, 66
Betazole, 272, 303
Black, James Whyte, 32
B-lymphocytes, 361, 374
Body temperature, 211, 213

BOL, 204, 205
Bovet, Daniele, 32
Burimamide, 5, 9, 10, 30, 31, 37, 41, 46, 50, 79, 81, 100, 115, 116, 143, 144, 203, 256, 271, 272, 275, 288, 290, 294, 332, 343, 356, 364, 366, 367, 396, 397, 400, 401, 402

Calcium-ion, 28
Carbachol, 44, 46, 47, 48
Cardiac function, 99
Catecholamine release, 336, 337
Central thermoregulatory pathways, 211, 215
Chemical comparison between H_2-receptor antagonists, 405, 406, 409
Chlorcyclizine, 212
Chlorpheniramine, 103, 107, 229, 290
Cholecystokinin, 133
Cholinergic stimulation, 45, 48
Cholinergic receptors, 243
Cholinergic responses, 46
Chronotropic response of rabbit atrial muscle, 143, 144
Cimetidine, 30, 31, 37, 41, 42, 43, 52, 72, 75, 88, 89, 91, 103, 107, 190, 192, 203, 204, 215, 216, 222, 224, 229, 240, 243, 246, 271, 332, 365, 396, 402, 403

415

Clonidine, 79, 255, 256, 257, 258, 259, 260, 261, 263, 265, 266, 304
cAMP, 37, 48, 58, 67, 79, 165, 167, 168, 169, 172, 174, 175, 176, 179, 188, 214, 228, 235, 271, 272, 273, 274, 275, 282, 285, 286, 289, 290, 293, 295, 299, 301, 302, 303, 304, 306, 307, 308, 309, 312, 314, 315, 316, 325, 326, 330, 331, 332, 338, 353, 362, 366, 367, 368, 370, 371
Cyclic nucleotides, 325
Cyclizine, 367

Dale, Henry Hallet, 32
dbcAMP, 58, 59, 60, 64, 67
Denervation super sensitivity, 172
Dextrobrompheniramine, 222, 224, 240, 243, 304, 306, 309, 311, 314
Diamine oxidase, 4
Digitalis-histamine interaction, 105, 107, 109
Diphenhydramine, 72, 73, 75, 81, 145, 153, 156, 157, 334, 335, 336, 365, 367
Dimaprit, 187, 189, 190, 191, 198, 201, 202, 203, 221, 222, 240, 265, 274, 275, 277, 288, 393, 396, 409
Dog gastric mucosa, 287, 291
Dog gracilis muscle, perfused, 116, 117, 118, 121, 122

Esophageal histamine receptors, 68

Gastric fistula cats, 83, 88, 89
Gastric fistula dogs, 82, 91, 93
Gastric microcirculation, 131, 136, 137
Gastric mucosal cells, 287, 294, 295
Gastric secretion, 11, 13, 35, 46, 57, 61, 66, 70, 74, 78, 79
Gastric mucosal arteriolar responses, 134
Gastrin, 24, 30, 31, 35, 37, 43, 45, 48, 58, 61, 63, 66, 67, 68, 71, 74, 78
Gastrin I, 71, 72
Gastrin receptor, 26, 28
cGMP, 327, 342, 343
Grossman and Konturek hypothesis, 27
Guanethidine-sympathectomized rats, 83, 85
Guinea pig atria, 81, 93, 148, 150, 153, 156
Guinea pig cortical slices, 174
Guinea pig gastric mucosa, 82, 93

Haloperidol, 243
Hippocampal slices, 175
Hippocampal slices guinea pig, 304
H_1 and H_2 receptors, 9, 10, 11
H_2 isoreceptors, 94
H_2 receptor mediated systems, 24
Histamine
  activation of axon reflex, 14
  allergy, 16
  anaphylaxis, 16
  antagonist, compound 929F, 2
  APUD system, 6
  binding site, 96, 201
  biosynthesis, 3
  cardiac responses to, 10
  catabolism, 3
  central actions of, 300
  centrally administered, 241
  chemical characterization, 377
  chemical evidence for the active form at H_1 and H_2 receptors, 384
  conformation, 380
  coronary vascular responses to, 10
  dication, 386
  depressor substances, 8
  distribution, 5
  drug-disease interactions, 99
  dynamic-structure-activity analysis, 406, 407
  effect on
    cardiovascular system, 8
    central nervous system, 15
    endocrine glands, 11
    exocrine glands, 11
    heart, 100–103, 109, 110, 271, 283
    peripheral nervous system, 14
  final-common-pathway hypothesis, 13
  gastric secretory response, 2
  historical perspective, 1
  in brain, 161, 162, 165, 235, 299, 314, 315
  increased capacity during tissue growth and repair, 14
  induced, 14, 31
  local vasodilator mechanisms, 14
  metabolic pathways, 4
  molecular mechanisms, 11
  monocation, 385
  nascent, 14
  nonmast cell-non APUD system, 6
  pathophysiologic role, preface, 13
  parietal cell stimulation, 38

Histamine *(contd.)*
  pharmacology, 1
    cardiovascular system, 8
    endocrine glands, 11
    exocrine glands, 11
    mechanisms, 12
    smooth muscle, 10
  physiology, 1, 23, 36
  protonation, 379
  release
    chymotrypsin, 6
    cobra venim, 6
    dextran, 6
    d-tubocurarine, 6
    48/80, 6
    ovomucoid, 6
    phospholipase, 6
    polyvinyl pyrrolidone, 6
    stilbamidine, 6
  storage, 5
  tautomerism, 379, 389, 391, 393, 396
  triple response, 8
  uptake, 48, 50
Histamine-induced conduction
    arrhythmias, 110
Histamine-induced drinking behavior, 219,
    220, 221, 222, 224, 225, 227, 228, 229,
    230, 231, 232, 233, 234, 236, 240, 243,
    245, 246
Histamine-mediated vasodilatation, 115,
    116, 118, 120, 127
Histamine sensitivity during growth, 36
Histamine stimulated acid secretion, 24, 57
Histaminergic fibers, 171, 174
Histaminergic pathways, 215
Histidine decarboxylase, 3, 4, 11 31, 36, 50
    163, 212, 300, 356
Histidine induced hypothermia, 213
Histidine loading, 212, 210
H-substance, 2
6-hydroxydopamine, 117, 118, 121, 122,
    124, 125
Hyposensitivity to histamine following
    reserpine treatment, 176, 178

ICI 63197, 58, 59, 66, 288
Imidazole acetic acid, 163, 258, 259, 263, 264,
    265, 266
Imidazole-n-methyltransferase, 4, 299
Inflammation, 351, 352, 353, 354, 358

Inflammation, role of histamine, 30, 31
in vivo microscopy, 132, 133
Isobutylmethylxanthine, 306, 308
Isolated canine fat cell model, 329
Isolated gastric glands, 37, 39, 40, 41, 48
Isolated lumen perfused whole stomach, 57
Isolated pareietal cells stimulation of, 38

Kahlson-Rosengren-Svensson Hypothesis,
    27

Lipid mobilization, 326, 327, 334, 335, 336,
    337, 344
Lipolytic response to histamine, 332, 338,
    341, 342, 343, 345
Lower esophageal sphincter (LES), 69, 70,
    71, 72, 73, 74, 75, 76, 77, 78
LSD, 185, 187, 188, 194, 196, 198, 199, 204,
    205, 206
T-Lymphocytes (CTL), 361, 362, 364, 365,
    367, 368, 369, 370

McN-A-1293, 212
Mast cell storage pool, 117
Mast cells, 6
Mepyramine, 9, 10, 11, 24, 30, 116, 118,
    119, 120, 123, 124, 126, 133, 135, 166,
    186, 192, 198, 212, 290, 315
Methapyrilene, 229, 240
1,4-methylhistamine, 163
2-methyl histamine, 101, 148, 167, 187, 221,
    240, 289, 290, 304, 332, 340, 367, 409
4-methyl histamine, 101, 116, 148, 187, 221,
    222, 240, 257, 265, 273, 274, 275, 277,
    282, 289, 290, 304, 305, 312, 313, 314,
    340, 367, 393, 409
1,4-methylimidazole acetic acid, 163
3-methyl-imidazole acetic acid, 200
α-methylnoradrenaline (αMNA), 262, 263
Methyltolazoline, 80, 91, 92, 93
Metiamide, 5, 24, 25, 26, 29, 37, 42, 57, 58,
    60, 62, 63, 64, 65, 66, 67, 71, 72, 73, 74,
    77, 79, 81, 84, 85, 87, 89, 90, 115, 116,
    118, 119, 126, 135, 143, 144, 145, 147,
    148, 150, 153, 156, 157, 166, 171, 203,
    256, 257, 258, 259, 260, 261, 262, 263,
    264, 265, 266, 271, 274, 277, 278, 288,

Metiamide *(contd.)*
  290, 294, 304, 306, 309, 311, 315, 332,
  334, 335, 336, 340, 342, 356, 357, 365,
  366, 367, 396, 400, 402, 403
Metiamide-histamine interaction, 25
Metiamide-pentagastrin interaction, 26
Microiontophoresis, 162, 164
Microvasculature, 8
Modification of behavioral and
  physiological components of body fluid
  homeostasis, 219
Monoamine oxidase, 4
Morphine, 215, 216

NE-induced cAMP accumulation, 341
NE-induced FFA release, 340, 341
Nephrectomized animals, 225
Nitroglycerin, 118, 119, 123
Nonmast cell storage pool, 117
Norepinephrine bitartrate, 118, 119

One cell hypothesis, 28, 29
Ouabain, 105, 106, 107, 108, 109
Oxyntic cells, 24, 25, 94
Oxotremorine, 215, 216, 217

Paraventricular nucleus, 241, 242, 246, 247,
  229, 230
Papaverine, 138
Parietal cell receptors, 37
Parietal cells, 12, 39, 40, 41, 45, 48, 285,
  286, 294
Pentagastrin, 25, 28, 43, 44, 45, 58, 59, 66,
  67
Pentagastrin-metiamide interaction, 28
Pentagastrin-stimulated acid secretion, 24
Phentolamine, 82, 93, 243
Phosphodiesterase inhibitors, 37

Potentiation of manganese ions, 29
Promethazine, 143, 240, 246, 274, 277, 282,
  290
Propranolol, 81, 224, 225, 240, 243, 245,
  334, 336
Prostaglandins, 285, 286, 288, 291, 293, 295
2-(2-pyridyl)ethylamine (PEA), 101, 116,
  221, 222, 274, 277, 282, 409
Pyrilamine, *see* Mepyramine
Rabbit, anethetized, 83
Rabbit atria, 148, 153, 156
Rabbit heart, 271, 283
Receptors in denervated vessels, 121
Renin-angiotensin system, 225
Richards, Alfred Newton, 32
Ro 44602, 212

Schild plot, 25, 41, 42, 43, 81
Secretin, 37
SKF 91487, 409
SKF 91581, 410
Supraoptic nucleus, 241, 242, 243, 244, 246,
  247

Tetrahydrozoline, 79, 80, 91, 92, 94
2-thiazolethylamine, 167
2-(2-thiazolyl)-ethylamine (Th EA) 101, 103
Tolazoline, 79, 80, 81, 82, 83, 84, 85, 86, 87,
  89, 90, 92, 93, 94, 95, 96, 97, 167
Tripelennamine, 229, 240, 340
Two cell hypothesis, 27, 28

Vascular smooth muscle, histamine
  receptors in, 115
Vasodilatation, 117, 119, 125, 133
Vasodilatation
  mechanisms of, 115
Vasodilatin, 8, 23